'We need look no further than ourselves to find microworlds ripe for exploration; each of us provides a surface that supports an interactive microbial population, the location and composition of which is dependent upon the structure and metabolism of the layers that compose our skin.'

Thus begins a book that surveys the world of the skin and its microflora, in health and disease, and in animals as well as man. The approach is essentially an ecological one, moving from the physical and chemical properties of the skin as a microbial habitat, through a consideration of the various major groups of microorganisms associated with it, to an account of the complex associations between these microorganisms.

The skin flora in health is introduced as a prelude to the understanding of microbial skin disease, and the mechanisms of pathogenicity are explored as the major groups of infective skin conditions are reviewed. The principles of treatment, disinfection and prevention receive proper attention, as does the important topic of hospital-acquired infection, where the skin is so often implicated.

The text is accompanied by numerous tables containing a wealth of practical and experimental detail, and is extensively referenced. This is a book that will be essential to dermatologists, medical microbiologists, veterinarians and research workers in these fields.

THE SKIN MICROFLORA AND MICROBIAL SKIN DISEASE

THE SKIN MICROFLORA AND MICROBIAL SKIN DISEASE

Edited by
W. C. NOBLE

Department of Microbial Diseases,
Institute of Dermatology,
United Medical and Dental Schools,
University of London, UK

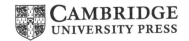

CAMBRIDGE
UNIVERSITY PRESS

PUBLISHED BY THE PRESS SYNDICATE OF THE UNIVERSITY OF CAMBRIDGE
The Pitt Building, Trumpington Street, Cambridge, United Kingdom

CAMBRIDGE UNIVERSITY PRESS
The Edinburgh Building, Cambridge CB2 2RU, UK
40 West 20th Street, New York NY 10011–4211, USA
477 Williamstown Road, Port Melbourne, VIC 3207, Australia
Ruiz de Alarcón 13, 28014 Madrid, Spain
Dock House, The Waterfront, Cape Town 8001, South Africa

http://www.cambridge.org

First published 1993
First paperback edition 2004

A catalogue record for this book is available from the British Library

Library of Congress cataloguing in publication data

The Skin microflora and microbial skin disease / edited by W. C. Noble.
p.   cm.
Includes bibliographical references and index.
ISBN 0 521 40198 4 (hardback)
1. Skin – Infections.   2. Skin – Microbiology.
[DNLM: 1. Skin – microbiology.   2. Skin Diseases, Infectious–
microbiology.   WR 220 S6285]
RL201.S62.   1992
616.5′01 – dc20   92-15538 CIP

ISBN 0 521 40198 4 hardback
ISBN 0 521 61206 3 paperback

Contents

List of contributors   *page* ix
Preface   xi
1 The basis of the skin surface ecosystem   *D. McEwan Jenkinson*   1
2 Nutrition of cutaneous resident microorganisms   *K. T. Holland*   33
3 Physical factors affecting the skin flora and skin disease   *M. E.*
   McBride   73
4 Coryneform bacteria   *J. J. Leyden & K. J. McGinley*   102
5 Coryneforms as pathogens   *J. J. Leyden & K. J. McGinley*   118
6 Staphylococci on the skin   *W. C. Noble*   135
7 Staphylococci as pathogens   *W. C. Noble*   153
8 Streptococci and the skin   *M. Barnham*   173
9 Other cutaneous bacteria   *W. C. Noble*   210
10 Fungi and fungal infections of the skin   *R. J. Hay*   232
11 Bacterial and fungal skin disease in animals   *D. H. Lloyd*   264
12 Viral skin disease in man   *P. Morgan-Capner*   291
13 Viral skin disease in animals   *D. H. Lloyd*   315
14 Microbial interactions on skin   *R. P. Allaker & W. C. Noble*   331
15 Adherence of skin microorganisms and the development of skin
   flora from birth   *R. Aly & D. J. Bibel*   355
16 Skin disinfection   *H. Kobayashi*   373
Index   387

Contributors

Robert P. Allaker
Skin Unit, Royal Veterinary College, University of London, Hawkshead Lane, North Mymms, Herts AL9 7TA, UK

Raza Aly
Departments of Microbiology & Dermatology, University of California, San Francisco, California 94143-0536, USA

Michael Barnham
Department of Microbiology, Harrogate General Hospital, Knaresborough Road, Harrogate HG2 7ND, UK

Debra J. Bibel
Department of Dermatology, University of California, San Francisco, California 94143-0536, USA

Roderick J. Hay
Department of Microbial Diseases, Institute of Dermatology, United Medical and Dental Schools, Guy's Hospital Campus, London SE1 9RT, UK

Keith T. Holland
Department of Microbiology, University of Leeds, Leeds LS2 9JT, UK

Hiroyashi Kobayashi
Division of Infection Control, University of Tokyo Hospital, 7-3-1 Hongo, Bunkyo-ku, Tokyo, Japan 113

James J. Leyden
Department of Dermatology, University of Pennsylvania, Clinical Research Building, 422 Curie Boulevard, Philadelphia, Pennsylvania 19104-6142, USA

David H. Lloyd
Skin Unit, Royal Veterinary College, University of London, Hawkshead Lane, North Mymms, Herts AL9 7TA, UK

Mollie E. McBride
Department of Dermatology, Baylor College of Medicine, One Baylor Plaza, Houston, Texas 77030, USA

David McEwan Jenkinson
91 St Albans Road, Edinburgh EH9 2PQ, UK

Kenneth J. McGinley
Department of Dermatology, University of Pennsylvania, Clinical Research Building, 422 Curie Boulevard, Philadelphia, Pennsylvania 19104-6142, USA

Peter Morgan-Capner
Department of Virology, Royal Preston Hospital, Sharoe Green Lane, Preston PR2 4HG, UK

William C. Noble
Department of Microbial Diseases, Institute of Dermatology, United Medical and Dental Schools, St Thomas' Hospital Campus, London SE1 7EH, UK

Preface

The seminal book by Mary J. Marples *The Ecology of Human Skin* and that of W. C. Noble and Dorothy A. Somerville *The Microbiology of Human Skin* were monographs – attempts to encapsulate all the knowledge on a limited topic. This approach, which also attempted a comprehensive bibliography, is no longer feasible, perhaps no longer desirable. The reasons for this stem in part from a vastly increased knowledge of the components of the human skin flora and their role in disease of organs or systems other than skin, and in part from a recognition of the similarities and dissimilarities of the skin flora of mammals other than humans. Accordingly, it seemed appropriate to ask a number of those active in research to contribute a chapter on their areas of special expertise and to provide access to classical and recent publications without attempting a complete bibliography.

This should not be taken to imply that all is now known; we have a detailed knowledge of some areas but are almost totally ignorant in others. We do not know, for example, the role, at the molecular level, of skin lipid in promoting or preventing colonization of skin, even whether some lipid components are important for the host or the microbe. We know in exquisite detail the metabolic products of testosterone metabolism that contribute to axillary odour but have no adequate taxonomy by which to classify the coryneforms that are responsible for the metabolism. We know the DNA sequence of the epidermolytic toxins produced by some strains of *Staphylococcus aureus* yet do not know why this species colonizes the skin in atopic dermatitis.

Investigation of the skin microflora has its own intrinsic interest: the ecology of skin is as varied as that of any macrohabitat; yet we need to be able to maintain and manipulate this habitat in a safe manner. Our ability to tolerate therapeutic immunosuppression or an indwelling catheter or prosthesis may depend on our ability to manage well the habitat that is also our physical interface with the rest of the world.

W. C. Noble
London

1

The basis of the skin surface ecosystem

D. McEWAN JENKINSON

The compelling challenge of exploration has, with the advent of space probes, been extended to include much closer investigation of a variety of distant planets and their potential to support life. As spaceships reveal more and more surface environments that are barren and hostile to human habitation, like that of the moon, the enormity of the search for planets suitable for colonization is emphasized.

There are, however, equally demanding and exciting investigative challenges, though requiring different technical skills, if the telescope is exchanged for the microscope. We need look no further than ourselves to find microworlds ripe for exploration; each of us provides a surface that supports an interactive microbial population, the location and composition of which is dependent upon the structure and metabolism of the layers that compose our skin.

Microorganisms float unseen in the air around us, often on 'flying saucers' of keratin a few microns in diameter, which, as we shall see later, are derived from the surfaces of different mammals. Some of these airborne microorganisms, for genetic survival, need to colonize the skin of other individual hosts of the same or different species. However, although mammalian skin surfaces are very large in comparison to those of the microbial 'spacecrafts', they are, in relative terms, distant and there are abundant alternative hostile surfaces, such as the soil, roads and pavements. Thus the microbes, assuming that they could have a view of their surroundings, are faced with a problem of a magnitude comparable to that of human colonization of large distant planets, but with the additional complication that the surfaces they seek move in random directions and often at high speed. Microorganisms, even if successful in reaching a mammalian surface on saucers without propulsion, then have to survive within a complex dynamic external ecosystem analogous to that on the surface of the earth.

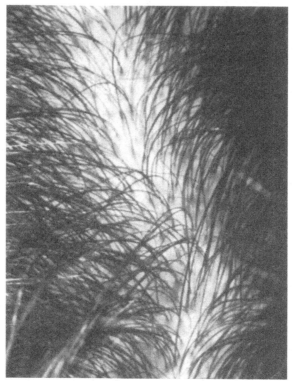

Fig. 1.1. A view of the haired skin surface of a human, illustrating the 'afforested' nature of the surface to be colonized.

In this chapter, the elements of the mammalian skin surface ecosystem will be considered in general terms, from the perspective of the microorganism.

Skin surface topography
The long-range perspective

Initial examination of mammals from a distance reveals a diversity in surface area, colour and contour. Comparison of a mouse with an elephant provides an obvious example. In most mammals the surface is covered with a layer of hair, which gives the skin an outward appearance comparable to an aerial view of afforestation (Fig. 1.1). The density, colour and degree of surface orientation (i.e. discerned whorling patterns), however, vary markedly between species, within individuals and even between body areas (Fig. 1.2). In some mammals, for example, the elephant, and in specialized body regions, such as the muzzle of the dog and palms of man, this hair cover is absent.

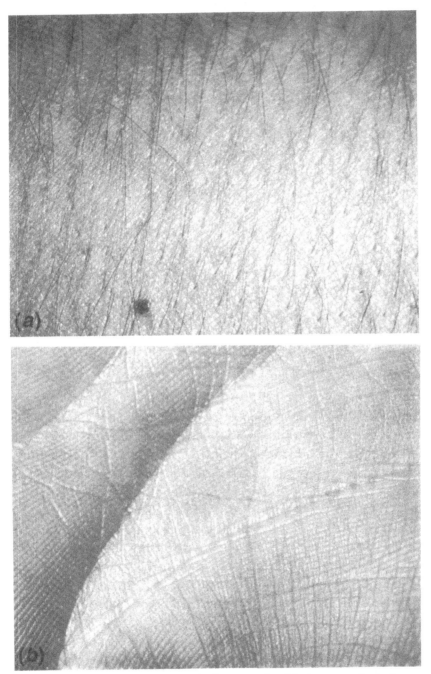

Fig. 1.2. (*a*) The surface of the human forearm. In this instance the hair cover is less dense and the surface of the skin can more readily be discerned. (*b*) The skin of the human palm is completely devoid of hair and the surface is therefore readily accessible.

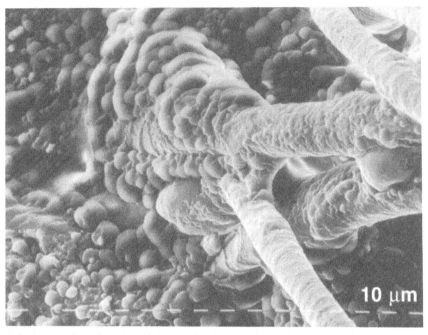

Fig. 1.3. A scanning electron micrograph of the surface of ovine skin after fixation and freeze-drying. This photograph illustrates that the hair pore is sealed by layers of a 'cement', which is probably hardened lipid.

The microscopic view

A closer look within the coat using a scanning electron microscope (Fig. 1.3) reveals that the hairs are covered with a 'cement-like' material, which seals the entry to the pores from which they emerge.[1] Debris, mainly fragments of loose or broken hairs, is also regularly observed. The zones between the hairs (Fig. 1.4) are composed of flat cells (squames), the margins of which are sealed by the same 'cement-like' material. The surface of glabrous skin likewise has an appearance reminiscent of a cemented 'crazy paving'. This is, however, not a completely barren terrain. The covering 'cement' is composed of a complex mixture of lipids, and its removal by application of lipid solvents, for example during the critical-point drying process, one of the preparative techniques for scanning electron microscopy, permits detection of microbial inhabitants. These microbes are most frequently found around the mouths of hair follicles (Fig. 1.5), although they are also present in the interfollicular region.

The colonizing organism will therefore land initially either on a protective hair cover, which it has to penetrate to reach the skin surface, or on a seemingly hostile defensive paving. In spite of the presence of microbes on this surface, there is little evidence from observation of the terrain that it is a suitable habitat for the growth and development of a micropopulation. The incoming

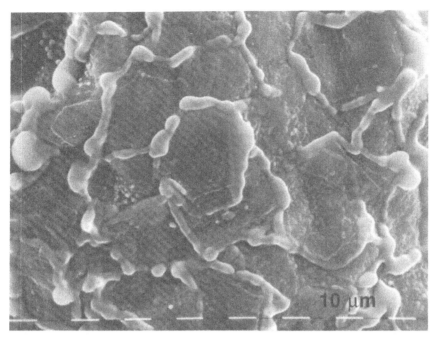

Fig. 1.4. A scanning electron micrograph of the follicular skin surface of bovine skin, after freeze-drying to preserve lipids. The surface, which resembles a cemented crazy-paving, provides a formidable barrier against invasion.

organism intending to inhabit this microscopic world would seem therefore to have to penetrate to an underlying zone. Even if successful, the difficulties it faces before it can settle and reproduce are, however, even more complex, as can be seen from study of the climate, underlying topography and chemical nature of this microworld.

Skin surface climate
Air movement

Before reaching the surface terrain, the floating microbe has, as it approaches the skin, first to negotiate a zone of air movement directed across the surface. An envelope of upward-moving air has been demonstrated surrounding the human body, including the more densely haired regions, by means of a Schlieren optical system.[2] Two to four times more microorganisms were detected in this zone of airflow than in the surrounding environment, and areas of high bacterial concentration were found at areas of low air movement, such as under the armpits and chin. A similar airflow has been demonstrated around the skin of domestic animals, although little is known about its role in the airborne transmission of particles. The air movement is unlikely to be

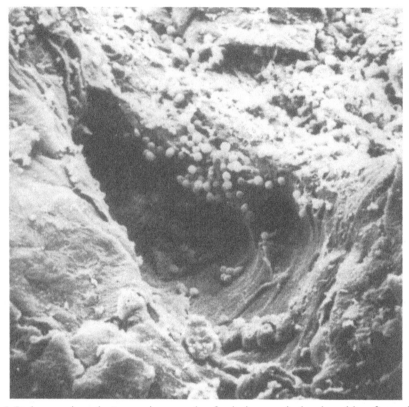

Fig. 1.5. A scanning electron micrograph of a hair pore in bovine skin after critical-point drying, a procedure which results in the removal of the surface lipids. Colonizing microorganisms can be located at the mouth of the pore, which can now readily be identified.

confined to the hair surface and it is possible that, especially in windy conditions, there could be significant air movement within the coat.

Skin temperature

The temperature of the skin surface fluctuates in response to both environmental and physiological changes, mainly as a result of dermal vascular responses. Skin temperature generally ranges from about 30 to 40 °C as the air temperature varies from 15 to 40 °C. However, extreme variations in ambient temperature and solar radiation can, via cutaneous receptors and the sympathetic nervous system, cause dramatic alterations in the cutaneous circulation and hence in surface temperature. For example the skin temperature of the Alaskan sled dog can approach 0 °C in subzero conditions.[3] Skin temperature, although often marginally higher over subcutaneous arteries, was found to be fairly uniform in cattle kept in the shade, but in strong sunlight there was as much as an 8 °C temperature difference between black and white areas, attributed to the more effective reflectance of the white hair.[4] Coat pigmentation can thus have an important contributory role in modifying the environmental factors influencing surface temperature. Physiological responses by the host, such as shivering and non-shivering thermogenesis, can significantly increase cutaneous blood flow and hence also influence skin temperature.[5-9]

Humidity

The environment on the skin is also likely to be a humid one. The cornified squames are hygroscopic and capable of absorbing 3–4 times their own weight of water from the atmosphere.[10] Surface humidity therefore, like temperature, probably varies appreciably, depending on the ambient conditions. The surface moisture level will also be influenced by transepidermal water movement from the blood to the skin surface and by sweating, a metabolic response to heat stress in some species. The water content at the skin surface is therefore temperature dependent.[11]

Gaseous composition

The composition of the gaseous environment within the surface layers of the skin has still not been clearly defined but there is again a dynamic state. Gases, with the exception of carbon monoxide, easily penetrate the skin by diffusion, depending on the differences in concentration or in vapour pressure inside and outside, and on their temperature and solubility in water and fat.[12] The epidermis does however, have a considerable barrier effect on diffusion,[13-15] including that of some gases; the loss of carbon dioxide from skin is, for example, 14 times less rapid than that from muscle. It is still not known whether gases such as oxygen and carbon dioxide concentrate in pockets within the outer layers of the skin, thereby providing regional differences in the gaseous microenvironment that may favour the growth of particular organisms. This is, however, a distinct possibility, which should not be overlooked in view of the distribution of the surface inhabitants that will be described later.

Skin structure

The presence of microorganisms at the surface, and the higher bacterial counts within the moving air immediately above it, indicate that the microenvironment is capable of supporting colonization. The evidence from the pictures of the surface terrain, however, leads to the conclusion that any such microbial reproduction is most likely to occur underneath the outer surface. The colonizing bacterium will therefore require to penetrate the outer defensive

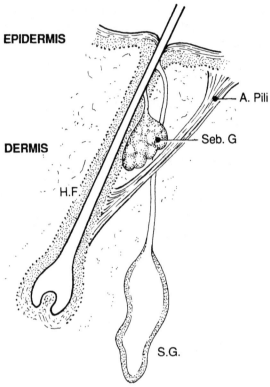

EPIDERMIS

A. Pili

DERMIS

Seb. G

H.F

S.G.

Fig. 1.6. A diagram illustrating the basic structure of the skin. The two main layers, the epidermis and the dermis, are shown. Within the dermis are the components of the basic hair follicle unit, which consists of a hair follicle with its hair (HF), an arrector pili muscle (A. Pili), a sebaceous gland (Seb G) and a sweat gland (SG) situated in the relative positions shown.

wall and enter the skin itself. Consequently, to appreciate the problems involved as the organism goes 'underground' to locate the zone favourable for growth and development, there is a need for knowledge of the structure of the skin.

This quest will begin by consideration of a perpendicular section through the skin to reveal the layers and structures that compose and underlie the surface. The basic components of the skin are illustrated in Fig. 1.6. The skin is divided into two main layers, the epidermis and the dermis. Within the dermis are the elements of what is termed the hair follicle unit. This consists of a hair follicle with its associated hair, an arrector pili muscle, a sebaceous gland and a sweet gland. In the embryo these organs develop from the epidermis and hence, although sited within the dermis, they are modified epidermal structures. Their functions will become apparent as the nature of the skin surface is considered in greater detail.

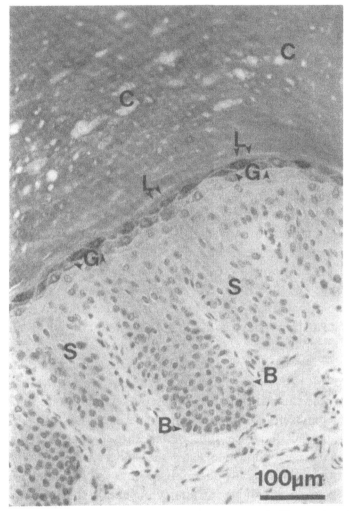

Fig. 1.7. A micrograph of the epidermis of the human fingertip illustrating the different epidermal layers; stratum basale (B), stratum spinosum (S), stratum granulosum (G), stratum lucidum (L) and stratum corneum (C). Haematoxylin and eosin stain.

The dermis

The dermis, which is subdivided into two regions, an upper stratum papillare and a lower stratum reticulare, provides, by means of constituent collagen and elastic fibres, a pliable framework for the vascular supply, which transports the nutrients for maintenance and growth, and the lymphatic system, which aids drainage. The physiology of the dermis is complex and, for a discourse on the skin surface, it is sufficient to emphasize that changes in the metabolism of this zone or in the nutrient supply can have profound effects on the growth and integrity of the epidermis and hair follicles and the functional ability of the skin glands. Further information on dermal function can be obtained from reviews.[16,17]

The epidermis

The structure of the epidermis is essentially the same in all mammals, although the number of layers present within it varies between glabrous and haired regions of skin, and to a lesser extent between species. In glabrous areas, such as sole of the human foot or the muzzle of domestic animals, the zones identified in Fig. 1.7 can be distinguished.[18–20] In such instances the total thickness can be of the order of 0.4–0.6 mm,[21] and papillomatous downgrowths (rete pegs) are prominent. However, in haired animals the stratum lucidum is generally absent, the stratum granulosum if present is usually found as a single, often intermittent, layer, and the stratum spinosum is much thinner. Thus, in species like the sheep and mouse the living epidermis is relatively thin and consists of only about 4–5 cell layers; in the sheep, for example, it has an overall thickness of the order of 17 μm under a stratum corneum some 2.5 times thicker.[22] Epidermal thickness thus apparently varies inversely with coat density and it can be considered, in general terms, that the more dense the coat the thinner the epidermis.

The cells in the basal layer are interconnected by desmosomes, which, however, do not provide a complete intercellular barrier. Mobile host cells such as mast cells and neutrophils can penetrate into the intercellular spaces of the stratum spinosum through which small molecules can also pass, as evidenced by the fact that tracer substances such as lanthanum and horseradish peroxidase have been shown to enter the epidermis from the dermis.[14,23] However, lanthanum generally does not penetrate into the interspace between the stratum granulosum and the stratum corneum. In this region, membrane-coating granules migrate towards the plasma membrane of the cells and discharge their lamellar content into the intercellular spaces.[24,25] The epidermis, therefore, acts not only as a cellular barrier to invasion but also limits possible entry by intercellular passage.

The epidermis is formed by mitotic division of cells in the stratum basale, which then migrate outwards, apparently in a columnar formation.[26] As they do so they differentiate and undergo a process called keratinization,[27] which results in the gradual formation of the surface zone of dead cells (the stratum corneum). The cells of this outer layer (squames) therefore contain an inert protein, keratin,[28,29] and provide the outer defensive layer seen in Fig. 1.4. The squames are ultimately shed from the outer surface into the atmosphere by a process termed desquamation.

The rate of epidermal turnover is variable and relatively slow. It takes about

12–14 days for complete transfer of a cell from the basal layer to the granular layer of the healthy epidermis.[30] The processes of cell production, differentiation and keratinization are influenced by a number of factors such as circulating and local humoral agents.[31, 32] Turnover is particularly affected during repair after injury, where increases in the thickness of the living epidermis (hyperplasia) and of the stratum corneum (hyperkeratosis) are often prominent. More detailed information on epidermal function can be obtained from reviews.[33–5]

Epidermal production is therefore a dynamic process that results in continual shedding of squames into the environment.[36–8] These act as 'flying saucers' for attached microbes and aid their general dissemination. The potential impact of this process can be gauged from the fact that, in an indoor environment, 75 per cent of the airborne particles contain protein and up to 1 per cent have been shown to be derived from skin. In public places with airflow systems the percentage can be much higher; in the London Underground for example, 10 per cent of the particles collected were squames.[39, 40]

Melanocytes with a dendritic appearance can be found in the basal region of the epidermis. These contain granules of a pigment (melanin), which upon stimulation by solar radiation can be transferred to the keratinocytes to give the skin a tanned appearance.[17, 41, 42] As a consequence these cells, as indicated earlier, have an influence on skin surface temperature. Also within the epidermis are free and specialized nerve endings that provide the host with information on the external environment.[43–8] These include tactile receptors, which when stimulated induce, via the nervous system, reflex and behavioural mechanisms designed to remove the source of the stimulus. Insects landing on the leg, for example, are liable to be swatted with the palm of the hand. In close association with the epidermal nerve fibres is another type of dendritic cell, the Langerhans cell.[49] This cell type is known to have an immunological function and to act as an antigen-presenting cell.[50] It thus has an important role in immune surveillance and in the early stages of immune reactions to foreign proteins,[51, 52] be they live organisms or toxins. The Langerhans cell may, in view of its close apposition to the nerve fibres, also have a role in signal presentation to the nervous system.

The hair follicle

The hairs that form the coat arise from the hair follicles. They are derived from cells at the base (the bulb) of the follicles, which also divide by mitosis, but, in contrast to the epidermis, grow outwards not as a sheet but in a single column. The cells in the column differentiate and keratinize to produce, in this instance, hairs, which are in effect cylinders of dead cells composed of keratin.

The histological structure of the hair follicle and its different layers is well documented and details of the anatomy of the hair follicle and the processes involved in the control of hair growth and development including the location and mode of action of the melanocytes that provide the hair colour, can be obtained elsewhere.[19, 20, 53-5] The hairs also provide 'early warning' of potential intruders by means of a palisade network of nerve fibres around the hair follicles, which sense tactile stimuli.[56-8] This sensory system and that of the epidermis, however, has a limited sensitivity, and inhabitants, such as mites, which exert a pressure below the required threshold, can evade detection. Whiskers on the face of animals are specialized hair follicles,[59] which are highly sensitive to tactile stimuli.

It is evident that the marked differences in the appearance of the coat between species are not due to variation in the basic mechanism of hair formation, although the presence or absence of colour is dependent on the nature of the melanocytes in the hair bulb. Mammalian coats can therefore now be described in terms of variations in the size, the distribution and the mode of emergence of the hairs, variables that are used to classify and distinguish them.

Hair follicle grouping The integument of species such as man, the pig, horse and cow, with the exception of the specialized glabrous regions such as the muzzle, contains a number of complete hair follicle units, as described in Fig. 1.6. The follicles are, however, not all of a uniform length and diameter, and the number per cm^2 of skin varies markedly from as few as 10–20 in the pig to over 2000 in some breeds of cattle. Thus the pig has a sparse coat composed of large hairs or bristles while the cow has a much denser coat of finer hairs. There are significant regional variations in coat density within species and over the body surface of individuals, as shown by comparison of the human arm with the scalp.

Other species, such as the dog, cat, sheep and camel, exhibit hair follicle grouping.[60] Here only a proportion of the follicles, the primary follicles, are components of complete units; the remainder, the secondary hair follicles, are smaller and have no associated arrector pili muscle or sweat gland. They may or may not have an accompanying sebaceous gland. As the purpose of the arrector pili muscle is to erect the hairs, it follows that the secondary hairs are not capable of erection; they form an underlying fur beneath the larger primary or guard hairs. The hair group, as seen in sections cut parallel to the skin surface, generally consists of a trio of primary hairs in close apposition to a number of secondary hairs. In some species, for example, the camel, the cluster is surrounded by a well-defined connective tissue sheath, which enables it to be readily delineated.[61] The ratio of primary (P) to secondary (S) hairs is highly variable between and within species; for example the P:S ratio in British sheep is about 1:3–1:6 compared with about 1:15–1:25 in the woolly merino breed,[62] giving rise to coat types of quite different density and appearance even within the same species.

Hair emergence patterns Further variations in the format and density of the surface coat arise from different patterns of hair emergence. In species that do not exhibit hair grouping the hairs emerge individually, although often grouped as trios (e.g. Meijéres trios in man). The pattern of emergence of grouped hairs, on the other hand, varies considerably between species. In the dog and cat, for example, they emerge as a group consisting of a primary hair surrounded by a variable number (3–7) of secondary hairs. Each group has an associated compound arrector pili muscle and sebaceous gland,[63] and a sweat gland in the same relative positions as in the hair follicle unit. In contrast, in the sheep, goat and camel, the primary hairs, each follicle of which is accompanied by its arrector pili muscle, sebaceous gland and sweat gland, emerge independently through separate pores but often as closely associated trios. The secondary hairs emerge through separate pores either individually or in groups or tufts in close association with these primary hairs. The number of secondary groups accompanying each primary follicle again can vary considerably.

The hair cycle It is evident that the colonizing organism can be presented with a variety of coat types depending on the species or body area upon which it lands. However, to survive it must also be capable of adapting to changes in the environment of the coat, even within a given body area, as coat density and hair dimensions vary with season to meet the thermoregulatory requirements of the host.[8]

Hair follicles undergo a cycle of growth that consists of three phases:[54, 64–6]

anagen – a stage of follicle regeneration and active hair growth;
catagen – a stage of follicle involution and shrinkage;
telogen – an inactive resting period.

During anagen there is rapid proliferation of the cells in the hair bulb. This process appears to be dependent on stimulatory signals from the hair papilla, a region of the dermis that invaginates into the base of the bulb. The 'intrinsic' factor responsible for triggering the growth phase of the cycle has still not been identified, although it is now known that hair growth is influenced by photoperiod and by circulating hormones. The duration of the anagen stage is highly variable, even between body areas of the same individual; on the human scalp it lasts about 3 years in contrast to the limbs where its duration is usually 3–6 months.

At the beginning of catagen, which is generally a rapid transition phase, the lowermost cells of the bulb degenerate and gradually the matrix cells over the papilla revert to an undifferentiated form; the underlying papilla becomes a free cluster of primordial germ cells. The outcome is the formation of a club hair, which ascends the follicle as a result of multiplication of the underlying matrix cells until the club reaches the level of attachment of the arrector pili muscle. There the club hair enters telogen, firmly fixed by spindle-shaped processes.

After a variable resting period of as much as 3–6 months, anagen recommences by the downward growth of a strand of cells that envelop the papilla. The new hair forms initially as a thin keratinized cupola, which differentiates in a separate shaft adjacent to the club hair. The club hair is eventually shed but not always immediately; club hairs can often be found lying alongside their successors and in some species they can remain for several cycles. The mechanism by which the club hair is released is still uncertain, although it almost certainly involves more than mechanical stimulation. Plucking stimulates regrowth and in laboratory animals is used to provide standardized conditions for experimental study. However, this system whereby a new hair grows before the shedding of the old one ensures that a hair covering is retained during moulting.

Hair replacement patterns and seasonal coat variation The patterns of hair replacement are not the same in all mammals but fall broadly into three categories, seasonal, mosaic and wave.

Wild mammals that have to cope with a wide range of ambient conditions exhibit patterns of seasonal hair replacement. Sheep and goats have an annual replacement cycle with a short anagen phase in summer and a long telogen phase during the winter, while cattle shed their coat twice per annum, in the spring and autumn.[67, 68] In cattle the hairs produced in summer are shorter and thicker than those produced in winter by the same follicles. This has the effect of reducing coat insulation in the summer to meet the demands of the increased ambient temperature. Coat insulation can also be reduced in species with grouped hairs by the provision of an undercoat of lower density in summer; in deer and goats not all of the secondary follicles contain a hair in summer.

A mosaic pattern, where the cycle of hair growth is not uniform over the body, is found in man. For example, the hairs on the scalp have a much longer anagen phase than those on the arm and hence there is considerable regional variation in the growth cycle.

Some laboratory rodents exhibit a wave pattern of hair growth, whereby anagen begins at one region of the body, usually the neck, and proceeds caudally over the body as a progressive wave of growth. Thus the hairs at different parts of the body are not at the same stage of the cycle whereas those within a given region are at a synchronous stage. Hair growth is apparently not affected by shaving but resting hairs can be stimulated into anagen if plucked. Plucking, therefore, as mentioned above, has been used in rodents as a means of synchronizing the cycle in specific body regions for experimental studies of factors that influence hair growth.

Colonizing microorganisms are therefore likely to face widely different microhabitats, depending on the species of mammal they land on, the location within each mammal and the time of year at which the landing takes place.

The chemical composition of the skin surface

It has already been established that the hairs and the squames of the stratum corneum are mainly composed of keratin, a substance unfavourable to microbial growth. The apparently hard intercellular cement also seems to be an unlikely source of nutrients for microbial growth and reproduction. Nevertheless the location of microorganisms on the skin (see Fig. 1.5) and in the zone immediately above it, indicates the presence of additional, and potentially nutritive, chemical substances. This is confirmed by analysis of skin washings, which have revealed the presence of lipids, proteins, minerals and hormones. Many of these have important biological functions within the body and, although their precise roles on the skin have still to be established, some of them have antimicrobial actions.[69, 70]

These substances appear to be derived from sweat and sebum, the products of the sweat and sebaceous glands, respectively, and to a lesser extent from the epidermis itself. The composition of these secretions is described in greater detail in Chapter 2. Here we are concerned more with their location, which appears to be between the squames of the stratum corneum. Microscopical examination of histological sections of frozen tissue stained for lipids with Sudan dye reveals a continuous column of staining from within the sebaceous gland, through the duct and pilosebaceous canal to the intercellular spaces of the outer stratum corneum (Figs 1.8 and 1.9). At least some of the sebaceous lipids therefore seem to percolate through the outer stratum corneum. Immunostaining of the bovine epidermis with an antiserum to cattle sweat proteins revealed that they too are present within the corneum.[71]

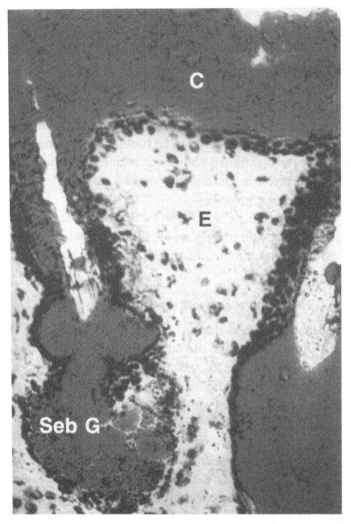

Fig. 1.8. A low-power view of a cryosection of sheep skin stained with Sudan IV for lipid and counterstained with haematoxylin. There is continual staining from the sebaceous gland (Seb G) to the stratum corneum (C). The living epidermis (E) does not exhibit a staining reaction.

It thus appears that sebum and sweat do not, as previously supposed, flow out across the skin but rather into the stratum corneum, probably as an emulsion.[72] This emulsion, which seems to permeate throughout the entire outer corneum, is the probable source of the intercellular 'cement'. As the epidermis grows outwards it seems reasonable to suppose that the intercellular emulsion dehydrates and hardens to provide a lipid seal between the outermost squames. Thus, although the modified emulsion apparently provides, at the surface, a barrier to entry into the corneum, it is, in its newly secreted form, a

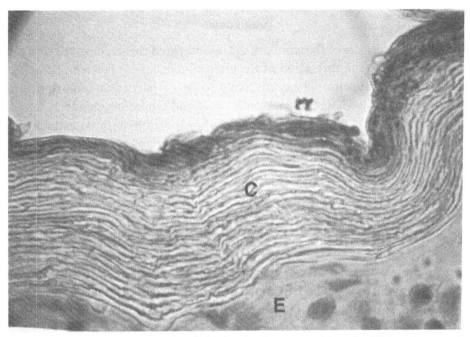

Fig. 1.9. Sudan IV staining for lipid in the human epidermis. This micrograph illustrates the presence of lipid between the layers of the outer stratum corneum (C). Living epidermis is marked (E).

potential growth medium for organisms capable of penetrating into it. The chemical composition of this mixture is, as will be seen later, highly variable between species and can alter considerably in response to host dietary changes and to alterations in the ambient environment. In hot climates, the composition of the sweat alters considerably during prolonged profuse glandular activity; in the horse, for example, the protein content of the sweat gradually falls during continuous sweating.[73]

In man and most of the haired mammals studied to date, the pH of the skin surface varies considerably but, overall, tends to be acidic,[74,75] an exception being the dog, which has an alkaline skin surface. The extremities, such as the muzzle, teat and the interdigital spaces in man, also tend to be more alkaline. In cattle, over the haired surface, pH is fairly uniform and not appreciably affected by environment except on exposure to very hot humid conditions, when it tends to become alkaline.[76] Skin pH can, however, exhibit regional patterns[77] and alter in response to factors such as season, ischaemic hypoxia and in disease states.[78-80] It seems probable that in healthy individuals the skin surface presents a growth medium with a pH that may vary between body regions but, due to localized buffering systems, is likely to be fairly constant overall in given locations.

Skin glands

Some of the products of the emulsion are, as indicated earlier, derived from the epidermis during the formation of the intercellular barrier layers in the outer layers of the spinosum. These are likely to be of particular importance in species such as the whale that lack both sweat and sebaceous glands. It seems, however, that in most mammals a significant proportion of the constituents of the intercellular emulsion is derived from the skin glands.

Sebaceous glands

The sebaceous glands are alveolar exocrine skin glands, which in haired regions are always associated with hair follicles as part of the unit (pilo-sebaceous glands), although, as described earlier, every hair does not have an associated gland. Their ducts open into the follicular canal, unlike those of the corresponding 'free' sebaceous glands in glabrous skin, which open directly to the skin surface. In some body regions the glands are simple lobes and in others a composite of identical lobes separated by trabeculae. Consequently they differ considerably in size and number between species and body areas. Each lobe consists of cells at varying stages of development and degeneration surrounded by a peripheral zone of low cuboidal cells. Sebum excretion is a relatively slow process, which, allowing for storage time within the hair follicle, takes some 6–9 days.[81,82]

Sebum is a complex mixture, which varies with age and diet and between species. It is rich in lipids that include essential fatty acids such as linoleic, which although nutrients can also, in specific circumstances, inhibit microbial growth. Some of the constituent fatty acids are volatile and may have a role in the attraction or repulsion of vectors of disease such as insects.

Sweat glands

The sweat glands are tubular exocrine skin glands, which contribute an aqueous fluid containing minerals and proteins to the surface emulsion. They are also generally found as part of hair follicle units but again, as described earlier, there is not always a gland associated with each hair. Glands in the anatomical position beside the hair follicle are termed 'epitrichial' or 'peritrichial' to distinguish them from the 'atrichial' glands in glabrous skin, which open to the surface directly through the epidermis. However, all sweat glands consist of a secretory fundus and a long duct. The fundus is composed of an inner layer of secretory cells surrounded by a single layer of myoepithelial cells and a sheath of fibrocytes.

The rate of sweat production and the magnitude of the response are highly variable between species. The profuse output in man and the horse promoted the traditional view that sweat glands are thermoregulatory organs. However, while this is true of primates, equids and some bovids, it is now evident that the magnitude of the output in most mammals is insufficient to lead to a significant lowering of body temperature in hot conditions.[83] Thus sweat is now believed to have a number of functions, an important one of which is in the maintenance of skin surface defence. Among the constituents of sweat are vitamins, immunoglobulins and hormones, biologically active substances, which as potential nutrients and inhibitors have an active role in determining the balance of the surface micropopulation. However, more detailed information on the effects of the constituents of the surface emulsion on the surface microflora and fauna is required.

The considerable range in sebum and sweat compositions between species could well be the outcome of a need to achieve within each of them an emulsion with satisfactory 'spreading' properties to enable complete skin coverage and an intact lipid cement; in rodents, which lack sweat glands on their body surface, it may be that there has been an evolutionary compensation in sebum composition to enable surface fluidity to be maintained.

Sweat and sebum secretion

The histological appearance of the sebaceous gland lobe led to the concept that sebum is derived from progenitor cells in the peripheral layer, which develop as they grow inwards towards the centre of the gland and ultimately disintegrate to form the secretion.[19,84] This process has been termed 'holocrine' secretion, which by definition implies that the entire secretion is simply the product of dead cells. However, it now seems more likely that the inner developing cells are derived only from precursors at the base of the lobe and that they grow outward as a column in a manner analogous to hair follicle growth.[85] Instead of producing a keratinized cylinder, in this instance the cell death results in a secretory product. The concept of holocrine secretion has also been challenged: evidence of intercellular transport through the basal layer into the sebum and the possibility of secretion during cell development indicate that the constituents of sebum are not all simply derived from dead cells and hence that sebum production is a more complex process than holocrine secretion.[86] This term could well become obsolete as new evidence on the mode of secretion emerges.

The historical concepts of secretory activity in the sweat gland are also based on light- and electron-microscopic observations of unstimulated glands.[87] The atrichial glands are believed to exhibit eccrine secretion whereby the sweat is produced by exocytosis without widespread disruption of the apical membrane. The epitrichial glands, on the other hand, are traditionally believed to also secrete in an apocrine manner. This process involves the formation of blebs at the apical portion of the secretory cell membrane, which are ultimately 'pinched off' into the glandular lumen.

Evidence from studies of stimulated sweat glands reveals that this traditional classification of sweat glands is no longer tenable and has led to the formulation of an alternative hypothesis – that the sebaceous and the sweat glands, both atrichial and epitrichial, have the same basic secretory mechanism.[86] It is considered that in both gland types the secretion is the product of two processes, cell death and secretion (including paracellular transfer), the relative importance of which can vary. Cell death, for example, is likely to dominate in the production of sebum and of sweat in species, such as the sheep, where there is low output and rapid secretory fatigue.[88] Secretory activity, on the other hand, may have a more dominant role in the rapid and profuse production of sweat in man and bovids. This hypothesis essentially promotes the view that the sebaceous and sweat glands, which are epidermal derivatives, function in a manner similar to that of the epidermis itself. The epidermis produces cells that are active during their period of differentiation, and when dead have a protective function on the skin. The idea that the glands similarly produce active secretory cells, which ultimately die to produce protective products on the skin, provides an attractive thesis for subsequent testing.

The acinar glands

It has been mentioned previously that some glabrous areas of skin contain sweat and sebaceous glands while others, like the skin of the elephant, have no glands at all. There is within the mammals a further variation to this general picture. In a number of mammals the skin of specialized glabrous areas on the face, for example the muzzle of cattle,[89, 90] contains an entirely different type of skin gland, an acinar gland, which has an appearance similar to that of salivary glands. These glands produce a mucus-rich fluid, which in such regions presumably replaces the sebum/sweat emulsion within the stratum corneum.

An extended definition of the skin surface

It is now evident that the outermost zone, the coat, acts on the one hand as a barrier to colonization from the environment but also provides a more stable microclimate for resident microorganisms. The epidermis provides in its outer layers a protected region with nutrients capable of supporting growth and development. Thus, when examining the dynamics of the skin surface ecosystem it is, for practical reasons, more appropriate to consider the skin surface as more than simply the outer margin exposed to the environment. Consequently the surface has been, for biological purposes, defined as the epidermis and the associated superficial hair coat. This definition will therefore be applied hereafter, when considering the inhabitants of the ecosystem.

Location of the surface inhabitants

It is now evident that the surface of healthy skin is capable of supporting life and that a diverse range of ectoparasites including microbes can and does utilize the environment within the outer stratum corneum and hair coat in spite of the defence mechanisms designed to restrict surface colonization and penetration to the dermis. Some of the inhabitants complete their life cycle on the skin and are considered to be residents while others, the transients (visitors), spend only a limited time there, mainly to feed.[91-3]

The residents

The resident organisms are not only faced with the host defences, they also have to contend with and overcome additional biological defence systems. They require to compete for nutrients with other resident inhabitants and also to combat direct challenges from them, for example, toxins produced by competitive species. The inhabitants have therefore adapted to meet the stringencies of the environment, including competitive inhibition, to provide a balanced ecosystem.[93-6]

A number of the surface inhabitants are mobile and specially equipped to penetrate the outer defences to enter the coat and attach to hairs (Fig. 1.10). Arthropods such as keds, mites and lice can enter and reside in this outer zone because they are small enough to escape detection by the 'early warning system' of nerves in the epidermis and around the hair follicles. Some are scavengers that feed on epidermal keratinized debris and exudate from wounds; these inhabitants can cause superficial damage to the epidermis,[97] which in healthy skin also seems to be subliminal to the host detection systems. Others, like *Demodex* spp., invade the epidermis or hair follicles also undetected until lowered host defences, as yet undefined, favour their proliferation to the extent that pathological conditions ensue.

Removal of successive layers of squames with adhesive tape has demonstrated that the microbial population of healthy skin is, as might be expected, located in the outer layers of the stratum corneum, which are permeated with the emulsion. The superficial position of the microbial habitat was established

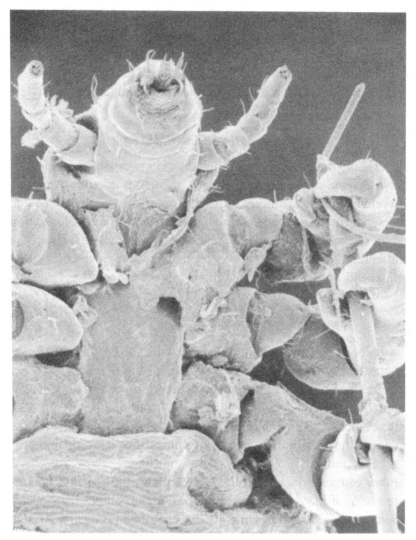

Fig. 1.10. Scanning electron micrograph of a louse attached to a hair from the bovine skin surface.

by the fact that between 75 and 95 per cent of all bacteria were located in the first four tape strips and there was a successive exponential decrease in bacterial number.[98–101] Electron microscopical studies have confirmed the peripheral location of the microbial population within the corneum and have shown that the mouths of the hair follicles are also important sites of microbial aggregation.[101–3] The inhabitants are, therefore, restricted to the outer few layers of the corneum and the pores of the hair follicles by the 'solid keratin wall', the disposition of the surface emulsion and the 'moving staircase' provided by the continually growing epidermis.

The microbial population seems to be distributed as mixed microcolonies between the layers of the outer stratum corneum; bacteria are often found in close association with yeasts or moulds.[93] Tape strips reveal that not all squames are colonized and it appears that the organisms live in symbiotic groups, probably in pockets where the thermal and gaseous microenvironment is favourable and the nutrient content of the emulsion is high. The overall size and balance of the surface population does, of course, alter if large fluctuations in host metabolism or the ambient conditions occur.[104] The delicacy of the balance is illustrated by the fact that increasing the ambient temperature to 30 °C raised the overall bacterial micropopulation on cattle skin by about 100-fold and modified the balance between species to the extent that residual changes were still detectable after a period of a week at 15 °C.[105] Nonetheless the skin population is a specialized one with only a limited number of inhabitants capable of continued growth and development. This is of advantage to the host because non-resident pathogenic bacteria face not only its defence systems but also considerable biological competition for survival.

Newly formed microorganisms produced within the stratum corneum adhere to squames[92] and are shed continuously into the wider environment by desquamation. The source of the 'flying saucers' of keratin with their attached organisms has therefore now been identified. What has not yet been fully explained, however, is how colonizing microbes, with no obvious means of propulsion, penetrate the coat and epidermal defences to reach the layers of intercellular emulsion. The healthy skin of the newborn[106] is rapidly colonized with bacteria soon after birth, a process not readily explained by transmission by larger mobile inhabitants, particularly visiting insects, that abrade or damage the epidermis. The resident bacteria presumably maintain a reproductive population against the continuously outward-moving epidermis by regular displacement of progeny to the lower layers of the corneum. This may be assisted by lateral movement of the emulsion within the corneum; radiolabelled substances applied to the skin spread across it within this layer.[107] However, the host, by this continuous outward movement, limits the size of the surface population and restricts its location to the periphery of the epidermis.

Viruses can proliferate within the living epidermis, where they induce pathological changes. However, it has still to be established whether or not they are capable of residing in the healthy epidermis. It is possible that viruses could reside in the basal cells in a latent uncapsulated form, restrained from replicating by local defence systems yet to be identified, until the advent of favourable conditions such as local immunosuppression. Cutaneous nerve endings or melanocytes are other possible host targets for viruses but the

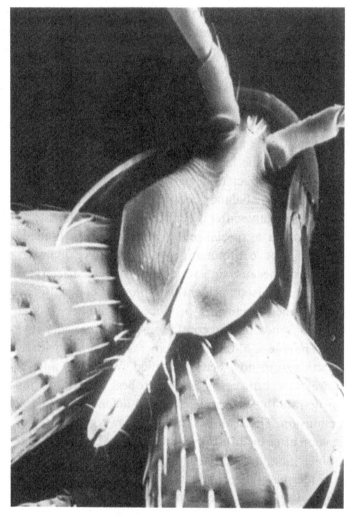

Fig. 1.11. Scanning electron micrograph showing the mouth parts of a flea. The proboscis is used in a manner analogous to a pneumatic drill to penetrate the skin.

outward epidermal growth makes the possibility of residence in the maturing keratinocytes unlikely because latent organisms would be extruded before having the opportunity to reproduce.

Viruses that replicate in the epidermis are most probably inoculated after a severe breach of the surface defences induced by events such as physical trauma or insect transmission. Prior damage has been shown to be a requirement for infection by orf virus,[108] and both immunocytochemical staining and reabrasion of the new epidermis over recently infected skin failed to provide evidence of viral retention in the newly healed skin.[109] The circumstantial evidence suggests that orf virus is not a resident of the epidermis, although it replicates within it. However, the possibility that it may be retained in an infective, encapsulated form within the coat for prolonged periods has not yet been eliminated. The advent of viral nucleic-acid probes may help resolve the question of whether or not viruses, such as orf, are latent residents of the surface or introduced visitors.

The transients

Most of the visitors to this ecosystem have developed specialized appendages to enable them to penetrate through the coat and epidermis to the underlying dermis, a source of nutrient fluid. While disrupting the surface defences they induce immune responses in the dermis and can cause local or systemic disease by transmitting pathogenic bacteria and viruses into or through the surface ecosystem.[110]

Various methods of skin penetration are employed. The bed bug, for example, is equipped with a stylet, which acts like a hypodermic needle, while that of the flea (Fig. 1.11) is applied with a vibratory action analogous to a pneumatic drill. The stable fly has a hardened proboscis with teeth that cut into the skin, while the tick has a combined cutting and piercing technique. Consequently the resulting damage is not uniform and can elicit variations in the host response.

Disruption of the surface defences

Breach or destruction of the surface defences also occurs as a result of abrasion, cuts, burns and the action of toxic chemicals. Colonization by microorganisms thus becomes easier and infection can follow as a result of the reduced defensive capacity at the surface and perhaps associated detrimental changes in dermal metabolism or immunosuppression.

However, less severe, often barely detectable, changes in the balance of the surface inhabitants can increase susceptibility to infection. These can be induced by alterations in host metabolism, for example by dietary change, and factors, such as maceration, scraping, clipping, shaving and solvent application, that modify the surface environment even though they do not sever the epidermis. For example, infection with *Dermatophilus* spp., which cannot be induced in cattle by applying the motile zoospores to untreated skin, was obtained after their application to skin that had been clipped or lightly wiped with solvent.[111] Washing the skin and occlusion of skin regions also influence the population dynamics of the skin surface bacteria.[112, 113]

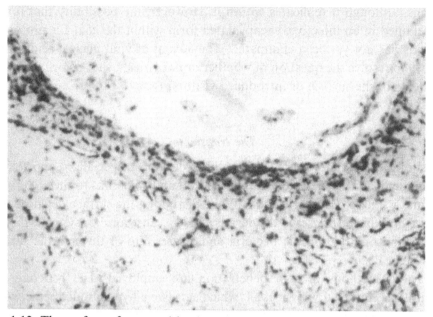

Fig. 1.12. The surface of a wound in sheep skin 12 h after damage. Dendritic cells, with major histocompatibility complex class II epitopes, can be seen aggregating at the exposed dermal surface. These rapidly provide the basis of a protective defence system within the dermis and act as a template for subsequent epidermal regeneration beneath it.

Repair mechanisms

Localized breach of the epidermis, however, presents only a transient opportunity for the invading pathogen because the host mounts a rapid response. In sheep, for example, epidermal damage induces an aggregation of dendritic cells with a surface reaction for class II molecules of the major histocompatibility complex. These cells, which appear to develop locally from lymphocytes, interdigitate to form a barrier at the outer margin of the exposed dermis.[114] This dendritic cell mass acts as a framework for a complex localized dermal immune defence system; T cells and neutrophils accumulate within it. It also acts as a template for a new layer of basal epidermal cells, which spread underneath it from the margins of the neighbouring undamaged epidermis to seal the gap and provide the basis of a new epidermis over the damaged zone (Fig. 1.12). The cellular mass is shed as a scab when the new underlying epidermis has matured. Infection induces a similar but more extensive reaction. Some helminth parasites, however, penetrate to the host dermis, where they escape detection because they have surface membranes compatible with those of the host tissues; they have, in effect, developed methods of immunodisguise to enable them to evade the host response.[115]

Conclusions

Mammalian skin has developed a number of peripheral defence systems designed to prevent or restrict invasion. Microorganisms arriving at the skin surface (defined as the epidermis and hair coat) require to elude an 'early warning' tactile system and penetrate to the floor of a bleak and often dense 'forest' of hairs. There they are faced with a 'cemented crazy paving', which most have to breach to reach a microenvironment suitable for colonization. Even if successful the incomer still has to adapt to a specialized microclimate, compete for nutrients with other inhabitants and be prepared for chemical warfare; an ability to combat chemical attack both by other organisms and the host is an essential requirement for survival. Even if successful they are effectively on a 'moving staircase', which restricts their inward spread and limits them to the coat and outer regions of the epidermis. It does, however, enable their progeny to leave the skin attached to 'flying saucers' of keratin, a mechanism that presumably increases their chances of locating and infecting other mammals.

The elaborate host defence mechanisms therefore restrict but do not prevent colonization; the skin surface supports a wide range of resident inhabitants and is visited by other organisms, in many instances briefly, to feed. A number of these visitors are equipped to penetrate the skin surface and obtain sustenance from dermal fluids. By causing breaches in the surface defences they probably facilitate entry of other organisms to the ecosystem.

Full definition of the ecosystem of healthy skin, including the mechanisms within it that increase susceptibility to infection and the systems involved in maintaining a balanced population, is still a long way off. However, further exploration of this miniature world will provide information on its inhabitants and on how they penetrate the host defences and succeed in colonizing this complex ecosystem. It is often stated that the risk of skin and other infections is increased when the body becomes 'run down'. This state has not yet been defined, as it represents the outcome of multifactorial influences on the body defences including those at the skin surface. Consequently, there is considerable scope for further exploration of this microworld by multidisciplinary biological teams, including microbiologists, before adequate measures to prevent infection by alien pathogens can be devised.

References

1 Jenkinson D McEwan, Lloyd DH. The topography of the skin surface of cattle and sheep. Br Vet J 1979; 135: 376–79.

2 Lewis HE, Foster AR, Mullan AR, Cox RN, Clark RP. Aerodynamics of the human microenvironment. Lancet 1969; i: 1273–77.

3 Irving L, Krog J. Temperature of skin in the Arctic as a regulator of heat. J Appl Physiol 1955; 7: 355–64.

4 Clark JA, Cena K. Die Anwendung von Thermovisions-Techniken bei Tiesen. Deut Tierarztl Wochenss 1972; 79: 292–96.

5 Johnson PC. Peripheral circulation. New York: John Wiley; 1978.

6 Bohr DF, Somlyo AP, Sparks HV Jr. The cardiovascular system. In: Handbook of physiology, Section 2. Baltimore: American Physiological Society/Williams & Wilkins; 1980.

7 Keatinge WR, Harman MC. Local mechanisms controlling blood vessels. Monographs of the Physiological Society No 37. Academic Press, London 1980.

8 Jenkinson D McEwan. Thermoregulatory function. In: Thody AJ, Friedman PS, eds. Scientific basis of dermatology. Edinburgh: Churchill Livingstone; 1986: 89–112.

9 Zucker IM. Reflex control of the circulation. London: Wolfe Medical; 1991.

10 Kligman AM. The biology of the stratum corneum. In: Montagna W, Lobitz WC Jr, eds. The epidermis. New York: Academic Press; 1964.

11 Spencer TS, Linamen CE, Akers WA, Jones HE. Temperature dependence of water content of stratum corneum. Br J Dermatol 1975; 93: 159–64.

12 Rothman S. Physiology and biochemistry of the skin. Chicago: University Press; 1955.

13 Middleton JD. Pathways of penetration of electrolytes through stratum corneum. Br J Dermatol 1969; 81: 56–61.

14 Elias PM, Friend DS. The permeability barrier in mammalian epidermis. J Cell Biol 1975; 65: 180–91.

15 Elias PM, Cooper ER, Korc A, Brown BE. Percutaneous transport in relation to stratum corneum structure and lipid composition. J Invest Dermatol 1981; 76: 297–301.

16 Montagna W, Bentley JP, Dobson RL. The dermis. In: Advances in biology of skin X. Oxford: Pergamon; 1970.

17 Jarrett A. Volume 3: the dermis and dendrocytes. In: The physiology and pathophysiology of the skin. London: Academic Press; 1974.

18 Breathnach AS. An atlas of the ultrastructure of human skin. London: Churchill; 1971.

19 Ross MH, Reith EJ, Romrell LG. Histology: a text and atlas. 2nd ed. Baltimore: Williams & Wilkins; 1989: 347–76.

20 Telford IR, Bridgman CF. Introduction to functional histology. New York: Harper & Row; 1990: 287–303.

21 Orland GF. Structure of the skin. In: Goldsmith LA, ed. Volume 1: Biochemistry and physiology of the skin. New York: Oxford University Press; 1983.

22 Lloyd DH, Amakiri SF, Jenkinson D McEwan. Structure of the sheep epidermis. Res Vet Sci 1979; 26: 180–82.

23 Hashimoto K. Intercellular spaces of the human epidermis as demonstrated with lanthanum. J Invest Dermatol 1971; 57: 17–31.

24 Matoltsy AG, Parakkal PF. Membrane-coating granules of keratinizing epithelia. J Cell Biol 1965; 24: 297–307.

25 Orland GF, Holbrook K. The lamellar granules of epidermis. Curr Prob Dermatol 1981; 9: 28–49.

26 Christophers E, Wolff HH, Laurence EB. The formation of epidermal cell columns. J Invest Dermatol 1974; 62: 555–59.

27 Matoltsy AG. Keratinization J Invest Dermatol 1976; 67: 20–25.

28 Matoltsy AG, Matoltsy MN. The membrane protein of horny cells. J Invest Dermatol 1966; 46: 127–29.

29 Elias PM, McNutt NS, Friend DS. Membrane alterations during cornification of mammalian squamous epithelia. A freeze-fracture tracer and thin-section study. Anat Rec 1975; 189: 577–94.

30 Weinstein GD, Van Scott EJ. Autographic analysis of turnover times of normal and psoriatic epidermis. J Invest Dermatol 1965; 45: 257–62.

31 Bergotresser PR, Taylor JR. Epidermal turnover time: a new examination. Br J Dermatol 1977; 96: 503–09.

32 Wilke MS, Hsu BM, Wille JJ, Pittelkow MR, Scott RE. Biologic mechanisms for the regulation of normal human keratinocyte proliferation and differentiation. Am J Pathol 1988; 131: 171–81.

33 Jarrett A. Volume 1: the epidermis. In: The physiology and pathophysiology of the skin. London: Academic Press; 1973.

34 Mali JWH, ed. Volume 6: keratinization and growth regulation. In: Current problems in dermatology. Basel: Karger; 1976.

35 Lloyd CW, Rees DA. Cellular controls in differentiation. London: Academic Press; 1981.

36 Noble WC. Dispersal of skin microorganisms. Br J Dermatol 1975; 93: 477–85.

37 Noble WC, Habbema JDF, van Furth R, Smith I, De Raay C. Quantitative studies on the dispersal of skin bacteria into the air. J Med Microbiol 1976; 9: 53–62.

38 Meers PD, Yeo GA. Shedding of bacteria and skin squames after handwashing. J Hyg Camb 1978; 81: 99–106.

39 Clark RP, Shirley SG. Identification of skin in airborne particulate matter. Nature 1973; 246: 39–40.

40 Clark RP. Skin scales among airborne particles. J Hyg Camb 1974; 72: 47–52.

41 Champion RH, Gillman T, Rook AJ, Sims RT. An introduction to the biology of the skin. Oxford: Blackwell Scientific; 1970.

42 Thody AJ, Friedman PS. Scientific basis of dermatology. Edinburgh: Churchill Livingstone; 1986: 36–57.

43 Weddell G, Palmer E, Pallie W. Nerve endings in mammalian skin. Biol. Rev. 1955; 30: 159–95.

44 Arthur RP, Shelley WB. The innervation of human epidermis. J Invest Dermatol 1959; 32: 397–411.

45 Montagna W. Cutaneous innervation. In: Advances in biology of skin, volume 1. Oxford: Pergamon; 1960.

46 Iggo A, Muir AR. The structure and function of a slowly adapting touch corpuscle in hairy skin. J Physiol 1969; 200: 763–96.

47 Cunnigham FC, Fitzgerald MJT. Encapsulated nerve endings in hairy skin. J Anat 1972; 112: 93–97.

48 Cauna N. Fine morphological characteristics and microtopography of the free nerve endings of the human digital skin. Anat Rec 1980; 198: 643–56.

49 Wolff K. The Langerhans cell. Curr Prob Dermatol 1972; 4: 79–145.

50 Bjercke S, Jannicke E, Braathen L, Thorsby E. Enriched epidermal Langerhans cells are potent antigen-presenting cells for T cells. J Invest Dermatol 1984; 83: 286–89.

51 Edelson RL, Fink JM. The immunologic function of skin. Sci Am 1985; 252: 34–41.

52 Bos JD, Kapsenberg ML. The skin immune system: its cellular constituents and their interaction. Immunol today 1986; 7: 235–40.

53 Straile W. A study of the hair follicle and its melanocytes. Develop Biol 1964; 10: 45–70.

54 Lyne AG, Short BF. Biology of the skin and hair growth. Sydney: Angus and Robertson; 1965.

55 Jarrett A. Volume 4: the hair follicle. In: The physiology and pathophysiology of the skin. London: Academic Press; 1977.

56 Weddell G, Miller S. Cutaneous sensibility. Ann Rev Physiol 1962; 24: 199–222.

57 Jenkinson D McEwan, Sengupta BP, Blackburn PS. The distribution of nerves, monoamine oxidase and cholinesterase in the skin of cattle. J Anat 1966; 100: 593–613.

58 Giacometti L, Montagna W. Adv Biol Skin 1969; 9: 393–98.

59 Straile W. Sensory hair follicles in mammalian skin: the Tylotrich follicle. Am J Anat 1960; 106: 133–47.

60 Jenkinson D McEwan. The skin of domestic animals. In: Rook AJ, Walton GS, eds. Comparative physiology and pathology of the skin. Oxford: Blackwell Scientific; 1965: 146–58.

61 Lee DG, Schmidt Nielsen K. The skin sweat glands and hair follicles of the camel (*Camelus dromedarius*). Anat Rec 1962; 143: 71–78.

62 Carter HB. The hair follicle group in sheep. Anim Breeding Abstracts 1955; 23: 101–16.

63 Lovell JE, Getty R. The hair follicle, epidermis, dermis and skin glands of the dog. Am J Vet Res 1957; 18: 873–85.

64 Montagna W, Dobson RL. Hair-growth. In: Advances in biology of skin IX. Oxford: Pergamon; 1967.

65 Ryder ML. Growth cycles in the coat of ruminants. Int J Chronobiol 1978; 5: 369–94.

66 Valkovic V. Human hair. Boca Raton, FA: CRC Press; 1988.

67 Dowling DF, Nay T. Cyclic changes in the follicles and hair coat in cattle. Austral J Agric Sci 1960; 11: 1064–71.

68 Ryder ML. Hair. London: Edward Arnold; 1973.

69 Hibbit KG, Cole CB, Reiter B. Antimicrobial proteins isolated from the teat canal of the cow. J Gen Microbiol 1969; 56: 365–71.

70 Hermann WP, Habbig J. Immunological studies on the proteins of human eccrine sweat. Arch Dermatol Res 1976; 255: 123–28.

71 Jenkinson D McEwan, Lloyd DH, Mabon RM. Location of the source of the soluble skin surface proteins of cattle by immunofluorescence. Res Vet Sci 1976; 21: 124–26.

72 Lloyd DH, Dick WDB, Jenkinson D McEwan. Structure of the epidermis in Ayrshire bullocks. Res Vet Sci 1979; 26: 172–79.

73 Kerr KG, Snow DH. Composition of sweat in the horse during prolonged epinephrine (adrenaline) infusion, heat exposure and exercise. Am J Vet Res 1983; 44: 1571–77.

74 Draize JH. The determination of the pH of the skin of man and common laboratory animals. J Invest Dermatol 1942; 5: 77–85.

75 Marples MJ. The ecology of human skin. Illinois: Charles C. Thomas; 1963.

76 Jenkinson D McEwan, Mabon RM. The effect of temperature and humidity on skin surface pH and the ionic composition of skin secretions in Ayrshire cattle. Br Vet J 1973; 129: 282–95.

77 Green M, Carol B, Behrendt H. Physiologic skin pH patterns in infants of low birth weight. Am J Dis Child 1968; 115: 9–16.

78 Abe T, Mayuzumi J, Kikuchi N, Arai S. Seasonal variations in skin temperature, skin pH, evaporative water loss and skin surface lipid values on human skin. Chem Pharm Bull 1980; 28: 387–92.

79 Harrison DK, Walker WF. Micro-electrode measurement of skin pH in humans during ischaemia, hypoxia and local hypothermia. J Physiol 1979; 291: 339–50.

80 Agosti M, Bruno R, Brugola L, Giacomelli D. Variation in skin pH in parasitic skin diseases (mange and lice) in beef cattle. Atti Soc Ital Sci Vet 1985; 37: 384–85.

81 Downing DT, Strauss JS, Ramasastry P, Abel M, Lee CW, Pochi PE. Measurement of the time between synthesis and surface secretion of sebaceous lipids in sheep and man. J Invest Dermatol 1975; 64: 215–19.

82 McMaster JD, Jenkinson D McEwan, Noble RC, Elder HY. Output of triglyceride from the sebaceous gland and to the skin surface of cattle. Res Vet Sci 1986; 41: 242–46.

83 Jenkinson D McEwan. Comparative physiology of sweating. Br J Dermatol 1973; 88: 397–406.

84 Rhodin JAG. Histology: a text and atlas. London: Academic Press; 1974.

85 Jenkinson D McEwan, Elder HY, Montgomery I, Moss VA. Comparative studies of the ultrastructure of the sebaceous gland. Tissue Cell 1985; 17: 683–98.

86 Jenkinson D McEwan. Sweat and sebaceous glands and their function in domestic animals. Adv Vet Dermatol 1990; 1: 229–51.

87 Schiefferdecker P. Die Hautdrusen des Menchen und der Saugetiere; ihre biologische und rassenanatomische Bedeitung sowie die Muscularis sexualis. Biol Zentrabl 1917; 37: 534–62.

88 Jenkinson D McEwan, Montgomery I, Elder HY. The ultrastructure of the sweat glands of the ox, sheep and goat during sweating and recovery. J Anat 1979; 129: 117–40.

89 Mackie AM, Nisbet AM. The histology of the bovine muzzle. J Agric Sci. 1959; 52: 376–79.

90 Majeed MA, Zaidi IH, Ilahi A. The nature of nasolabial gland secretion (NLGS) in large domestic ruminants. Res Vet Sci 1970; 11: 407–10.

91 Somerville-Millar DA, Noble WC. Resident and transient bacteria of the skin. J Cut Pathol 1974; 1: 260–64.

92 Andrews MLA. The life that lives on man. London: Faber & Faber; 1976.

93 Lloyd DH. The inhabitants of the mammalian skin surface. Proc R Soc Edinb 1980; 79B: 25–42.

94 Selwyn S. Natural antibiosis among skin bacteria as a primary defence against infection. Br J Dermatol 1975; 93: 487–93.

95 Adler J. The sensing of chemicals by bacteria. Sci Am 1976; 234: 40–7.

96 Marsh PD, Selwyn S. Studies on the antagonism between human skin bacteria. J Med Microbiol 1977; 10: 161–70.

97 Britt AG, Cotton CL, Pitman IH, Sinclair AN. Effects of the sheep chewing louse (*Damalinia ovis*) on the epidermis of the Australian Merino. Austr J Biol Sci 1986; 39: 137–43.

98 Röckl H, Muller E. Beitrag zur Lokalisation der Mikroben der Haut. Arch Klin Exp Dermatol 1959; 209: 13–29.

99 Williamson P, Kligman AM. A new method for the quantitative investigation of cutaneous bacteria. J Invest Dermatol 1965; 45: 498–503.

100 Noble WC, Somerville DA. Microbiology of human skin. London: WB Saunders; 1974.

101 Lloyd DH, Dick WDB, Jenkinson D McEwan. Location of the microflora in the skin of cattle. Br Vet J 1979; 135: 519–26.

102 Montes LF, Wilborn WH. Anatomical location of normal skin flora. Arch Dermatol 1970; 101: 145–59.

103 Malcolm SA, Hughes TC. The demonstration of bacteria on and within the stratum corneum using scanning electron microscopy. Br J Dermatol 1980; 102: 267–75.

104 McBride ME, Duncan WC, Knox JM. The environment and the microbial ecology of human skin. Appl Environ Microbiol 1977; 33: 603–8.

105 Lloyd DH. The effect of climate on the microbial ecology of the skin of cattle and sheep [PhD thesis]. University of Glasgow; 1978.

106 Sarkany I, Gaylarde CC. Skin flora of the newborn. Lancet 1967; i: 589–90.

107 Jenkinson D McEwan, Hutchinson G, Jackson D, McQueen L. Route of passage of cypermethrin across the surface of sheep skin. Res Vet Sci 1986; 41: 237–41.

108 Jenkinson D McEwan. Histopathological studies of ovine orf. Vet Dermatol Newslett 1989; 12: 18–20.

109 McKeever DJ, Jenkinson D McEwan, Hutchinson G, Reid HW. Studies of the pathogenesis of orf virus infection in sheep. J Comparat Pathol 1988; 99: 317–28.

110 Orkin M, Maibach HI. Cutaneous infestations and insect bites. In: Dermatology series, volume 4. New York: Marcel Dekker; 1985.

111 Lloyd DH, Jenkinson D McE. The effect of climate on experimental infection of bovine skin with *Dermatophilus congolensis* Br Vet J 1980; 136: 122–34.

112 Bibel DJ, Lovell DJ, Smiljanic R. Effects of occlusion upon population dynamics of skin bacteria. Br J Dermatol 1976; 95: 607–12.

113 Hartmann A. Restriction of washing and its effect to the normal human skin flora. Arch Dermatol Res 1978; 263: 105–10.

114 Jenkinson D McEwan, Hutchison G, Onwuka SK, Reid HW. Changes in the MHC Class II dendritic cell population of ovine skin in response to orf virus infection. Vet Dermatol 1991; 2: 1–9.

115 Chappel LH. The biology of the external surfaces of helminth parasites. Proc R Soc Edinb 1980; 79B: 145–72.

2

Nutrition of cutaneous resident microorganisms

K. T. HOLLAND

Introduction

Investigators concerned with the nutrition of microorganisms usually start their research with the question, 'What chemicals does this microorganism require to grow?' Perhaps a better question would be, 'What chemicals does this microorganism utilize in its environment?' To obtain formal proof of the nutrition of cutaneous microorganisms in the skin environment has been an impossibility for many reasons. There is the ethical problem of obtaining samples of both the cutaneous populations and human skin. Experiments on laboratory animals, although offering some hope, are severely limited because the skin microflora is different from that of man. For example, there are no propionibacteria or *Malassezia furfur* on animal skin, yet these micro-organisms are widely distributed over human skin. Also, and related, are the different macromorphological structures of animal and human skin. Animal skin is haired and lacks the sebaceous gland systems with large follicles and small vellus hairs. Even those animals bred hairless have skin that is distinctly different from human skin. Another complication is that the sampling of the skin environment and the subsequent chemical and biochemical analyses of presumptive nutrients can be misleading. The molecules used as nutrients by the resident microflora may well not be present in the sample because they have been used to exhaustion; some of the molecules in the sample may well be end-products of metabolism of the microbial population, for example acetate and propionate from *Propionibacterium acnes* fermentation. Analysis of skin-surface lipids, sweat and their emulsion have yielded an amazing array of chemicals. However, to predict which chemicals are used by what microorganism is more a matter of personal conviction rather than certain knowledge. Strictly there can be no such value as an 'average' composition of sweat, as this varies between individuals, and between sites and sampling

Table 2.1. *Substances recovered from sweat*

Less than 0.1 mg/l	0.1–0.99 mg/l	1.0–9.9 mg/l	10–99 mg/l	More than 99 mg/l
Iodine	Bromide	Potassium	Chloride	Glycine
Magnesium	Fluoride	Sodium	Phosphate	Ornithine
Manganese	Calcium	Copper	Sulphate	Serine
Cadmium	Iron	Methionine	Alanine	Urea
Lead	Zinc	Taurine	Arginine	Mucoprotein
Nickel	Cystine	Glutamine	Citrulline	Lactic acid
Acetylcholine		Cysteine	Histidine	
Vitamins		Creatinine	Isoleucine	
		Uric acid	Leucine	
			Lysine	
			Phenylalanine	
			Threonine	
			Tyrosine	
			Valine	
			Asparaginic acid	
			Glutamic acid	
			Asparagine	
			Arginine	
			Ammonia	
			Urocanic acid	
			Glucose	
			Pyruvic acid	

occasions on the same individual. Thus the standard deviation in the concentration of each amino acid in a population of normals is about 50 per cent of the mean value and, even in a single individual followed over 12 months, the standard deviation is 45 per cent of the mean. The values shown in Table 2.1 are for the composition of sweat at the skin surface, thus including some epidermal components, and are derived from data collated from a number of publications.[1]

From a very general point of view the relationship between a microorganism's behaviour, physiological response and expressed phenotype is dependent on, amongst other factors, the types of available nutrients and their concentration. Furthermore, these physiological responses operate within an open system rather than a closed one; that is, the environment is dynamic and changing, with a throughput of nutrients, production and loss of microbial biomass, and excretion and loss of bacterial metabolites and extracellular products.

Classical bacterial growth kinetics predict that the growth of a population is dependent on temperature, which is considered to be reasonably steady compared with other factors, on pH, on the concentration of the limiting nutrient, and on the presence and concentration of inhibitors. Clearly, over time the limiting nutrient concentration may change and this will affect the population's rate of growth.[2] In addition, it is more than possible that nutrient limitation will change from one nutrient to another, producing not only a change in growth rate but also a major phenotypic change in the cells.[3] Changes in inhibitor concentration, or their gain or loss, will also have these effects. Nutrition, then, has major influences on the type of population, its density, its turnover rate and its expressed phenotype.

The nutritional requirements, which are represented by carbon and energy source, oxygen, nitrogen source, phosphate, sulphur and many ions and vitamins, are determined at a minimal level by the genotype of the cell. This is expressed, in the majority of cases, not by the internal enzymatic constitution but by the ability to transport the particular molecule across the cytoplasmic membrane into the cell. Large molecules, polymers and polar molecules do not permeate across the lipophilic membrane and require transport-specific protein groupings. Sensitivity to inhibitors is dependent also on the cell being able to transport the molecule into the intracellular target site. Interestingly, the skin environment has many lipophilic molecules that should permeate the cell membrane without specific transporters and these molecules may well be both nutrients and inhibitors.

From the foregoing it is clear that the nutritional requirements of the cells of any species have a range from a minimum to a maximum where the minimum can be determined in vitro experimentally whereas the maximum could be imponderable. What seems intuitively correct is that the minimal nutritional requirements of the particular microorganism represent those chemicals that are normally and consistently present in the natural environment in which that microorganism resides.

All the resident microflora of human skin are chemoorganotrophs and require organic nutrients. Oxidation of these nutrients produces the cells' energy requirements, and carbon is incorporated into the cell biomass from organic molecules.

Organic molecules may also be required because the pathways for their synthesis are not present. It is easy to design in vitro investigations to determine the reasons for the absolute requirement for a specific molecule. Inward transport of the molecule can be determined by suspending the cells in buffer with an energy source such as glucose, exposing them to a radiolabelled molecule of interest, and after a short incubation, separating them from the suspending fluid, and then determining the radiolabel held by them. Confirmation of transport and dismissal of cell-wall surface adsorption of the test molecule can be undertaken with some technical difficulty by repeating the experiment with protoplasts of the cells. If the molecule is transported into the protoplast, then the synthetic pathway for the molecule may or may not be encoded by the genotype. However, if it is not transported, then it is clear that it must be capable of being synthesized within the cell. Confirmation of an incomplete synthetic pathway can be obtained by analysing the cell extract for the enzymes that are involved in the synthesis of the molecule.

All these approaches first rely on more technically simple methods to determine nutrient requirements. Initial information is gained by observation of the lack of recovery, or reduced recovery, of microorganisms from the skin using commercially available nutrients. An example would be the inability to isolate *M. furfur* from skin samples using media without a lipid supplement. From this point, two major approaches may be taken. Cells suspended in buffer can be exposed simultaneously to a range of suspected nutrients and, after incubation, the fluid phase analysed for their reduction in concentration. This method has several problems. It indicates what can be used not what is required, and because of competition between molecules for the same transport system, spurious results may be obtained. The other approach is to test the ability of a synthetic medium with a full range of possible nutrients to support the growth of the cells when a single component nutrient is omitted. The results cannot be interpreted with confidence because some molecules may substitute for others. A typical example is the group of aromatic amino acids. Furthermore, as already mentioned, the remaining compounds may cause reduced growth because of transport competition.

A more dependable strategy, but more time consuming, is sequential omission. Clearly, as more compounds are omitted, growth yield may decrease because of overall reduction in carbon and nitrogen, which can be redressed by increasing the concentration of the remaining molecules. This approach should determine the minimal requirements. These findings will only be relevant to the environment in which they have been tested. For instance, uracil and pyruvate are not required by *Staphylococcus aureus* when grown in the presence of oxygen. However, under anaerobic conditions both are required. Further complications arise in regard of the criteria used for nutrient requirement. If requirement only refers to that for cell growth, then the methods of sequential omission will suffice. However, if the requirements include those for extracellular protein, enzyme, toxin and virulence factor production, then the minimal requirements may well not suffice. Again, using *S. aureus* as an example, the production of toxic-shock syndrome toxin (TSST-1) can be modulated by the environmental Mg^{2+} concentration, with low and

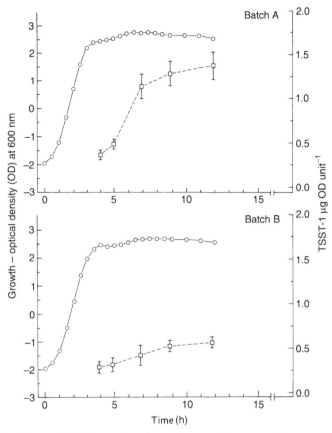

Fig. 2.1. The effect of different batches of a medium on the growth and toxin production by *Staph. aureus*. ○, growth; □, toxin (TSST-1, toxic-shock syndrome toxin-1).

high concentrations being partially inhibitory.[4] This will be dependent on other environmental characteristics. No better example can be found than the variance in extracellular enzyme production in different batches of the same commercial medium, an example of which is given in Fig. 2.1. *Staphylococcus aureus* showed identical, as far as could be measured, growth kinetics and yet the production of extracellular TSST-1 was very different in the two batches of brain–heart infusion (D. Taylor & K. T. Holland, unpublished).

The remainder of the chapter will be concerned with chemicals and their role as either, or both, nutrients and inhibitors. The emphasis will be on the resident normal microflora, namely the staphylococci, propionibacteria, the less taxonomically defined aerobic coryneforms and *M. furfur* (*Pityrosporum ovale*). Since the last edition of *Microbiology of Human Skin* in 1981,[1] there has been little progress in the field of nutrition of the cutaneous microflora. The

Table 2.2. Summary of nutrient requirements of cutaneous microorganisms

Microorganism	Carbohydrate can be used as a C/E[a]	Amino acids C/E[a]	Amino acids Minimal number required	NH₄ as sole nitrogen source	Vitamin number required	Nucleotides	Lipid essential	Relationship with oxygen
Micrococcus spp.	+	+	1–3	(+)	1–3	–	–	Aerobic
Staphylococcus spp.	+	+	1–13	(+)	2–5	[+]	–	Facultative anaerobic
Propionibacterium spp.	+	+	8?	–	3	–	–	Microaerophil[b]
Aerobic coryneforms	+	+	+?	(+)	(+)	–	(+)	Aerobic and facultative anaerobe
Malassezia furfur	+	?	?	?	?	?	+	Aerobe
Acinetobacter spp.	(+)	+	–	+	–	–	–	Aerobe
Escherichia coli	+	+	–	+	–	–	–	Facultative anaerobe
Serratia spp.	+	+	–	+	–	–	–	Facultative anaerobe
Proteus spp.	+	+	–	+	–	–	–	Facultative anaerobe
Providencia spp.	+	+	–	+	–	–	–	Facultative anaerobe
Pseudomonas spp.	+	+	–	+	–	–	–	Aerobe, anaerobic respiration
Enterobacter spp.	+	+	–	+	–	–	–	Facultative anaerobe

[a] Carbon/energy source; [b] usually isolated anaerobically; ?, not known; ( ), for some isolates only; [ ], required when growing under anaerobic conditions.

Table 2.3. *Extracellular enzymes produced by the cutaneous microorganisms*[5, 36, 44-5, 79-83]

Microorganisms	Lipase	Esterase	Protease	Keratinase	Haemolysin	DNAse	PO$_4$ase	Neuraminidase	Hyaluronate lyase	Nitrate reduction
Staphylococcus										
aureus	+	+	+		+	+	+	−	−	(+)
simulans	+	+	(−)		+	+	+	−	−	+
xylosus	(+)	(+)	(−)		(−)	(−)	(+)	−	−	(+)
cohnii	(+)	+	(+)		(−)	(−)	(+)	−	−	−
saprophyticus	+	+	(−)	+	+	+		−	−	(+)
haemolyticus	+	+	(−)	+	+	−		−	−	−
warneri	+	+	(−)	+	(+)	+		−	−	(+)
hominis	+	+	(−)	+	(+)	+	+	−	−	(+)
epidermidis	+	+	+	+	(+)	+		−	−	(+)
capitis	+	+	(−)	+	(+)	+		−	−	(+)
saccharolyticus								−	−	
auricularis	+	+	(−)		(−)	+	−	−	−	(+)
Micrococcus										
luteus	−		+	+	−	−	−	−		
lylae	(+)		+	+	−	−	−	−		
sedentarius	−		+	+	−	−	−	−		
varians	−		+	+	−	−	−	−		
roseus	−		−	−	−	−	−	−		
kristinae	−		−	+	−	−	−	−		
nishinomiyaensis	(+)		+	+	−	−	−	−		
Propionibacterium										
acnes	+		+	−	(+)	+	+	+	+	+
avidum	+		+	−	+	+	−	−	−	
granulosum	+		−	−		+	−	−	+	
Aerobic coryneforms:										
lipophilic	+		−		−	(+)	(+)			(+)
Brevibacterium	−	−	+	+		+				
Corynebacterium	+	−	+	−	−	−	(+)	−		(+)
Acinetobacter spp.		−	−			−		−	−	−
Escherichia coli		−	−			−		−	−	+
Enterobacter spp.			+			+		−	−	+
Proteus spp.	+		+			+		−	−	+
Providencia spp.			−			−		−	−	+
Pseudomonas spp.	+	−	+		−	+	−	−	−	+
Serratia spp.	+	+	+			+	−	−	−	+
Malassezia furfur	+		+			+	−	−	−	−

+, produced by all isolates; (+), produced by most isolates; (−), produced by some isolates.

majority of the work cited will be post-1975. This date was chosen because from this time the taxonomies of the staphylococci and micrococci were greatly improved. In data from before that year, it is difficult to relate information on nutrition of these groups to their recent nomenclature. The reader is referred to *Bergey's Manual of Systematic Bacteriology* for general information about physiological tests that have a nutritional basis, for example, sugar fermentations.[5]

It is worth noting that there is more information on the nutrition of staphylococci, micrococci and propionibacteria than on the other common members of the skin microflora, namely the aerobic coryneforms and *M. furfur*. There are various reasons for this. The staphylococci and micrococci have received much attention by taxonomists, and the staphylococci, not just *S. aureus*, are of increasing medical importance in modern times. The interest in propionibacteria has been promoted by their possible role in acne.

The attempt in this chapter is to present a comparison of the similarities and differences of nutritional requirements amongst the skin inhabitants. It is hoped that this will stimulate further enquiry into this field of study and indicate that our present knowledge is far from adequate. The subjects considered are water-soluble substances – extracellular enzymes, inorganic ions, oxygen, carbon/energy source, nitrogen source and vitamins – and lipids.

Table 2.2 summarizes the nutrient requirements of the cutaneous micro-organisms. All the inhabitants are chemoorganotrophs, requiring organic nutrients and using oxidation of these to obtain energy. The minimum requirements are known for only a few Gram-positive bacteria. However there is more information on the vitamin requirements of the cutaneous microflora. The information in Table 2.2 highlights the dependence of the Gram-positive microflora, the resident and dominant group, on at least one vitamin. There is no requirement for vitamins or indeed an organic nitrogen source by the Gram-negative group. This reinforces the view that the Gram-negative group have evolved in a habitat different from the skin.

Water-soluble substances

Extracellular enzymes

At this juncture, it is worth giving an introduction to extracellular enzymes that are produced by microorganisms. It is generally agreed that extracellular enzymes are required to scavenge for nutrients by making available low molecular-weight compounds, which can be transported across the cell

Table 2.4. *Potential nutrients produced by the activities of*
extracellular enzymes

Enzymes	Substrate	Use	Nutrients
Lipase	Water-insoluble compounds with ester bonds, e.g. triglycerides	Carbon/energy Biotin deficiency	Glycerol Fatty acids Fatty acids
Protease	Proteins and peptides	Carbon/energy and nitrogen source	Peptides and amino acids
Phosphatase	Phosphorylated organic molecules	Carbon/energy Phosphate source	Dephosphorylated sugars Phosphate
DNAse	DNA	Carbon/energy Phosphate source Base source	Sugar Phosphate Purines and pyrimidines
Neuraminidase	Sialic acid	Carbon/energy	Sugars Polyalcohols
Hyaluronate lyase	Hyaluronic acid and related polymers	Carbon/energy	Sugars

membrane. These arise from high molecular-weight polymers which cannot enter the cell. Extracellular enzymes are those produced within the cell and specifically exported through the cytoplasmic membrane. In the case of the Gram-negative bacteria these extracellular enzymes are held within the periplasmic space by the outer cell membrane, and are only released with cell death when the outer membrane is damaged. However, some Gram-negative cells have specific mechanisms for translocating the enzyme through the outer membrane.[6] Gram-positive bacteria are known for their extracellular enzyme production, and these enzymes, in the main, are released into the surrounding environment. However, some enzymes remain bound to the cell wall as well as being released into the environment. Such is the case with the phosphatase of *S. epidermidis*.[7] There are two useful reviews on extracellular enzymes.[8,9] Control of production of these enzymes is complicated and interesting. Some are growth linked and are produced in a constant ratio to cell biomass; the role of these would appear to be essential, regardless of the fluctuations in the external environment. Other enzymes are not growth linked and their production in the cell is controlled by the cell sensing the external environment. Many extracellular enzymes are repressed by the presence of glucose, and proteases can be repressed by amino acids in the environment. It is a

Table 2.5. *Salt tolerance of cutaneous microorganisms*[5, 38, 44, 82, 84]

Microorganism	Growth up to % NaCl
Staphylococcus	
aureus	15
simulans	15
xylosus	10
cohnii	15
saprophyticus	10
haemolyticus	10
warneri	10
hominis	10
epidermidis	10
capitis	10
saccharolyticus	?
auricularis	15
Micrococcus	
luteus	7.5
lylae	7.5
sedentarius	7.5
varians	7.5
roseus	7.5
kristinae	10
nishinomiyaensis	< 7.5
Propionibacterium	
acnes	?
avidum	?
granulosum	?
Aerobic coryneforms:	
lipophilic	9
Brevibacterium	15
Corynebacterium	10
Acinetobacter spp.	?
Escherichia coli	Low
Enterobacter spp.	Low
Proteus spp.	Low
Providencia spp.	Low
Pseudomonas spp.	Low
Serratia spp.	8.5
Malassezia furfur	?

reasonable assumption that the difference in control of production of these enzymes implies a different functional role.

Table 2.3 gives the range of extracellular enzymes produced by the skin microflora. Virulence factors such as haemolysins, some of which are not enzymes, produced by, for example, *S. aureus*, have been included, even though their function is involved in the defence against host cellular attack. Host cell lysis may release nutrients and expose the internal polymers to other enzymatic attack to increase nutrient availability. In many cases, it is not clear whether haemolysis as seen on media is due to a specific haemolysin(s) or whether red blood-cell lysis has been caused by other enzymes, or indeed whether the lysis is enzymatic.

The skin has polymers, including lipids, polysaccharides and proteins, and mixed polymers of various structures; the skin microflora produces extracellular enzymes that degrade these polymers to release smaller, manageable nutrients. The substrates, end-products and suggested functions of these enzymes are given in Table 2.4. End-products of all the enzymes would appear to have a direct nutritional value. However, one of the end-products of lipase activity, free fatty acids, may be inhibitory and this issue will be discussed under lipids below.

The two most common enzymatic activities produced by the skin microflora are lipase and protease. In most cases, it is not known whether the bacteria that are capable of degrading soluble protein and keratin produce enzymes for each substrate. It is clear that keratinases will attack soluble proteins and that a protease which attacks soluble proteins generally has no keratinase activity. Also, it is common for bacteria to produce more than one protease, as do *S. aureus*, *S. epidermidis* and *P. acnes*.[7, 10, 11] Overall there is no highly consistent pattern of production of the various enzymes by the cutaneous microflora. This implies either that there are various ecological niches in or on the skin, or that there may be cross-feeding, or that for much of the time the skin has a supply of monomers for the nutrition of the bacteria that do not produce extracellular enzymes.

The definitive role and importance of the extracellular enzymes of the cutaneous microorganisms will only be determined when enzyme-deficient mutants, which are otherwise isogenic with the wild-type strain, are made and tested in suitable model systems.

Inorganic ions

The inorganic ions required by the cutaneous microflora will be similar to any other human-associated prokaryote and consequently little time will be spent on this subject. The majority of ions are required in micromolar external concentrations and when transported into the cell are cofactors of enzymes. Higher concentrations (millimolar) of phosphate are required for synthesis of DNA, RNA, phospholipids and polymers such as teichoic acid. Some of the cutaneous bacteria, including staphylococci, coryneforms and propioni-bacteria (see Table 2.3), produce extracellular phosphatases that hydrolyse phosphate from a variety of organic molecules and polymers. Magnesium is also required in higher concentrations for cytosolic enzymes and it functions to stabilize the energy-transducing ATPase system in the cytoplasmic membrane. Sulphur, present in redox enzymes, is probably assimilated via sulphate. The sulphur present in methionine and cysteine is taken up directly, in the form of the amino acids, or more likely as small peptides containing these amino acids.

Bacterial taxonomists often use the reduction of nitrate by a bacterium as one of many taxonomic criteria. However, this test does not distinguish between the microorganism reducing nitrate for assimilating nitrogen, or using the nitrate as an electron acceptor for energy transduction. Some cutaneous bacteria (see Table 2.3) do reduce nitrate. At present, in many cases, it is not known whether this is energetically favourable. Furthermore, it is unclear whether there is enough nitrate in the habitat for such a function.

The ions are nutrients and as such will have an effect on the growth rate of the microorganisms if they are in limiting concentration. Consequently, their availability may determine the population density at a skin site.

It has been shown with *S. aureus* that the concentration of a particular ion can modulate the production of extracellular toxins, although it is possible that this effect is controlled via growth rate.[4,12] These effects may be exhibited by other cutaneous bacteria. It is known that phosphate limitation in an environment can increase phosphatase production by *S. aureus* and other staphylococci, and, conversely, excess phosphate represses phosphatase production.[13,14]

Ions can influence the growth and physiology of microorganisms by affecting the osmotic strength of the surroundings. Increasing the ionic strength of the medium increases the osmotic strength and reduces the environment's water activity. Therefore, ions may influence growth, particularly of the Gram-negative cells (apart from *Serratia* spp.) that attempt to colonize the skin, because the skin may have a low water activity. Gram-positive bacteria can grow in an environment with a low water activity and, consequently, have a high salt tolerance (Table 2.5). The osmotic pressure of the experimental media used to obtain the data in Table 2.5 would be higher than that obtained with the stated concentration of NaCl because other solutes present would have an osmotic influence. No information is available, as yet, on the priopionibacteria, many of the aerobic coryneforms or *M. furfur*.

Gram-negative bacteria, in general, show poor adaptation to high environmental osmotic pressures and have low internal turgor pressures

Table 2.6. *Utilization of sugars and polyalcohols by staphylococci and micrococci.*[5]

Compound	S. aureus	S. simulans	S. cohnii	S. xylosus	S. saprophyticus	S. haemolyticus	S. warneri	S. hominis	S. capitis	S. epidermidis	S. auricularis	S. saccharolyticus	Micrococcus spp.
Glucose	+	+	+	+	+	+	+	+	+	+	+	+	+
Lactose	+	+	(+)	(+)	+	(+)	(+)	(+)	–	(+)	(+)	–	–
Maltose	+	–	+	+	+	+	+	(+)	–	+	+	–	(+)
Mannitol	+	+	+	+	+	(+)	+	–	+	–	–	–	(+)
Fructose	+	+	+	+	+	(+)	+	(+)	+	+	+	+	+
Galactose	+	–	(+)	(+)	(+)	(+)	(+)	(+)	–	(+)	–	–	+
Mannose	+	+	–	+	–	–	(+)	(+)	+	(+)	(+)	+	–
Ribose	+	(+)	(+)	(+)	(+)	(+)	(+)	(+)	–	(+)	(+)	–	(+)
Sucrose	+	+	(+)	(+)	+	+	+	+	+	+	(+)	–	+
Trehalose	+	+	+	(+)	+	+	+	+	–	(+)	+	+	–
Turanose	+	–	+	(+)	+	(+)	(+)	+	–	(+)	(+)	–	–
Glycerol	+	+	+	+	+	+	+	+	+	+	+	–	+
Arabinose	–	–	–	(+)	–	–	–	–	–	–	–	–	(+)
Xylose	–	–	–	+	+	–	–	–	–	–	–	–	(+)
Xyliitol	–	–	(+)	(+)	+	–	(+)	+	–	–	–	–	–
Meleziose	–	–	–	–	–	–	(+)	+	–	(+)	–	–	–
Cellobiose	–	–	–	–	–	–	–	–	–	–	–	–	–
Gentibiose	–	–	–	–	(+)	–	–	–	–	–	–	–	–
Sorbitol	–	–	–	–	–	–	–	–	–	–	–	–	(+)
Inositol	–	–	–	–	–	–	–	–	–	–	–	–	–
Salicin	–	–	–	–	–	–	–	–	–	–	–	–	–
Adonitol	–	–	–	–	–	–	–	–	–	–	–	–	–
Dulcitol	–	–	–	–	–	–	–	–	–	–	–	–	–
Arabitol	–	–	–	–	–	–	–	–	–	–	–	–	–
Erythritol	–	–	–	–	–	–	–	–	–	–	–	–	–
Erythrose	–	–	–	–	–	–	–	–	–	–	–	–	–
Raffinose	–	–	–	–	–	–	–	–	–	–	–	–	–
Melibiose	–	–	–	–	–	–	–	–	–	–	–	–	–
Fucose	–	–	–	–	–	–	–	–	–	–	–	–	–
Rhamnose	–	–	–	(+)	–	–	–	–	–	–	–	–	(+)
Lyxose	–	–	–	–	–	–	–	–	–	–	–	–	–
Sorbose	–	–	–	–	–	–	–	–	–	–	–	–	–
Dextrin	–	–	–	–	–	–	–	–	–	–	–	–	–

( ), not all isolates can utilize the compound.

(0.8–5 atm). Gram-positive bacteria have higher internal turgor pressures, 15–20 atm, and can adapt to an increase in the environmental osmotic pressure. The primary regulatory solute is K^+ and then there are secondary systems of synthesis of osmoprotectants.[15]

Protons are important ions in the environment because their concentration determines the local pH and, consequently, the growth yield and growth rate of the resident microbial populations. The bacterial cells maintain a near-neutral pH regardless of the external pH.[16] This pH homeostasis is essential for cell viability. Environmental pH values that are acidic or alkaline depress growth because there is a requirement for the cell to expend energy, otherwise used for biomass production, in order to regulate the internal cell pH against the proton gradient that is set up between the internal and external pHs.

The pH of the skin is acidic pH 5–6 and the total cutaneous microflora, it can be assumed, is viable at these pH values.[17,18] No systematic study has looked at the physiological aspects of the microflora under controlled pH conditions, apart from those of propionibacteria grown in a continuous culture model (in which only one isolate of each species was studied). The propionibacteria grew between pH 4.5 and 8.0, with optima between pH 5.5 and 6.0;[19] *Propionibacterium acnes* was acid tolerant, growing between pH 4.5 and 7.5, whilst pH values between 5.0 and 8.0 supported the growth of *P. avidum* and *P. granulosum*. Changes in growth rate and biomass were equally related to change in pH with *P. acnes* and *P. avidum*. However, highest yields of *P. granulosum* occurred at pH 7.5, even though the highest growth rate was at pH 6.0 (Fig. 2.2).

Proton concentration (pH) can affect the production of extracellular enzymes. In the same study,[19] low levels of lipase, protease, phosphatase and hyaluronate lyase were detected in continuous culture at pH values near the extremes of the pH growth range, owing to both low production and high denaturation. It is more than likely that this would occur with the other members of the cutaneous microflora that produce extracellular enzymes. Indeed, no TSST-1 and little hyaluronate lyase were detected when *S. aureus* was grown at pH 5.5, although the growth yield was depressed by only 33 per cent compared to growth at pH 7.4, at which large amounts of TSST-1 and hyaluronate lyase were produced (D. Taylor & K. T. Holland, unpublished).

The extremes of the pH in which the other cutaneous bacteria can grow are greater than those of the propionibacteria. Consequently, environmental pH values in the 4.5–6.0 range will differentially affect the production of extracellular enzymes in addition to the growth of the various groups of microorganisms. For example, high production of lipase by propionibacteria occurs at low pH, in contrast to the absence of staphylococcal lipase at pH 5.0

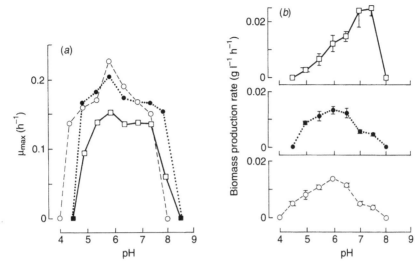

Fig. 2.2. The effect of pH on the growth of propionibacteria. (*a*) Effect of pH on the maximum specific growth rate of *P. acnes* (○), *P. avidum* (●) and *P. granulosum* (□). (*b*) Effect of pH on biomass production at 0.33 μ_{max} of *P. acnes* (○), *P. avidum* (●) and *P. granulosum* (□). The bars represent 95 % confidence limits about the mean.

and below. Only when the pH was raised to about 6.5 did staphylococcal lipase production approach that of the propionibacteria. These experiments were carried out in a base medium with added pooled homogenized and sterilized sebaceous glands.[20] Situations can be envisaged where, at low pH, growth of propionibacteria occurs with little or no extracellular enzyme production, and other skin residents would remain viable but not grow. At slightly higher pH values the propionibacteria reach maximum growth rate with high extracellular enzyme production, and the other residents grow slowly with little extracellular enzyme production. At higher pH the propionibacteria are disadvantaged, with lower growth rates and reduced extracellular enzyme production, and now the other resident microorganisms grow quickly and produce maximum amounts of extracellular enzymes. Therefore, the pH of microenvironments on the skin may play a decisive role in determining which microorganisms remain in residence.

The findings of Puhvel and coworkers mentioned above[20] could explain those of Marples and colleagues.[21] Using different antibiotics to inhibit selectively the main groups of microorganisms on the skin, Marples' team showed that only when the propionibacteria were inhibited did the free fatty acid levels on the skin decrease, and they therefore concluded that the lipases of the propionibacteria were the main source of activity, cleaving sebaceous triglycerides to di- and monoglycerides, and to free fatty acids and glycerol. It is probable that the staphylococcal lipases play a more prominent role when the local skin pH rises to above pH 6.0.

Oxygen

Table 2.2 above includes information on the oxygen requirements of the cutaneous microorganisms. Within these are strict aerobes, such as the brevibacteria, lipophilic coryneforms and micrococci, and many facultative anaerobes such as the staphylococci. The latter use oxygen as the terminal electron acceptor in their electron transport-linked phosphorylation system and in the absence of, or with any limitation by, oxygen rely on substrate-level phosphorylation, namely fermentation. It should be noted that *S. saccharolyticus* grows very poorly under aerobic conditions and in this respect resembles the propionibacteria. As mentioned previously, it is possible that anaerobic respiration may be used when there is limitation by oxygen and in the presence of nitrate or fumarate, which serve as electron acceptors. Examples of bacteria using nitrate and fumarate are the Gram-negative bacteria listed in Table 2.3. Staphylococci can utilize nitrate.[22]

The relationship between oxygen and propionibacteria is a contentious and interesting one. Efficient recovery of propionibacteria from skin samples on agar media is carried out under anaerobic conditions, which suggests that these bacteria are anaerobes. More recent work supports that of Evans and Mattern,[23] that growth will occur aerobically. These bacteria can grow in a medium with 100 per cent air saturation, but at a reduced rate compared to growth under anaerobic conditions.[24] Interestingly, at low oxygen concentrations in continuous culture, about 10 per cent air saturation, the biomass concentration is significantly increased above that found during growth under anaerobic conditions, but the growth rate is not.[24] This indicates the utilization of oxygen as a terminal electron acceptor, with a gain of energy per oxidized molecule over that obtained from substrate-level phosphorylation via the propioniate pathway. This conclusion is supported by similar results on using a defined synthetic medium, where porphyrin-like substances are evident only in oxygenated cultures (E. M. Gribbon & K. T. Holland, unpublished); by biochemical evidence for electron transport-linked phosphorylation;[25] by the increase in enzymes that protect against toxigenic oxygen species, such as superoxide anion, peroxides, or hydroxyl radicals, in the presence of air;[26] and by the near total loss of production of acetate, propionate and other fermentation end-products when air is present.[26] Taking into consideration the arguments set out above, it is probably wiser to regard the cutaneous propionibacteria as microaerophiles rather than anaerobes.

The presence or absence of oxygen affects extracellular enzyme production. Levels generally decrease with elevation of oxygen tension for the propionibacteria, whilst with *S. aureus*, the most intensely studied staphylococcus, the opposite occurs.[24,27] Three extracellular enzymes of *S. simulans* were completely repressed during anaerobic growth.[28]

The presence of oxygen can influence directly other nutritional requirements, as exemplified by the requirements for uracil and pyruvate under anaerobic conditions of the majority of staphylococci.[29] This can be explained by the failure of *S. aureus* to use its dihydroorotate oxidase to synthesize uracil. This membrane oxidase, whilst oxidizing dihydroorotate, uses oxygen as the electron acceptor. Therefore, in the absence of oxygen the reduction of dihydroorotate cannot occur, uracil synthesis decreases and the level of the oxidase is increased owing to the lack of depression by uracil. The addition of uracil to media under anaerobic conditions overcomes the nutritional deficit and represses the synthesis of the oxidase.[30] Under anaerobic conditions pyruvate is required for the production of acetyl-coA, which is necessary for lipid synthesis, because the majority of pyruvate is drained off to lactate by the high activity of lactate dehydrogenase.[30]

Carbon/energy source
Sugars and polyalcohols

In the design of synthetic media it is normal to include a chemical that is specifically used by microorganisms for carbon assimilation and energy supply. Classically this has been a sugar and, as often as not, glucose. However, many bacteria, including the cutaneous types, can (and are more likely to) use peptides and amino acids in their habitat. Furthermore, with the exceptionally high content of lipid in the skin environment, it might be expected that lipids would also be used as carbon/energy sources. Although there is good evidence that specific amino acids are used as carbon/energy sources, there is little evidence to support the view that lipids are used for the assimilation of carbon and/or oxidized for energy transduction. The Gram-negative bacteria, such as *Escherichia coli*, can use fatty acids, and *Serratia* spp. have lipases that hydrolyse triglycerides to fatty acids, and these can be oxidized.[31] As will be seen later, other bacteria can use the short-chain fatty acids, such as acetate, propionate and butyrate.

Contained in Table 2.6–2.8 is information on sugars and polyalcohols that can be used by the cutaneous bacteria. The majority of this information has been abstracted from relevant sections of *Bergey's Manual of Systematic Bacteriology*.[5] The data are most probably not exhaustive because they have

Table 2.7. *Utilization of sugars and polyalcohols by propionibacteria, corynebacteria, brevibacteria and lipophilic coryneforms*[5, 44-5, 84]

Compound	P. acnes	P. avidum	P. granulosum	C. xerosis	C. minutissimum	B. epidermidis	Lipophilic coryneforms[a]	
Glucose	+	+	+	+	+	+	+	+
Lactose	−	+	−	−	−	+	(+)	
Maltose	(+)	(+)	+	−	+		(+)	(+)
Mannitol	(+)	+	+		+			
Fructose	+	+	+	+	+		(+)	
Galactose	+	+	(+)	+			(+)	
Mannose	+	+	(+)	+	(+)			
Ribose	+	+	(−)					
Sucrose	−	+	+	+	+	+	(+)	(+)
Trehalose	−		+	−	−		(+)	
Turanose								
Glycerol	+	+	+				−	(+)
Arabinose	−	+	−	−				
Xylose	−	(+)	−	−	−			
Xylitol								
Melezitose	−	+	(+)					
Cellobiose	−	−	−					
Gentibiose				+				
Sorbitol	(+)	−	−					
Inositol	(+)	+	−					
Salicin	−	+	−	+				
Adonitol	+	+	−					
Dulcitol	−	+	−					
Arabitol		−	−					
Erythritol	+	−	−					
Erythrose								
Raffinose	−	+	(+)	−				
Melibiose	−	+						
Fucose	−	−	−	−				
Rhamnose	−			−				
Lyxose		−						
Sorbose	−							
Dextrin				−				

[a] Information in left-hand column from Smith[44] and in right-hand column from McGinley et al.[45]
( ), not all isolates can utilize the compound.

Table 2.8. Utilization of sugars and polyalcohols by Gram-negative bacteria[5, 85]

Compound	Ps. aeruginosa	E. coli	Enterobacter spp.	Proteus spp.	Providencia spp.	Serratia spp.	Acinetobacter spp.
Glucose	+	+	+	+	+	+	
Lactose	−	+	+	−	−	−	
Maltose	+	+	+	+	+	+	
Mannitol	+	+	+	−	+	+	
Fructose	+					+	
Galactose	−	+					
Mannose	−	+					+
Ribose	+					+	
Sucrose	−	(+)	+	+	−	+	
Trehalose	−	+	+	(+)	−	+	
Turanose							
Glycerol	+	+	+		−	+	+
Arabinose	−	+	+	−	−	−	+
Xylose	−	+	+	+	−	−	
Xylitol							
Melezitose			+				
Cellobiose	−	−	+	−	−	(+)	
Gentibiose							
Sorbitol	−	+	+	−	−	+	
Inositol	−	−	+	(+)	+	(+)	
Salicin		+	+		(+)	+	
Adonitol		−	+	−	+	(+)	
Dulcitol		+	−	−	+		
Arabitol		+	+	−	+	−	
Erythritol	−						
Erythrose							
Raffinose		(+)	+	−	−	−	
Melibiose		(+)	+	−	−	−	
Fucose	−					+	
Rhamnose	−	(+)	+	−	(+)	−	
Lyxose							
Sorbose							
Dextrin							

( ), not all isolates can utilize the compound.

come from physiological tests assaying for acid production in media with added sugars, etc. Negative results in these tests, especially with strict aerobes, may not, in some cases, necessarily indicate that these test microorganisms cannot utilize the sugar. Furthermore, these tests have been designed, along with others, to allow species and strain differentiation, and substrates that are more relevant to the skin environment have not necessarily been selected.

The arrangement of sugars in the Tables 2.6–2.8 is based on those used to identify the staphylococci, and those that are most commonly utilized are arranged at the top of the table. Lack of information is indicated by the absence of a symbol and a symbol in parentheses shows that not all isolates of the species can use the compound. The distribution of sugar utilization is similar amongst the Gram-positive bacteria. However, the propionibacteria can also use many of the compounds listed in the lower half of Table 2.7. The significance of these data is not certain, if indeed there is any biological significance. It is possible that the propionibacteria have evolved in a different ecological niche from the other bacteria, one where there is a wider variety of carbon/energy substrates. The propionibacteria are the most common bacteria inhabiting the pilosebaceous ducts, whilst most other groups of bacteria are more associated with the skin surface.

The sugar utilization patterns of the Gram-negative bacteria are much wider than for the Gram-positive group (Table 2.8), and this indicates that the Gram-negative bacteria have evolved in different environments than the skin, for example in the gut and aqueous environments. Here, the range of carbon/energy sources would change and be varied.

The extracellular enzymes produced by the cutaneous microflora that make available sugars, etc. are lipase, hyaluronate lyase and neuraminidase (see Table 2.4).

Amino acids

Amino acids, but more particularly di- and tripeptides, can be utilized by the cutaneous flora as carbon/energy sources. No exhaustive study has been carried out to identify which amino acids can be used as carbon/energy sources for all the different species of the microflora. Many of the Gram-negative group, for example, *Pseudomonas* spp. and *Serratia* spp., can use a wide range of amino acids, whilst others, along with the Gram-positive group, may use a more limited range. However, in most cases this has not been ascertained, although it is known that media containing amino acids or peptides, but not sugar, support growth. This is certainly the case with the micrococci, staphylococci, lipophilic coryneforms, *P. acnes* and *P. avidum*. Of interest is the use of arginine by the two major groups of bacteria on the skin,

Table 2.9. *Various carbon/energy sources for Gram-negative bacteria*[5, 82, 86-7]

Compound	*Ps. aeruginosa*	*E. coli*	*Enterobacter*	*Proteus* spp.	*Providencia* spp.	*Serratia* spp.	*Acinetobacter* spp.
Lactate	+	+				+	+
Pyruvate	+					+	+
Acetate	+	+				+	+
Malate	+	+					+
Citrate	+	−	+	(+)	+	+	−
Succinate	+	+					+
Fumarate	+	+					+
α-ketoglutarate	+						+
Fatty acids	+				+	+	+
Alcohols							
Amides	+						
Amines	+					+	+
Cyclohexanol							
Quinate						+	+
Benzoate	+					+	

( ), not all isolates can utilize the compound.
This information is not exhaustive.

staphylococci and propionibacteria. Arginine use as a carbon/energy source was associated with staphylococci that had a limited host range.[32] *Staphylococcus saprophyticus* and *S. sciuri* do not require arginine for growth and they are found primarily on the skin of lower mammals. Those strains that are auxotrophic can revert to arginine independence. These bacteria have flexibility to deal with changing environments containing different amounts of arginine. Niche-specific species such as *S. aureus*, *S. simulans*, *S. capitis* and *S. warneri*, which have stable auxotrophic arginine characteristics, also have multiple amino acid and vitamin requirements. These nutritional requirements lock the microorganisms into a particular habitat. Some *S. epidermidis* isolates show auxotrophy reversion and consequently this species is found over a wider range of habitats. They are more uniformly spread over various skin sites. There is evidence that the nutrition of *P. acnes* and *P. avidum* is different from that of *P. granulosum* with respect to the carbon/energy sources used by these bacteria on skin. *Propionibacterium acnes* and *P. avidum* are protease producers and can use arginine as a carbon/energy source, whilst *P. granulosum* does not produce a protease and cannot use arginine.[33] In addition, lipase production by *P. granulosum* is growth linked and that of *P. acnes* and *P. avidum* is not.[34] Furthermore, only growth of *P. granulosum* is sugar or glycerol dependent.[33] These data can be interpreted as showing reliance by *P. acnes* and *P. avidum* on their proteases to scavenge for peptides and amino acids, especially arginine, for carbon/energy requirements, whereas *P. granulosum* relies on its lipase to hydrolyse triglycerides to glycerol, which is its carbon/energy source. Rebello and Hawke suggested that this was the function of the lipase of *P. acnes*, but this seems unlikely, because that lipase is not growth-linked.[35] Also, the addition of up to 3 mg/ml oleic acid, monoolein, diolein or triolein did not improve the yield of *P. acnes* grown in continuous culture in eight amino acids and four vitamins with or without glucose (E. M. Gribbon & K. T. Holland, unpublished). This indicates that for this one isolate the lipids are not carbon/energy sources.

Other carbon/energy sources

Besides sugars, amino acids and peptides, the cutaneous microflora can use other organic molecules as carbon/energy sources. Information available is listed in Table 2.9. Some of these substances may be found on skin and are, therefore, relevant to the nutrition of the resident microflora. Many of the microorganisms can use carboxy acids and soluble short-chain fatty acids. Those bacteria that are facultatively anaerobic or microaerophilic produce some of these compounds when fermenting. For example, propionibacteria produce mainly acetate and propionate, and these could act as carbon/energy

Table 2.10. Amino acid requirements of Micrococcus spp.[37]

Species (and number of isolates)

Amino acid	M. luteus (58)	M. lylae (21)	M. sedentarius (24)	M. varians (49)	M. roseus (19)	M. kristinae (19)	M. nishinomiyaensis (20)
Alanine		S	S		S	S	S
Glycine		S	R	R			RS
Serine							
Cysteine	RS		RS	S	S		RS
Valine		S	RS			RS	S
Aspartate						S	RS
Asparagine							
Methionine	RS	RS	RS	RS	S	S	S
Threonine					S		
Isoleucine		RS	RS		S	S	RS
Lysine			RS				S
Leucine			RS			S	S
Glutamate							RS
Phenylalanine		RS	RS			S	S
Tyrosine	RS	R	RS		S	S	S
Tryptophan			S	S		RS	RS
Histidine		RS	S		S	S	S
Arginine		RS	RS				S
Proline			RS			S	S

Not every isolate of a species requires or is stimulated by the amino acid noted with R (required) and/or S (stimulated).

Table 2.11. *Amino acid requirements of* Staphylococcus *spp.*

Amino acid	Species (and number of isolates)												
	S. aureus			S. simulans	S. xylosus	S. cohnii	S. saprophyticus	S. haemolyticus	S. warneri	S. hominis	S. capitis	S. epidermidis	
	(50)	(1)	(1)	(12)	(100)	(39)	(68)	(100)	(34)	(209)	(42)	(169)	(1)
Alanine	RS			RS				RS	RS	RS	RS	RS	
Glycine	RS	S		RS				RS	RS	RS	RS	RS	R
Serine	RS			RS			S	RS	RS	RS	RS	S	
Cysteine	RS	R	R				RS	RS	RS	RS	RS	RS	R
Valine	RS	R		RS		RS	RS	R*	R*	RS	R*	RS	R
Aspartate		R		S					RS		S		
Asparagine													
Methionine	RS			RS			RS	RS	RS	RS	R*	RS	
Threonine	RS			RS		RS		RS	RS	RS	R*	RS	
Isoleucine				RS		S		RS	RS	RS	R*	RS	
Lysine				S									
Leucine	RS			RS			S	RS	RS	RS	R*	RS	
Glutamate		R		RS									
Phenylalanine	RS			RS			RS	RS	RS	RS	S	RS	
Tyrosine	RS			RS			RS	RS	RS	RS	RS	RS	
Tryptophan	S			RS		R		RS	RS	RS	RS	RS	
Histidine	RS			RS				R*	R*	R*	R*	R*	
Arginine	R*	S		R*	RS	RS		R*	R*	R*	R*	R*	R
Proline	RS	R		RS	RS	RS	RS	RS	RS	RS	RS	RS	R

Based on references 38, 39 and 41.
Not every isolate of a species requires or is stimulated by the amino acid noted with R (required) and/or S (stimulated).
* Indicates all isolates behave uniformly.

sources for the micrococci and brevibacteria. There is the possibility that cross-feeding occurs, although it is unlikely that there is an absolute dependency amongst the microflora.

There is in vitro evidence that RNA can be used as a carbon/energy source and/or possibly a nitrogen source, because the growth of *P. acnes* yield can be increased in a medium without sugar but with RNA. Furthermore an increasing yield of cells was correlated with an increasing input of RNA into the medium.[36]

Finally, as would be expected, the Gram-negative bacteria have a wider range of carbon/energy substrates than the Gram-positive bacteria, again indicating the different habitats in which they have evolved.

Nitrogen source

One distinguishing feature of the bacterial residents of human skin is the requirement for organic nitrogen by the vast majority of Gram-positive bacteria. The exceptions are some strains of *Micrococcus luteus* and *M. varians*. The amino acids required for growth and those which are stimulatory are given in Tables 2.10–2.12. In these tables the amino acids are ordered according to their relationship to their synthetic biochemical pathways. The information for the micrococci and staphylococci has been obtained by single omission experiments and, therefore, the minimum requirements for a microorganism cannot be deduced.[37,38] The most common amino acids required by the micrococci are arginine, cysteine, methionine and tyrosine; the other aromatic amino acids are often required or stimulatory. *Micrococcus sedentarius*, *M. luteus* and *M. nishinomiyaensis* are the most fastidious species, requiring up to eleven, six and six amino acids, respectively, whilst the other species require up to three amino acids.

Far more information is available on *S. aureus*, and a minimal medium with only cysteine, ammonium ions, salts and a carbon/energy source has been devised.[39] Using sequential omission of amino acids, 2 of 18 strains of *S. aureus* could be grown on four amino acids, namely cysteine, aspartate, glutamate and proline. The addition of arginine and glycine to this base medium enabled 14 strains to be grown. This medium would support the growth of *S. aureus* in continuous culture with the production of toxins and extracellular enzymes.[40] Using a similar approach, *S. epidermidis* has been grown on six amino acids (Table 2.11).

Within the staphylococci there is great variation in amino acid requirements, and the variation also occurs within the species. Indeed for *S. aureus* there have been 15 different defined media mentioned in the literature since 1970. The

Table 2.12. *Amino acid requirements of* Propionibacterium *spp.*

Amino acid	P. acnes (52[a])	(16[a])	(1[b])	P. avidum (10[a])	(10[a])	P. granulosum (19[a])	(6[a])
Alanine	+	+		+	+	+	+
Glycine	+	+		+	+	+	+
Serine	+	+		+	+	+	+
Cysteine	+	+	+	+	+	+	+
Valine	+	+	+		+	+	+
Aspartate		+			+		+
Asparagine	+	+			+	+	+
Methionine	+	+	+	+	+	+	+
Threonine	+	+			+	+	+
Isoleucine	+	+	+	+	+	+	+
Lysine	+	+			+	+	+
Leucine	+	+	+		+	+	+
Glutamate		+			+		+
Phenylalanine	+	+	+	+	+	+	+
Tyrosine	+	+		+	+	+	+
Tryptophan	+	+	+	+	+	+	+
Histidine	+	+		+	+	+	+
Arginine	+	+	+	+	+	+	+
Proline	+	+			+	+	+
Glutamine	+			+		+	
Hydroxyproline		+			+		+

Based on references 33 and 41.
[a] No attempt made to minimalize the number of amino acids in the medium in these studies.
[b] E. M. Gribbon and K. T. Holland (unpublished).

most common amino acid requirements are arginine, proline, valine and one of the aromatic amino acids. Many amino acids are stimulatory, as is also the case for the micrococci. Overall there is a greater demand for amino acids by the staphylococci than by the micrococci. The least demanding staphylococci are *S. xylosus*, *S. cohnii* and *S. saprophyticus*.

The three species of propionibacteria will grow with 18 amino acids present in the medium.[33,41] *Propionibacterium avidum* is the least demanding and will grow on 12 amino acids.[41] However, using a sequential omission of amino acids, growth in continuous culture of one isolate of *P. acnes* has been achieved with eight amino acids (Table 2.12) (E. M. Gribbon & K. T. Holland, unpublished). Therefore, it is likely that most if not all strains of *P. acnes* and

Table 2.13. *Vitamin requirements of Micrococcus spp.*[37]

Vitamin	M. luteus	M. lylae	M. sedentarius	M. varians	M. roseus	M. kristinae	M. nishinomiyaensis
Biotin	RS			S			
Nicotinic/nicotinamide	S	RS	RS	RS	RS		RS
Pantothenic acid	S	RS	RS	S	S		RS
Pyridoxine							
Thiamine	S	RS		S	RS		S
Riboflavin	S			S		S	
Folic acid	RS			S			

Not every isolate of a species requires or is stimulated by the vitamin noted with R (required) and/or S (stimulated).

P. granulosum will grow on less than 18 amino acids, and *P. avidum* isolates may well grow on fewer than 8 amino acids.

Where there are some data on the amino acid requirements of micrococci, staphylococci and propionibacteria, it is arginine, cysteine, methionine, valine and an aromatic amino acid that are commonly required. This would indicate that those amino acids, free or as peptides, are consistently available in the skin environment.

There is no information on the amino acid requirements of the cutaneous brevibacteria, corynebacteria, lipophilic coryneforms and *M. furfur*.

It is worth noting again that, at least in in vitro models, amino acids can reduce the growth of bacteria because of the competition amongst the amino acids that occurs for the same transport system to take the amino acid into the cell. It seems unlikely that this would present a problem in the natural environment, as the bacteria have evolved there and would be selected to have the efficient ratio of various transporter proteins in their cytoplasmic membranes.

Lastly, the microorganisms that possess proteases and keratinases (see Table 2.3) can make available peptides and amino acids from soluble proteins and keratins present in the environment. Also, those microorganisms not possessing these attributes may benefit from the efforts of those of their coinhabitors that do produce these enzymes.

Vitamins and micronutrients

The data on vitamin requirements are more reliable than those on other nutrients. This is because, first, the vitamins cannot substitute for each other's functions and, secondly, there are fewer vitamins to study compared to the number of amino acids and the vast array of potential carbon/energy sources.

As with the amino acids, the Gram-negative bacteria have no requirements for vitamins, whilst the micrococci, staphylococci, propionibacteria and some of the aerobic coryneforms require a limited number of vitamins. Once again there is no information on *M. furfur*. Tables 2.13–2.15 give the data on vitamin requirements of the bacteria and indicate those vitamins that are essential and those that are stimulatory.[33, 37, 41–3] The information on aerobic coryneforms has not been included because, first, *Corynebacterium minutissimum* and *C. xerosis* have no requirements, and secondly, the vitamin requirements of the lipophilic isolates, which have a vitamin demand, have not been defined, though all or some of the following are needed; riboflavin, nicotinamide, thiamine, pantothenate and biotin.[44, 45] The JK group of corynebacteria have

Table 2.14. *Vitamin requirements of* Staphylococcus *spp.*[42]

Vitamin	S. aureus	S. cohnii	S. haemolyticus	S. hominis	S. simulans	S. saprophyticus	S. warneri	S. capitis	S. epidermidis
Biotin		R*	R	R*	R	R*	R*	R	R
Nicotinic/nicotinamide	R*	R*	R*	R*	R*	R*	R*	R*	R*
Pantothenic acid		R			R				
Pyridoxine		R		R				R	
Thiamine	R*	R*	R*	R*	R*	R*	R*	R*	R*
Riboflavine									
Folic acid									

Not every isolate of a species requires or is stimulated by the vitamin noted with R (required) and/or S (stimulated).
* Indicates all isolates behave uniformly.

Table 2.15. *Vitamins and micronutrients required by* Propionibacterium spp.

Vitamin	P. acnes (41)	P. acnes (33)	P. acnes (a)	P. avidum (41)	P. avidum (33)	P. granulosum (41)	P. granulosum (33)
Biotin	S	S	R	S	S	S	S
Nicotinic/ nicotinamide	S	R	R		R		R
Pantothenic acid	R	R	R	R	R	R	R
Pyridoxine		R[b]	R				
Thiamine	S		R	S		S	
Riboflavin							
Folic acid							
Pyruvate	S			S		S	
Lactate	S			S		S	
α-Ketoglutarate	S			S		S	
Succinate	S						
Tween 80 (oleate)	S			S		S	
Adenosine	S			S		S	
Cytosine							
Guanine				S			
Thymidine							
Uracil							

( ), reference number (*a*, E. M. Gribbon & K. T. Holland (unpublished)).
[b] Required by some isolates.

been defined as lipophilic coryneforms with antibiotic resistance, and they have the same nutrition as the other lipophilic coryneforms.[46]

There is a variation in the demand for certain vitamins within a species or genus. However, there is a near consistent requirement for biotin, nicotinamide, pantothenate and thiamine amongst all these bacteria, where there are data. This is strong circumstantial evidence that these vitamins are available in the skin habitat, and at concentrations that are not limiting. If they were at limiting concentrations, then there would be competition amongst the groups of bacteria, and the range of isolates at any skin site would probably be reduced. It is possible that biotin is at a limiting concentration because, as will become evident later, fatty acids can substitute for biotin in media for the growth of some bacteria.

Adenine, guanine, pyruvate, lactate, α-ketoglutarate and succinate were stimulatory for the propionibacteria.[41] However, it is possible that these chemicals would not be stimulatory if the concentrations of the various amino acids were balanced for growth. Good growth in continuous culture could be

obtained in a medium containing glucose, eight amino acids and four vitamins
(E. M. Gribbon & K. T. Holland, unpublished).

Lipids

The fascination for investigation of lipids when studying skin is extremely
high, and this is most likely due to the large amounts of lipid on skin, the
variety of which is immense. Microbiologists and dermatologists have tussled
with the problems of appreciating the interaction of the resident and transient
microbial flora for many years. By far and away the most studied skin lipids
with regard to effects on microorganisms have been the triglycerides and the
products of lipase action, namely the di- and monoglycerides, glycerol and
especially the longer-chain fatty acids. The literature is awash with information
on both the stimulatory and inhibitory roles of the free fatty acids. Table 2.16
summarizes the information on this subject. Gram-negative bacteria, such as
E. coli, can take up and oxidize free fatty acids and this has been mentioned in
the section on carbon/energy sources. In the context of the majority of work
on free fatty acids and the cutaneous microorganisms, the concentrations of
the molecules have been in the low μg/ml range, which would be insufficient in
concentration to act as a carbon/energy source.

Lipids as nutrients

Only two groups of microorganisms have, in in vitro models, an absolute
demand for lipids, and they are the aerobic lipophilic coryneforms and *M.
furfur*.[44–50] The growth of lipophilic coryneforms is stimulated by oleic,
elaidic, isovaccenic and erucic acids and only slightly stimulated by linolenic,
linoleic and palmitoleic acids. However, some strains were slightly inhibited
by linolenic and linoleic acids.[51] *Malassezia furfur* required myristate or
palmitate, and oleate was stimulatory.[48] The micrococci and Gram-negative
bacteria have no requirement for oleate or any other free fatty acids. The
synthetic, semisynthetic and complex media that have been used to isolate and
study these bacteria do not require a lipid supplement.

The situation with the staphylococci and propionibacteria is less straightforward. The vast majority of staphylococci, except *S. aureus*, have a
requirement for biotin, and in its presence in vitro, oleic acid is not required for
growth. However, in the absence of biotin, oleate at 100 μg/ml will substitute
for biotin and will allow the growth of staphylococci that otherwise would
require biotin.[42] Therefore, in the skin environment the oleate present may be
an important nutrient for the staphylococci, assuming the biotin concentration
is low or limiting.

Table 2.16. *The effects of medium- and long-chain fatty acids on cutaneous microorganisms*

| Microorganism | Oleic acid | | | | Other fatty acids |
| | Essential | | Stimulating | | |
	Biotin present	Biotin absent	Biotin present	Biotin absent	Inhibitory
Micrococcus spp.	−	?	−	?	+
Staphylococcus spp.	−	+	−	+	+
Propionibacterium spp.	−	?	+	?	+
Lipophilic aerobic coryneforms	+		+		±
Gram-negative bacteria	−	−	−	−	+
M. furfur	+		+		?

Propionibacteria are generally recovered from skin samples on complex media without addition of oleate or Tween 80, and these bacteria can be recovered in a synthetic medium without a lipid source with high efficiency.[33] Many in vitro physiological studies have used media without a lipid supplement.[19, 24, 26, 33, 34, 41, 52] In an eight amino-acid medium with four vitamins, including biotin, the addition of oleic acid, monoolein, diolein or triolein did not effect growth of *P. acnes* in continuous culture at pH 5.7 (E. M. Gribbon & K. T. Holland, unpublished). The weight of evidence indicates that oleate or any other lipid source is not required for the growth of these bacteria. However, it is possible that the oleate requirement would only be demonstrated in a medium without biotin, and as yet this has not been tested. There is evidence that oleate is stimulatory in vitro.[40, 52] There are further in vivo investigations indicating that lipids are important to the colonization of skin by propionibacteria. These are, first, the increase in population density of propionibacteria during the years of puberty, when the sebaceous units enlarge and the sebum excretion rate increases simultaneously.[54, 55] Secondly, a loss of propionibacteria occurs from thin human skin grafted on to mice but not from full-thickness human skin similarly grafted; the thin skin has few or no sebaceous glands and therefore low sebum levels.[56] Thirdly, there is an association of propionibacteria only with human skin and guinea-pig perianal glands, both of which have triglycerides; other animals that lack triglycerides are not colonized by propionibacteria.[56] Fourthly, treatment for acne with 13-*cis*-retinoic acid reduces the rate of sebum excretion and the size of the sebaceous glands, and this is associated with a reduction in propionibacterial populations.[57-60] Finally, the distributions of the propionibacteria are associated with the distribution of sebaceous glands and the amount of triglycerides and their hydrolysis products, namely fatty acids.[61,62] The distribution of *P. granulosum* in lipid-rich areas and dependence on lipid seems more stringent than that of *P. acnes*.[55] This may not be caused by a dependence on lipid as a nutrient at low concentration, but more likely on its dependence on lipid and glycerol for a carbon/energy source (see carbon/energy above). There seems little doubt that lipids, especially triglycerides and oleate, are important factors in the environment for the colonization of skin by propionibacteria. It is known that there is an association between the distribution of rates of sebum excretion and the population densities of propionibacteria. However, it is possible that the bacterial population density is more dependent on the size of the pilosebaceous units.[62] Provided there is a threshold level of lipid, then the overriding factor controlling the population size of the propionibacteria will be the volume of the follicle. The findings of Kearney and coworkers[63] were similar for the *Micrococcaceae* and the propionibacteria and yet, in the investigation of Nordstrom and Noble,[55] there was no evidence that the staphylococci were dependent on sebaceous glands or their lipid product. This illustrates our incomplete knowledge of the in vitro nutrient requirements of the various bacteria. Clearly there is a need for caution against emphasizing the importance of one factor, such as a nutrient, in modulating microbial colonization of skin.

Lipids as inhibitors

Nearly all the data on the inhibition of microorganisms by lipids have been concerned with medium- and long-chain fatty acids, and the difference in sensitivity of the normal and transient microflora to these lipids. Based on this work there is a considerable weight of opinion that it is this differential sensitivity of the transient and resident microflora to particular fatty acids that mainly determines which microorganisms colonize the skin. The most active inhibitors are straight-chain species of lauric and myristic acids, with some effects by capric and palmitic and the di- and triunsaturated C_{18} species, linoleic and linolenic acids respectively.[51,53,64-72] Although there is not perfect consistency amongst the various investigations, it is clear that the lauric and myristic fatty acids and the equivalent monoglycerides inhibit most bacteria, whether they are transient or resident on skin. Also, the differential sensitivities between the transient and resident bacteria reside with linoleic and linolenic acids, the transient bacteria being more susceptible.[53,70,73] The majority of the investigations have been with the transient species, *Staph. aureus* and

Streptococcus pyogenes. The Gram-negative bacteria do not appear to be particularly more sensitive to the fatty acids than the Gram-positive bacteria. Consequently, it is unlikely that the presence of fatty acids is the key factor in determining the low carriage rate of Gram-negative bacteria on human skin.

The susceptibility of the transient bacteria to linoleic acid is pH dependent.[72] It has been reported that oleate, not normally considered an inhibitor by most investigators, is inhibitory to *Staph. aureus* and *Strep. pyogenes*, but not to coagulase-negative staphylococci and propionibacteria, at low pH 5.5.[69] This pH is considered to be about the average for many areas of the human skin.

There is varation of sensitivity to the fatty acids amongst both transient and resident bacterial skin flora. *Propionibacterium granulosum* has been reported to be more sensitive to linolenic and linoleic acids than is *P. acnes*.[68] Whether this one factor, amongst others, determines the limited distributions of *P. granulosum* on human skin compared with that of *P. acnes*, has yet to be ascertained.

The mechanism by which the lauric and myristic fatty acids inhibit microorganisms has not been formally proved, though the consensus is that the target site is the cytoplasmic membrane of the cell, where they cause melting of this structure, and in consequence, a lowering of the selectivity of the movement of molecules, both inward and outward. The possible mode of action of the linoleic and linolenic fatty acids is the production of aldehydic antibacterial molecular species via autooxidation.[66] If this occurs in the skin environment, and if there are anaerobic microenvironments, it is possible that the residents, which are not resistant to these fatty acids, may be protected.

There are in vitro experiments which indicate that lipid substances are a factor in preventing bacteria, such as *Staph. aureus* and *Strep. pyogenes* from permanently colonizing human skin, although these lipids may not necessarily be fatty acids. The persistence of *Staph. aureus* and *Strep. pyogenes* inoculated on to skin varies amongst people and the persistence of these bacteria is greatly influenced by the presence of lipid.[65,71,74] This was shown by removing lipid from the skin by acetone washing before inoculating with bacteria. Inhibitors including glycosphingolipids and to a lesser extent glycolipids have been shown to be present on the skin of mice by extracting and testing them in vitro.[75] As yet unexplained, these mice, which were fed on an essential fatty acid-deficient diet, supported a 100-fold higher cutaneous microbial population than mice fed on a normal diet. Furthermore, the mice receiving a fatty acid-deficient diet commonly carried *Staph. aureus* on their skin whilst the other group of mice did not. It is possible that the higher population densities of bacteria on the skin were due to increased skin hydration, caused by the increased transepidermal water flux. It is known that fatty acid deficiency affects the barrier function of the skin. This investigation, as noted by its instigators, indicated the lack of knowledge of the factors controlling the microbial population of skin. It may be of relevance that the glycosphingo-lipids and glycolipids found to be inhibitory on mice skin can be found on human skin.[76]

Lipases and fatty acids

Many of the cutaneous microorganisms produce lipases that degrade tri-glycerides present in nascent sebum to di- and monoglycerides, glycerol and free fatty acids. The lipase of *P. acnes* hydrolyses a range of triglycerides, including trilaurin and triolein, with trilaurin being hydrolysed faster.[77] In addition to glycerol, the end-products of hydrolysis are fatty acids – lauric acid, which is an inhibitor, and oleic acid, a growth stimulant. Therefore, it would appear that *P. acnes* has a mechanism for inhibiting its own colonization of the skin. A possible explanation for this paradox lies in the work of Nordstrom and Noble, who showed an association between the colonization density of *P. acnes* and the particular skin-surface lipid profiles of young individuals.[55] There were both inhibitory and stimulatory fatty acids in all lipid samples. However, an increase in skin colonization by *P. acnes*, which was associated with increasing age, was also associated with a reduction in the inhibitory C_{14} fatty acid. Therefore, the variation in the population density of the cutaneous microorganisms on different people at the same site might be explained, first, by the amount of triglyceride produced at the site, and secondly by the balance between the amounts of the inhibitory and stimulatory fatty acids.

It is likely that a similar interaction occurs with all the other cutaneous microorganisms that produce lipase. It is also possible that the inhibitory fatty acids are reduced in concentration locally on the skin as a result of their utilization by *M. furfur* and, therefore, there is a dependence of the other cutaneous microflora on the presence of *M. furfur*. Indeed there is an association of *M. furfur* and propionibacterial population densities.[78]

Conclusion

This chapter has concentrated on the nutrition of the resident microflora of human skin. Residents such as the staphylococci and propionibacteria have been studied in some detail in vitro. The knowledge of the microorganisms and data based on in vivo studies are scanty. Apart from the data acquired on the nutritional and inhibitory effects of lipids, studies have been segmented into generic groups, with little or no comparative experiments that include the majority of the cutaneous microorganisms. Investigations have been undertaken from the intellectual standpoint of determining the differences for taxonomic and differential purposes, rather than their similarities resulting from their evolution in the same environment. Nutrient and inhibitory factors on the skin must be important, along with other environmental considerations, in determining the type and density of particular microorganisms at a specific skin site on one individual compared to another. It is evident that there is much to be done to be confident in our understanding of the interaction of the microbial flora with our skin. Furthermore, it is imperative to improve our knowledge to the extent that we can predict the effect of ever-increasing amounts and varieties of orally and topically applied preparations on our important microbial guests.

References

1 Noble, WC. Microbiology of human skin. London: Lloyd-Luke; 1981.
2 Herbert D, Elsworth R, Telling RC. Continuous culture of bacteria; a theoretical and experimental study. J Gen Microbiol 1956; 14: 601–22.
3 Harder W, Dijkhuizen L. Physiological responses to nutrient limitation. Ann Rev Microbiol 1983; 37: 1–23.
4 Mills JT, Parsonnet J, Tsai Y-C, Kendrick M, Hickman RK, Kass EH. Control of production of toxic-shock-syndrome toxin-1 (TSST-1) by magnesium ion. J Infect Dis 1985; 151: 1158–61.
5 Murray RGE, Brenner DJ, Bryant MP et al. Bergey's manual of systematic bacteriology. London: Williams & Wilkins; 1986.
6 Wandersman C. Secretion, processing and activation of bacterial extracellular proteases. Mol Microbiol 1989; 3: 1825–31.
7 Cove JH, Holland KT, Cunliffe WJ. Growth yield, phosphatase and protease production by *Staphylococcus epidermidis* in batch and continuous culture. In: Jeljaszewicz J, ed. Staphylococci and staphylococcal infections [Stuttgart: Gustav Fischer]. Zentralbl Bakteriol 1981; (suppl 10): 169–73.
8 Randall LL, Hardy SJS. Export of protein in bacteria. Microbiol Rev 1984; 48: 290–98.
9 Randall LL, Hardy SJS, Thom JR. Export of protein: a biochemical view. Ann Rev Microbiol 1987; 41: 507–41.
10 Vesterberg O, Wadstrom T, Vesterberg K, Svensson H, Malmgren B. Studies on extracellular proteins from *Staphylococcus aureus*: I. separation and characterization of enzymes and toxins by isolectric focusing. Biochem Biophys Acta 1967; 133: 435–45.
11 Ingham E, Holland KT, Gowland G, Cunliffe WJ. Studies of extracellular proteolytic activity produced by *Propionibacterium acnes*. J Appl Bacteriol 1983; 54: 263–71.
12 Taylor D, Holland KT. Effect of dilution rate and Mg^{2+} limitation on toxic shock syndrome toxin-1 production by *Staphylococcus aureus* grown in defined continuous culture. J Gen Microbiol 1988; 134: 719–23.
13 Shah DB, Blobel H. Repressible alkaline phosphatase of *Staphylococcus aureus*. J Bacteriol 1967; 94: 780–81.
14 Okabayashi K, Futa M, Mizuno D. Localization of acid and alkaline phosphatases in *Staphylococcus aureus*. Jap J Microbiol 1974; 18: 287–94.

15 Csonka LN. Physiological and genetical responses of bacteria to osmotic stress. Microbiol Rev. 1989; 53: 121–47.

16 Booth IR. Regulation of cytoplasmic pH in bacteria. Microbiol Rev 1985; 49: 359–78.

17 Noble WC. Observations on the surface flora of the skin and on the skin pH. Br J Dermatol 1968; 80: 279–81.

18 Holland DB, Cunliffe WJ. Skin surface and open comedone pH in acne patients. Acta Dermatoven Stockh 1982; 63: 155–58.

19 Greenman J, Holland KT, Cunliffe WJ. Effects of pH on biomass, maximum specific growth rate and extracellular enzyme production by three species of cutaneous propionibacteria grown in continuous culture. J Gen Microbiol 1983; 129: 1301–07.

20 Puhvel SM, Reisner RM, Sakamoto M. Analysis of lipid composition of isolated human sebaceous gland homogenates after incubation with cutaneous bacteria: thin-layer chromatography. J Invest Dermatol 1975; 64: 406–11.

21 Marples RR, Downing DT, Kligman AM. Control of free fatty acids in human surface lipids by *Corynebacterium acnes*. J Invest Dermatol 1971; 56: 127–31.

22 Burke KA, Brown AE, Lascelles J. Membrane and cytoplasmic nitrate reductase of *Staphylococcus aureus* and application of crossed immunoelectrophoresis. J Bacteriol 1981; 148: 724–27.

23 Evans CA, Mattern KL. The aerobic growth of *Propionibacterium acnes* in primary cultures from the skin. J Invest Dermatol 1979; 72: 103–36.

24 Cove JH, Holland KT, Cunliffe WJ. Effects of oxygen concentration on biomass production, maximum specific growth rate and extracellular enzyme production by three species of cutaneous propionibacteria grown in continuous culture. J Gen Microbiol 1983; 129: 3327–34.

25 Midgley M, Mohd Noor MA. The interaction of oxygen with *Propionibacterium acnes*. FEMS Microbiol Lett 1984; 23: 183–86.

26 Cove JH, Holland KT, Cunliffe WJ. The effects of oxygen on cutaneous propionibacteria grown in continuous culture. FEMS Microbiol Lett 1987; 43: 61–65.

27 Taylor D, Holland KT. Production of toxic shock syndrome toxin-1 by *Staphylococcus aureus* under aerobic and anaerobic conditions and the effect of magnesium ion limitation. Rev Infect Dis 1989; 11 (Suppl 1): 151–55.

28 Donham MC, Heath HE, Leblanc PA, Sloan GL. Characteristics of extracellular protein production by *Staphylococcus simulans* biovar *staphylolyticus* during aerobic and anaerobic growth. J Gen Microbiol 1988; 134: 2615–21.

29 Evans JB. Anaerobic growth of *Staphylococcus* species from human skin: effects of uracil and pyruvate. Int J System Bacteriol 1976; 26: 17–21.

30 Lascelles J. Anaerobic growth requirements of staphylococci and the enzymes of pyrimidine synthesis. Ann NY Acad Sci 1974; 236: 96–104.

31 Nunn WD. Two carbon compounds and fatty acids as carbon sources. In: Neidhardt FC, Ingraham JL, Brooks Low K, Magasanik B, Schaechter M, Umbanger HE, eds. *Escherichia coli* and *Salmonella typhimurium* cellular and molecular biology, Washington DC: American Society for Microbiology; 1987: 285–301.

32 Emmett M, Kloos WE. The nature of arginine auxotrophy in cutaneous populations of staphylococci. J Gen Microbiol 1979; 110: 305–14.

33 Holland KT, Greenman J, Cunliffe WJ. Growth of cutaneous propionibacteria on synthetic medium; growth yields and exoenzyme production. J Appl Bacteriol 1979; 47: 383–94.

34 Greenman J, Holland KT. Effects of dilution rate on biomass and extracellular enzyme production by three species of cutaneous propionibacteria grown in continuous culture. J Gen Microbiol 1985; 131: 1619–24.

35 Rebello T, Hawke JLM. Skin surface glycerol levels in acne vulgaris. J Invest Dermatol 1978; 70: 352–54.

36 Smith RF. Role of extracellular ribonuclease in growth of *Corynebacterium acnes*. Can J Microbiol 1969; 15: 749–52.

37 Farrior JW, Kloos WE. Amino acid and vitamin requirements of *Micrococcus* species isolated from human skin. Int J System Bacteriol 1975; 25: 80–82.

38 Emmett M, Kloos WE. Amino acid requirements of staphylococci isolated from human skin. Can J Microbiol 1975; 21: 729–33.

39 Dobson BC, Archibald AR. Effect of specific growth limitations on cell wall composition of *Staphylococcus aureus* H. Arch Microbiol 1978; 119: 295–301.

40 Taylor D, Holland KT. Amino acid requirements for the growth and production of some exocellular products of *Staphylococcus aureus*. J Appl Bacteriol 1989; 66: 319–29.

41 Ferguson Jr DA, Cummins CS. Nutritional requirements of anaerobic coryneforms. J Bacteriol 1978; 135: 858–67.

42 Cove JH, Holland KT, Cunliffe WJ. The vitamin requirements of staphylococci isolated from human skin. J Appl Bacteriol 1980; 49: 29–37.

43 Cove JH, Kearney JN, Holland KT, Cunliffe WJ. The vitamin requirements of *Staphylococcus cohnii*. J Appl Bacteriol 1983; 54: 203–08.

44 Smith RF. Characterization of human cutaneous lipophilic diphtheroids. J Gen Microbiol 1969; 55: 433–43.

45 McGinley KJ, Labows JN, Zeckman JM, Nordstrom KM, Webster GF, Leyden JJ. Analysis of cellular components, biochemical reactions and habitats of human cutaneous lipophilic diphtheroids. J Invest Dermatol 1985; 85: 374–77.

46 McGinley KJ, Labows JM, Zeckman JM, Nordstrom KM, Webster GF, Leyden JJ. Pathogenic JK group corynebacteria and their similarity to human cutaneous lipophilic diphtheroids. J Infect Dis 1985; 152: 801–06.

47 Leeming JP, Notman FH. Improved methods for isolation and enumeration of *Malassezia furfur* from human skin. J Clin Microbiol 1987; 25: 2017–19.

48 Shifrine M, Marr AG. The requirements of fatty acids by *Pityrosporum ovale*. J Gen Microbiol 1963; 32: 263–70.

49 Faergemann J, Fredriksson T. Age incidence of *Pityrosporum orbiculare* on human skin. Acta Dermato Veneriol Stockh 1980; 60: 531–33.

50 Midgley G. Comparison of *Pityrosporum* (*Malassezia*) isolates by morphology and immunoelectrophoresis. Br J Dermatol 1985; 113: 783–84.

51 Smith RF. Fatty acid requirements of human cutaneous lipophilic corynebacteria. J Gen Microbiol 1970; 60: 259–63.

52 Greenman J, Holland KT, Cunliffe WJ. Effects of glucose concentration on biomass, maximum specific growth rate, extracellular enzyme production by three species of cutaneous propionibacteria grown in continuous culture. J Gen Microbiol 1981; 127: 371–76.

53 Puhvel SM, Reisner RM. Effect of fatty acids on the growth of *Corynebacterium acnes in vitro*. J Invest Dermatol 1970; 54: 48–52.

54 Leyden JJ, McGinley KJ, Mills OH, Kligman AM. Age-related changes in the resident bacterial flora of the human face. J Invest Dermatol 1975; 65: 379–81.

55 Nordstrom NKM, Noble WC. Application of computer taxonomic techniques to the study of cutaneous propionibacteria and skin-surface lipid. Arch Dermatol Res 1985; 278: 107–13.

56 Kearney JN, Hornby D, Gowland G, Holland KT. The follicular distribution and abundance of resident bacteria on human skin. J Gen Microbiol 1984; 130: 797–801.

57 Webster GF, Ruggieri MR, McGinley KJ. Correlation of *Propionibacterium acnes* populations with the presence of triglycerides on non-human skin. Appl Environ Microbiol 1981; 41: 1269–70.

58 King K, Jones DH, Daltry DC, Cunliffe WJ. A double-blind study of the effects of 13-*cis*-retinoic acid on acne, sebum excretion rate and microbial populations. Br J Dermatol 1982; 107: 583–90.

59 Leyden JJ, McGinley KJ. Effect of 13-*cis*-retinoic acid on sebum production and *Propionibacterium acnes* in severe nodulocystic acne. Arch Dermatol Res 1982; 272: 331–37.

60 Leyden JJ, McGinley KJ, Foglia AN. Qualitative and quantitative changes in cutaneous bacteria association with systemic isotretinoin therapy for acne conglobata. J Invest Dermatol 1986; 86: 390–93.

61 McGinley KJ, Webster GF, Leyden JJ. Regional variations of cutaneous propionibacteria. Appl Environ Microbiol 1978; 35: 62–66.

62 McGinley KJ, Webster GF, Ruggieri MR, Leyden JJ. Regional variations in density of cutaneous propionibacteria: correlation of *Propionibacterium acnes* populations with sebaceous secretion. J Clin Microbiol 1980; 12: 672–75.

63 Kearney JN, Ingham E, Cunliffe WJ, Holland KT. Correlations between human skin bacteria and skin lipids. Br J Dermatol 1984; 110: 593–99.

64 Kabara JJ, Swieczkowski DM, Conley AJ, Truant JP. Fatty acids and derivatives as antimicrobial agents. Antimicrob Agent Chemother 1972; 2: 23–28.

65 Aly R, Maibach HI, Shinefield HR, Strauss WG. Survival of pathogenic microorganisms on human skin. J Invest Dermatol 1972; 58: 205–10.

66 Gutteridge JMC, Lamport P, Dormandy TL. The antibacterial effect of water-soluble compounds from autoxidising linolenic acid. J Med Microbiol 1976; 9: 105–09.

67 Kabara JJ. Structure-function relationships of surfactants as antimicrobial agents. J Soc Cosmet Chem 1978; 29: 733–41.

68 Ko HL, Heczko PB, Pulverer G. Differential susceptibility of *Propionibacterium acnes*, *P. granulosum* and *P. avidum* to free fatty acids. J Invest Dermatol 1978; 71: 363–65.

69 Ushijima T, Takahashi M, Ozaki Y. Acetic, propionic and oleic acid as the possible factors influencing the predominant residence of some species of *Propionibacterium* and coagulase-negative *Staphylococcus* on normal skin. Can J Microbiol 1984; 30: 647–52.

70 Lacey RW, Lord VL. Sensitivity of staphylococci to fatty acids: novel inactivation of linolenic acid by serum. J Med Microbiol 1981; 14: 41–49.

71 Aly R, Maibach HI. Correlation of human *in vivo* and *in vitro* cutaneous antimicrobial factors. J Infect Dis 1975; 131: 579–83.

72 Naidoo J. Effect of pH on inhibition of plasmid-carrying cultures of *Staphylococcus aureus* by lipids. J Gen Microbiol 1981; 124: 173–79.

73 Heczko PB, Lutticken R, Hryniewicz W, Neugebauer M, Pulverer G. Susceptibility of *Staphylococcus aureus* and group A, B, C, and G streptococci to free fatty acids. J Clin Microbiol 1979; **9**: 333–35.

74 Aly R, Maibach HI, Mandel A, Shinefield HR. Factors controlling the survival of *Staphylococcus aureus* on human skin. Zentralbl Bakteriol Parasit Infekt Hyg I abt 1976; Suppl 5: 941–46.

75 Bibel DJ, Miller SJ, Brown BE, Pandey BB, Elias PM, Shinefield HR, Aly R. Antimicrobial activity of stratum corneum lipids from normal and essential fatty acid-deficient mice. J Invest Dermatol 1989; 92: 632–38.

76 Miller SJ, Aly R, Shinefield HR, Elia PM. *In vitro* and *in vivo* anti-staphylococcal activity of human stratum corneum lipids. Arch Dermatol 1988; 124: 209–15.

77 Ingham E, Holland KT, Gowland G, Cunliffe WJ. Partial purification and characterisation of lipase (EC 3.1.1.3) from *Propionibacterium acnes*. J Gen Microbiol 1981; 124: 393–401.

78 Leeming JP, Notman FH, Holland KT. The distribution and ecology of *Malassezia furfur* and cutaneous bacteria on human skin. J Appl Bacteriol 1989; 67: 47–52.

79 Gemmell CG. Extracellular toxins and enzymes of coagulase-negative staphylococci. In: Easmon CSF, Adlam C, eds. Staphylococci and staphylococcal infections, volume 2. London: Academic Press; 1983: 809–27.

80 Mikx FHM, DeJong MH. Keratinolytic activity of cutaneous and oral bacteria. Infect Immun 1987; 55: 621–25.

81 Marshall J, Holland KT, Gribbon EM. A comparative study of the cutaneous microflora of normal feet with low and high levels of odour. J Appl Bacteriol 1988; 65: 61–68.

82 Grimont PAD, Grimont F, de Rosnay HLC, Sneath PHA. Taxonomy of the genus *Serratia*. J Gen Microbiol 1977; 98: 39–66.

83 Gramoli JL, Wilkinson BJ. Characteristics and identification of coagulase-negative, heat-stable deoxyribonuclease-positive staphylococci. J Gen Microbiol 1978; 105: 275–85.

84 Sharpe ME, Law BA, Phillips BA. Coryneform bacteria producing methane thiol. J Gen Microbiol 1976; 94: 430–35.

85 Baumann P, Doudoroff M, Stanier RY. A study of the *Moraxella* group II. oxidative-negative species (genus *Acinetobacter*). J Bacteriol 1968; 95: 1520–41.

86 Warskow A, Juni E. Nutritional requirements of *Acinetobacter* strains isolated from soil, water and sewage. J Bacteriol 1972; 112: 1014–16.

87 Bojar RA, Holland KT, Leeming JP, Cunliffe WJ. Azelaic acid: its uptake and mode of action in *Staphylococcus epidermidis* NCTC 11047. J Appl Bacteriol 1988; 64: 497–504.

3

Physical factors affecting the skin flora and skin disease

M. E. McBRIDE

The physical character of the skin, the tough dry exterior, signifies its major function, that of protection from the environment. Less obvious is the complex cellular environment, which provides a site for interaction between the tissue and such physical assaults as heat, hydration and light, the object of which is to maintain an internal physiological homeostasis. It is remarkable that despite wide variations in environmental conditions, the skin has the capacity to maintain a stable microbial ecosystem.[1,2] It is the purpose of this chapter to assess the importance of physical factors, in the skin and from the environment, in maintaining normal microbial colonization and in changes resulting in infection. Previous reviews have provided insight into the importance of skin structure, hydration, temperature, pH, oxygen and carbon dioxide gradients.[3-9] Much has been learned of other physical properties of the skin, such as optical, electrical and mechanical properties,[10-12] but their relationship to microbial colonization has received less attention. Hydrophobicity is of importance for adherence,[13] yet its relationship to colonization of the skin surface and microbial invasion is poorly understood. Thus, knowledge of the biophysical properties of the skin in relation to microbial colonization has lagged behind progress in other areas, and many of these aspects present challenges for future investigation. Microbial colonization of the skin will be discussed in relation to the skin structure, pH, temperature, hydration, oxygen and carbon dioxide, and light. The physical factors involved in adherence will also be reviewed.

Skin structure

The physical structure of skin is of primary importance in microbial colonization. Anatomical observations, using light and electron microscopy,[14,15] distinguish two layers, the outer epidermis and the inner dermis. The epidermis consists of a continuously renewing epithelial cell population, the keratinocytes, arising from a basal or germination layer and continually differentiating towards the skin surface. The morphological changes observed within the cells are a result of the evolution of the keratinizing process and these are used to designate layers within the epidermis. Keratinocytes gradually lose their nuclei and viability; they become flattened, dry, and cornified to form the outermost layer, the stratum corneum. The horny cells of the stratum corneum (corneocytes) provide the tough dry exterior of the skin surface and form the principal barrier between the environment and the body.

This classical anatomical description of the skin has been augmented over the past decade by major technological advances. Immunohistochemical techniques, using monoclonal and polyvalent antibodies to various cell components,[16] have provided structural localization of different keratins.[17] This, in conjunction with the development of keratinocyte culture systems producing stratified squamous epithelium in vitro,[18] has enabled further identification of cell structures and an understanding of the factors necessary for epidermal differentiation. Keratinocytes are now known to have a multiplicity of complex functions, which encompass metabolic, endocrine and immunological activities.[19] Of particular significance to microbial colonization is the lipid secretion of lamellar bodies. These are secretory organelles found in cells of the spinous and granular layers of the epidermis that secrete lipids into the intercellular spaces, providing a further dimension to the anatomical structure.[20] These lipid domains are responsible for the barrier properties of the stratum corneum that control hydration and permeability.[21] Furthermore, they provide a hydrophobic surface and the lipids themselves have been shown to have antimicrobial properties.[22]

The dermal layer of the skin comprises connective tissue, tendons, elastic fibres, fat and collagen; it provides support for blood vessels, nerves and other specialized structures such as hair follicles, and glands. It also exercises a complex regulatory function, controlling epidermal differentiation and development of appendages.[23]

Specialized structures of the skin are the hair follicle, which along with the sebaceous glands forms the pilosebaceous unit, and the apocrine and eccrine glands. The apocrine glands have specific anatomical locations in man: they are concentrated in the axillae and in the perineum, are not found in any other region, and remain underdeveloped until puberty. The glands comprise a secretory coil, which is embedded deep in the dermis, and a straight tubular duct through which sweat is carried to the hair follicle and from there to the skin surface.[24] Apocrine sweat has been studied extensively in lower mammals and is responsible for pheromones and hence is related to territorial marking and mating behaviour. Study of apocrine sweat from man has been hindered by the difficulty in obtaining samples uncontaminated by other skin secretions. It is believed to be a colourless, odourless liquid when first excreted, but is enzymatically changed by the human microflora to odoriferous compounds that are responsible for body odour.[25, 26] The study of pheromones in man is still in its infancy, and the relationship of skin bacteria to pheromone production is speculative at the present time. There is no information relating apocrine secretion to microbial colonization, but the demonstration of lysozyme in apocrine ducts may be relevant to protection against microbial invasion.[27] Sebaceous glands are found on most of the skin surface excluding the palms of the hands and the soles and dorsum of the feet. They predominate on the face and scalp, with densities ranging from 400 to 800 glands/cm² of skin.[28] The clusters of acini that make up the bulk of the gland are responsible for sebum production; they are derived from renewing epithelial cells formed along a basement membrane, which gradually differentiate and produce lipid, forming globules that can be seen in the cytoplasm. When fully differentiated, the cells appear to consist entirely of lipid, they disintegrate and the lipid is forced into the duct.[14] The ducts are lined with stratified squamous epithelium that is continuous with the epithelium of the hair follicle and is constantly shedding keratinaceous cells. The duct, therefore, contains a mixture of lipid and cornified cells, which is forced into the hair follicle. The activity of sebaceous glands changes with development, being active at birth then relatively inactive until puberty. When peak activity is reached, sebum production then remains constant throughout life.[29] There is considerable variability in the size of the glands between individuals and between anatomical sites in any one person; this variability is related to the size of the hair follicle and others factors in the dermis.[29]

Hair follicles are distributed over the entire body surface, with the exception of the palms of the hand and the soles and dorsum of the foot. They develop in embryo from both dermal and epidermal components, resulting in an epidermal structure that extends into the dermis.[14] The distribution of hair follicles is physiologically controlled by dermal factors, forming a fixed pattern and occurring at regular intervals on the skin surface,[23] and there is variation in structure between follicles.[29] The nature of the keratinizing process in the hair follicle – whether or not it is a continuation of the process on the skin surface – has been a source of controversy. Descriptions of the epithelial cells in the hair follicle now distinguish two layers of epidermal cells, the outer root sheath, whose matrix cells reside in the hair bulb, and the innermost cells, which are derived from matrix cells in the peripheral part of the hair bulb. During the renewing process, the outer cells become multilayered and keratinized at about the level of the opening of the sebaceous duct; the innermost cells remain a single layer but move upward towards the cell surface, differentiate and desquamate, and thus are a major contributory factor in delivering the horny cells into the hair follicle.[30] This anatomical site, the pilosebaceous unit, has particular relevance to microbial colonization and infection.[29]

The cutaneous microflora is comprised predominantly of coagulase-negative species of *Staphylococcus*,[31] aerobic Gram-positive non-spore forming bacilli, commonly referred to as coryneforms,[32] and anaerobic *Propionibacterium* and *Malassezia* (*Pityrosporum*) spp.[33,34] In considering the relationship of the cutaneous microflora of normal skin to the structure of the epidermis, studies show that the majority of microorganisms are present in two sites – within the outermost layers of the stratum corneum and in the hair follicle. These observations have been made from various techniques: Price's classical skin scrubbing experiments, which showed that most bacteria could be recovered from the initial scrub samples;[35] skin stripping with cellulose tape through successive layers of the epidermis, which confirmed these observations;[36,37] histological sections of normal skin, which show bacteria between the squames of the superficial layers of the stratum corneum; and scanning electron microscopy, which provides visual evidence of microorganisms on the surface of epithelial cells in the stratum corneum.[38] Bacteria with coccal and bacillary morphology, representing the principal genera of the resident flora, have been observed. Ultrastructural studies have shown that most bacteria exist in microcolonies.[4] The number of organisms in these microcolonies was estimated by comparing populations from skin scrubbing experiments with counts obtained from contact plates.[39] Further studies comparing the number of epithelial cells or fragments in a skin scrub sample with total bacterial populations have given values as high as 10^4–10^5. Large variations were noticed between individuals and from different anatomical sites in any one individual.[40] A significant positive correlation was found between epithelial cells and microbial populations in scrub samples,[41] and it has been observed in all these studies that there are seemingly stable individual differences in desquamation rates as well as microbial populations. Little is known of the relationship between normal desquamation and the constancy of normal flora; factors involved in corneocyte exfoliation have been reviewed,[42] but the role of microorganisms was not addressed. Bacterial products have been shown to increase the detachment of keratinocytes in fibroblast cultures formed in vitro.[43]

Abnormal keratinization and hyperproliferation result in physical changes in the stratum corneum that may be relevant to microbial colonization, although this aspect has not been given much consideration. Structural changes are evident in erythrasma, the larger spaces between keratinocytes containing microorganisms.[44] In psoriasis[45] and in conditions such as seborrheic dermatitis and atopic eczema, increased prevalence of colonization by *Staphylococcus aureus* has been reported.[46–48] Various mechanisms have been postulated,[49] but the specific effect of structural differences has not been studied.

The hair follicle is the site of the largest concentration of microorganisms.[38] Not all hair follicles are colonized and factors responsible for follicular colonization are poorly understood because exact figures are difficult to obtain.[50, 51] The question of whether the follicle merely provides physical space and colonization is a random event, or whether there is a relationship between the different types of follicles, is unresolved. The follicle, however, does provide a specialized physicochemical environment, probably one with changes in oxygen tension and pH that would contribute to microbial proliferation.[29] Furthermore, the relationship of colonization to the cycle of hair growth has not been examined. Another structural aspect of follicular colonization is the relationship between microbial species and the anatomical depth of colonization. By combining information from histological sections and microbial counts, the anaerobic species, *Propionibacterium*, were found to be more uniformly distributed in the follicle closer to the skin surface than *Staphylococcus* spp.[50] which colonized the lower portion of the follicle in greater numbers. In a study of plasmid profiles of coagulase-negative staphylococcus from successive skin strippings of the epidermis, a variety of profiles were present on the surface, but with successive strippings the numbers of profiles diminished and became more consistently anatomically localized,[52] suggesting follicular colonization (which also supports the view that staphylococci colonize the deeper levels of the hair follicles).

Colonization of the follicle has received considerable attention in relation to sebum production and the pathogenesis of acne.[29] Abnormal keratinization in the hair follicle, leading to occlusion and subsequent inflammation, has been postulated as a critical step in the development of acne lesions,[53] although this is a multifactorial disease in which the chemical and hormonal factors have received more attention than the physical. Folliculitis is a common dermatological condition that can be caused by a variety of microorganisms: *Staphylococcus aureus*, *Streptococcus pyogenes*[54] and *Malassezia furfur*.[55] Gram-negative folliculitis characteristically follows antibiotic treatment of acne.[56] Factors responsible include proliferation of a critical mass of pathogens,[57] occlusion of the follicular opening by keratinaceous material,[58] and excessive hydration.[59] The last may be a factor in 'hot-tub' folliculitis, commonly caused by *Pseudomonas aeruginosa*.[60] Hot-tub temperatures are optimal for proliferation of *Ps. aeruginosa*, which is of environmental origin and can reach critical population densities for infection.

On changing from a microscopic view of the anatomical localization of microflora to macroscopic view, regional anatomical variations in population densities are well recognized.[3,5,61] While the anatomical distribution of the pilosebaceous unit is of significance in the regional variation in flora,[62] other localized anatomical sites – the more occluded areas of skin, such as the axillae, groin and the interdigital toe space – provide specialized ecological niches and altered environmental conditions that encourage the growth of organisms not found on exposed flat surfaces.[63] The normal axillary flora has been described as consisting of large populations of predominantly either staphylococcal or coryneform bacteria.[64] Toe webs also are heavily colonized with bacteria, including Gram-negative bacteria,[65] and have a greater prevalence of dermatophytes and potentially pathogenic microorganisms.[66] Physical factors contributing to this specialized microflora, such as increased hydration and temperature, will be discussed later in this chapter. The scalp is a specialized microbial ecosystem with high population densities of staphylococci, propionibacterium and pityrosporum. The role of the type and density of hair follicles and increased keratinization have been considered to be factors in colonization. The question whether or not dandruff is a hyperproliferative disease or of microbiological origin with *M. furfur* as an aetiological agent, or both, has been discussed.[67] Other factors that may contribute to the high microbial populations are increased temperature, because hair provides warmth, and the concomitant increase in moisture.

pH

Since the classical experiments of Marchionini in 1929,[68] demonstrating the acid pH of the skin, the concept of the 'acid mantle' as a protection against microbial invasion, has persisted. Early descriptive studies by Anderson,[69] Arbenz,[70] and Beare and coworkers[71] showed the acidity of the skin surface. This information has been thoroughly reviewed by Behrendt and Green[72] and by Noble.[5] These studies have shown that the pH of skin is close to neutrality at birth, but becomes acid within 1 week and on normal exposed skin remains constant throughout life. The pH range varies between 4.0 and 8.0 between individuals and between skin sites; higher values have been recorded in the axillae at the onset of puberty and in occluded areas. Some of the variations result from methods used to measure pH, and the importance of methods has been emphasized by Noble.[5]

Eccrine sweat is believed to be the main contributor to the acid pH of the skin. Eccrine glands are distributed in all areas of the skin, although they are more concentrated on the palms of the hands, soles of the feet, the forehead and the axillae. The eccrine sweat gland is composed of a secretory coil where the sweat is initially formed, and an excretory portion, the distal duct. In the secretory coil, sweat is isotonic, with a pH close to neutrality, but as it passes through the distal duct, Na, K and Cl ions are selectively reabsorbed, which results in a hypotonic solution and a lower pH of approximately 5.0. The sweat is acidified by either reabsorbing bicarbonate ions or secreting H^+. Other components of sweat that have been implicated in acidity are lactate, which is the end-product of glycolysis, amino acids, and ammonia, which may play a part in buffering the acidity. The production of sweat is under both thermal and neurological control and can be stimulated by an increase in the internal and skin surface temperature and by cholinergic agents, either emotionally or artificially. The different sites appear to be under different regulatory control: the forehead, axillae, palms and soles of the hands and feet respond primarily to emotional control, while glands of the remainder of the skin surface respond primarily to thermal stimuli. The rate of sweating has a demonstrable effect on the pH: an increase in production allows less time for the sweat to remain in the distal duct (where reabsorption takes place) and hence the sweat has a pH between 6.5 and 7.0.[73]

Although eccrine sweat has been considered to be responsible for the acidic pH of the skin and antimicrobial activity, bacteria can be cultured in it.[74] Furthermore, the presence of other secretions, apocrine and sebum, cannot be ignored and obviously contribute to skin pH, although the part played by each is difficult to assess. The hypothesis that acid pH prevents microbial growth on the skin has received a great deal of attention, even though most of the bacteria making up the normal flora do not have a strict pH requirement and can grow over a broad pH range. Early studies showed that skin sites with higher pH values had larger populations,[75] but later studies have not supported this.[76] Attempts have been made to show a relationship between pH and the skin flora by artificially changing the pH of the skin. An early study by Arnold demonstrated increased bacterial populations on the hands after soaking in an alkaline solution.[77] More recently, a study comparing the effects of repeated washing with a soap with pH close to neutrality with those of synthetic detergents with acid pH showed a slight increase in skin pH (0.3 pH units) after a 4-week exposure to soap as opposed to detergent. The increase in pH was accompanied by an increase in *Propionibacterium* spp. but not in numbers of *Staphylococcus epidermidis*.[78, 79]

The advent of the detergent skin-scrub method[80] changed many of the previous concepts of skin populations. This method combined detergent and a pH that permits the release and dispersal of microcolonies from the stratum corneum. Thus, skin populations were found to be larger than previously believed. It was postulated that an increase in pH altered the electrostatic charge and permitted the release of greater numbers of organisms from the skin surface. The question can be raised whether an increase in skin pH causes proliferation of the skin flora or the change in electrostatic charges releases the flora from the skin surface. The presence of positively and negatively charged ions from eccrine sweat may be the operating factor in the attractive and repellent forces between bacteria and skin surface, as the electrophoretic mobility of microorganisms is affected by pH.[81,82]

Certain specialized skin sites, such as the axillae, groin and toe webs, have both larger microbial populations and higher pH values. As these sites are occluded there is difficulty in studying the effect of skin pH on their microflora as a separate entity, because pH is intrinsically linked to both temperature and hydration, each of which affect the flora. Experimental studies correlating pH with the microflora have been done on skin occluded by plastic wrap. Under these conditions, temperature, hydration and pCO_2 increase as well. Hartman[83] confirmed earlier studies by Marples,[84] and Aly and co-workers,[85] who reported an increase in the mean total populations of colony-forming units (cfu) from the skin of the forearm from 1.8×10^6 cfu/cm^2 to 4.5×10^6 after 5 days of occlusion; the pH shifted from 4.38 to 7.05. The composition of the flora changed as well, resulting in a larger proportion of lipophilic coryneforms.

A study of three sites on the foot – dorsal, sole and the fourth toe cleft – has shown that the microbial density from each site directly correlated with skin pH.[86] The smallest populations were on the dorsal surface (mean log values, 3.08 cfu/cm^2) followed by the soles (5.61 cfu/cm^2) and the toe clefts (7.02 cfu/cm^2). The mean pH for the dorsal surface and the soles was 5.23 and 6.25. While the soles have highest concentration of eccrine glands, the toe cleft can be considered to have the specialized environment of an occluded site. These investigators point out that it is difficult to determine whether the increase in pH results from the by-products of microbial growth or whether a neutral pH is responsible for greater microbial proliferation.[87] End-products of carbohydrate utilization result in an acid pH, and while proteolytic degradation may also contribute to a lower pH by the release of amino acids, some proteolytic skin organisms can split urea, which would increase alkalinity.

The role of skin pH in protection against infection still remains to be established. Correlations between conditions with altered or abnormal sweating and increased susceptibility to infection have been examined.

Newrick and colleagues[88] studied the microflora of the foot in diabetics with impaired sweating and found no difference between these patients and a control group. They concluded it was unlikely that a change in microbial flora is involved in the propensity of the diabetic neuropathic patient for foot ulceration. The pH of the feet was not recorded. In patients with hereditary palmoplantar keratoma, who are prone to dermatophyte infections, the pH of the soles of 69 patients ranged between 5.5 and 5.9;[89] these investigators postulated that, as the pH optima of the proteases of dermatophytes were in the alkaline range,[90] the theory that an increased skin pH would lead to infection in these patients was negated, although a study has now shown that the optimum pH for the enzymatic activity of a protease from *Trichophyton mentagrophytes* is 5.5,[91] and another protease from candida was active at a pH of 4.5.[92] This supports the view that the pH of skin may facilitate or prevent infection in ways other than by stimulating or suppressing growth of pathogens; the specific pathogenic mechanism, such as the production of an enzyme or toxin, may be pH dependent. This has been shown to be the case in toxic shock syndrome, where the optimum pH for toxin production is at neutrality.[93]

In summary, the assumption that the acid mantle prevents bacterial colonization by inhibiting microbial growth is an oversimplification. It is more likely that pH alters electrostatic forces at the microbe–skin interface, which permits aggregation and attraction. Furthermore, it potentially provides a specific environment for pathogenic events that have strict pH optima.

Temperature

Although the core body temperature, that of the internal organs, is 37 °C, the temperature of the skin surface can vary as much as 20 °C. In the normal host, anatomical site and the temperature of the environment are the most important factors responsible for this variation. As shown in Fig. 3.1, the distal aspect of the limbs, the farthest from the core, experience the greatest effect from environmental temperatures.[94] Ranges in temperatures cited for different anatomical sites are shown in Table 3.1. Other environmental factors that affect body temperature are clothing and excercise.[5] Exercise increases body temperature and, in a hot climate, may lead to heat prostration from critically high body temperatures.[95] Although the environment can alter the skin temperature, there are limits beyond which skin damage occurs; extremes of heat (above 42 °C) and cold (less than 20 °C) cause pain, and these nervous stimuli usually result in avoidance behaviour.[96] Behavioural modification is a powerful force that tends to equalize hostile environmental conditions.

Table 3.1. *Skin temperatures of different anatomical sites*

Site	Temperature
Forehead	33.40
Clavicle	33.60
Above umbilicus	34.20
Lumbar region	33.30
Arm (biceps)	32.85
Palm of hand	32.85
Kneecap	32.35
Leg (calf)	32.20
Foot (sole)	30.20
Big toe	30.95

Adapted from: Rothman S. Physiology and biochemistry of the skin. University of Chicago Press, 1954.

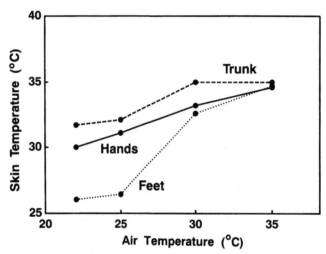

Fig. 3.1. Variations in skin temperature with different environmental temperatures (*adapted from*: Dubois EF. Heat loss from the human body. Bull NY Acad Med 1939; 15: 143).

The skin provides a barrier for maintaining a stable body temperature by two mechanisms, convection, which is the dispersal of heat through the skin from the blood vessels,[97,98] and sweating. A change in the temperature, either at the skin surface or internally in the hypothalamus, provides a nervous response that triggers vasodilation in the case of overheating or constriction for excessive cold. The nervous stimulus from the hypothalamus also stimulates the eccrine glands to secrete sweat. As well as heat lost from the loss of body liquid, the evaporation of the increased moisture on the skin surface has a cooling effect, which lowers the body temperature. In dry atmospheric conditions, the cooling effect of sweating is greater than in high humidity, where the evaporation rate is lower, resulting in greater discomfort in conditions of high humidity.[99]

The temperature of the skin obviously plays a part in maintaining a stable environment for the microbial ecosystem. Although the normal daily habits of most individuals necessitate continual cycling from periods of activity to inactivity, resulting in fluctuations in skin temperature, most of the organisms which make up the normal flora do not have strict temperature requirements. Most species of staphylococci, for example, will grow at between 20–40 °C (although the optimum is closer to 35 °C). If skin temperature can bring about changes in the microflora, it is more likely to do so indirectly: that is, the increase in temperature induces sweating and the resultant increase in moisture has a greater effect than the temperature alone. The combined effect of temperature and humidity in the axillae, groin, and toe webs probably contributes to the large microbial populations there. These sites are usually occluded by clothing, which further provides optimal conditions for microbial growth.

Skin temperature may play a more important part in skin invasion by pathogens. Many skin pathogens – dermatophytes and fungi responsible for skin infections such as chromomycosis (phaeohyphomycosis) – have temperature optima of 25 °C;[100] hence the lower temperature of the skin surface may provide a more hospitable environment. Species of *Mycobacterium* causing granulomatous skin diseases have temperature optima at 30 °C (such as *M. marinum*[101] and *M. haemophilum*).[102] Under these circumstances, skin temperature may be a significant factor in infection.

Of more recent interest has been the increased understanding of heat-shock proteins (hsp).[103] These are produced by virtually all cells in response to an increase in temperature, the range of which is dependent on the natural temperature of the species involved; their function is to repair damage caused by heat. The genetics of these proteins has been the object of much research: all organisms produce proteins encoded by the hsp-70 and hsp-90 families, which are considered to be of the greatest physiological significance in repairing cellular damage from heat.[104] Theoretically, heat damaged protein is repaired by a protein–protein interaction mediated by heat-shock proteins.[105] Furthermore, these proteins can be produced by conditions of stress other than heat. Of particular interest is the observation that heat-shock proteins are immunodominant antigens, which have been shown to produce specific antibodies and may provide protection. An immunological response to heat-shock proteins from *M. leprae* and *M. tuberculosis* has been reported.[106] It is also of interest to speculate whether heat-shock proteins play a part in changes that take place in dimorphic fungi with temperature. *Staphylococcus aureus* and *S. epidermidis* produce such proteins when temperatures increase from 30 to 40 °C.[107] These are temperature variations that can occur on the skin surface. It is interesting, therefore, to speculate on the role played by heat-shock proteins in protection against staphylococcal skin infections. Epidermal cells also produce these proteins,[103] and one may ask under what circumstances an antibody response to these could contribute to autoimmune disease.

Hydration

The presence of moisture on skin is one of the principal factors affecting cutaneous microbial populations. This is reflected by variations in populations under normal conditions from different anatomical sites, showing low numbers on exposed dry surfaces, as compared to higher values in occluded areas, such as the axillae, groin and toe web.[3, 4, 63]

Both physiological and environmental factors are responsible for skin surface hydration. Physiologically, water on the skin surface is derived from two sources, from the skin itself by transepidermal water loss (TEWL)[108] and from sweat produced by the eccrine glands.[73] In conditions of increased humidity, the skin has the ability to absorb water, a function that is controlled by the stratum corneum, specifically by the lipids that form the lipid domains. Treatment of the skin with lipid solvents results in a loss of this regulatory function and an increase in TEWL.[109] The lipid content and type responsible for this activity have been defined,[110] and it has been shown that after lipid removal, the concurrent water loss is a stimulus for lipid synthesis.[111] Conversely, prolonged drying has been shown to increase TEWL;[112] thus water is continually being supplied to the skin surface through a variety of complex mechanisms. Furthermore, changes in environmental temperature affect sweat production, and atmospheric humidity controls the rate of water evaporation from the skin surface. Therefore, on exposed sites the skin can be relatively dry, but in occluded areas the skin surface moisture is maintained.

Experiments in which hydration has been increased by occlusion[113] have shown an increase in microbial populations,[114] in particular of Gram-negative bacteria and lipophilic coryneforms (Fig. 3.2). Studies in which human subjects were sequestered in environmentally controlled chambers with temperatures raised to 95 °C and a relative humidity of 95 per cent showed an increase in microbial populations (Fig. 3.3) and Gram-negative prevalence. High temperatures alone, without increased humidity, had no effect.[115]

Excessive hydration, brought about by bathing, has often been considered

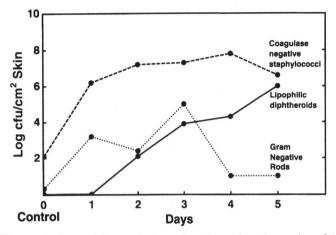

Fig. 3.2. Changes in bacterial populations (in colony-forming units, cfu) during 5 days occlusion under plastic wrap (*adapted from*: Aly R. Effect of occlusion on microbial population and physical skin conditions. In: Noble WC, ed. Sem Dermatol 1982; 1: 139).

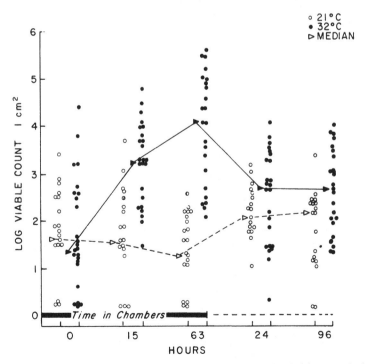

Fig. 3.3. The effect of temperature and humidity on microbial skin populations (*from*: Duncan and colleagues[115]).

as beneficial to health in general,[116] and skin diseases in particular.[117] Within the past decade, hot tub use has become popular and outbreaks of folliculitis associated with *Pseudomonas aeruginosa* have been reported.[68] Harmful effects of excessive hydration in military personnel serving in tropical countries have been observed: soldiers of the British army serving in South East Asia had an increased prevalence of foot infections in climates with high temperatures and humidities.[118] In Vietnam, 'immersion foot' was described, an infection by *Trichophyton mentagrophytes* resulting from wearing sodden boots.[119] Similarly, coal miners are subject to foot infections related to wet occlusion.[120] is a major factor in the excoriation of buttocks in infants wearing diapers (nappies), which frequently leads to infection.[121]

Corynebacterium minutissimum, the aetiological agent of erythrasma,[122] and a variety of coryneform bacteria that have been isolated from lesions of the hair in trichomycosis axillaris[123–26] and trichomycosis pubis,[127] are only evident in occluded sites, that is, the groin and axilla and the pubis, respectively. The moisture of these enclosed sites is considered to promote microbial growth, as these infections do not occur on exposed skin surfaces. Paronychia, infection of the nail fold,[128] caused by a variety of organisms (*Staphylococcus aureus*, *Streptococcus pyogenes* and *Candida albicans*) is usually initiated by trauma, such as nail biting or finger sucking; hydration has also been implicated and there are indications of occupationally associated prevalence related to hydration.[129]

Mechanical properties

The mechanical properties of skin have not received the interest and attention accorded to anatomical and chemical aspects, despite its protective role. The dermis provides mobility and elasticity by the different types of collagen and elastic fibres, which are structurally arranged to maintain underlying support, mobility and contour of the epidermis.[130, 131] The stratum corneum has varying degrees of elasticity depending on age, sex and anatomical site.[132] Hydration of the stratum corneum is the most significant variable in changes of elasticity and there is a direct correlation between hydration and elasticity.[108, 133] There is no evidence to date that mechanical or elastic properties of the skin affect microbial colonization. Friction, however, is an important factor in mechanical damage to the stratum corneum. This is considered as a factor in erythrasma, where adjacent skin surfaces in the groin produce friction,[134] and infection in infants resulting from wearing diapers.[135] Different diaper materials cause variable amounts of friction, which in conjunction with excessive hydration, lead to alterations in TEWL, pH, and skin damage, with an increased potential for infection.[121]

Oxygen and carbon dioxide

Although the skin surface is in contact with atmospheric oxygen, the oxygen in the epidermis originates from the arterial capillaries in the dermis. The partial pressure of carbon dioxide (pCO_2) in the epidermis correlates with that of arterial blood, but the partial pressure of oxygen (pO_2) is lower in the epidermis than in arterial blood. Skin, therefore, offers resistance to oxygen diffusion or, alternatively, oxygen is being used by the cells of the epidermis[136] or perhaps by microorganisms. Conversely, CO_2 passes through the epidermis with considerably less resistance and there is a higher pCO_2 in the skin than in atmospheric conditions.[137] It has been suggested that the higher pCO_2 results, in part, from CO_2 produced from metabolic activities of keratinocytes.[138]

The relative concentrations of oxygen and carbon dioxide in the skin are obviously of importance for the normal microbial colonization because the skin flora consists of anaerobes – e.g. *Propionibacterium* spp. – and strict aerobes such as *Brevibacterium* spp.; although staphylococci, coryneforms and many Gram-negative bacteria are facultative. It is well known that lowered pO_2 stimulates growth of many bacteria, including species of staphylococci, even though it is inhibitory to dermatophytes and fungi.[139] The perplexing feature of normal flora is the ability of anaerobes, for example *P. acnes*, to proliferate close to the skin surface, in contact with atmospheric oxygen. It has also been observed that, on primary cultivation from skin samples, *Propionibacterium* spp. can grow in mixed culture with staphylococci, but not on subculture.[140] It is appropriate to view this finding in context of a self-contained ecosystem such as a biofilm. The concept of biofilms has received increasing interest and been found to have growing relevance in biology and medicine in recent years.[141] Biofilms can be defined as the attachment of an aggregation of mixed organisms and their metabolic products to a surface, forming the development of a self-enclosed system where nutrients and gases diffuse into the system and metabolites accumulate and alter the microenvironment.[142] In this setting, a gradient in pO_2 would exist at different levels in the biofilm. Considering microcolonies of the skin in this context, it is possible to envisage variations in concentrations in gases that would allow growth in seemingly unlikely sites.

Experimental studies relating pO_2 and pCO_2 to microbial populations have used occlusion. Under occlusion pO_2 decreases and pCO_2 increases; this is accompanied by changes in the microbial flora, with increased populations. As mentioned above, these conditions induce other physical changes such as increased hydration, and therefore population increases cannot be solely attributed to the change in relative concentrations of these two gases.[143]

Physical factors in adherence of microorganisms to skin

Adherence is the initial step in colonization of surfaces, whether in the formation of a normal ecosystem or in an invasive pathogenic process. Studies on the adherence of microorganisms to skin have, thus far, emphasized chemical factors.[144-46] Physical factors, however, have been recognized in microbe–surface interaction that may be particularly relevant to the attachment of microorganisms to the skin, because forces of a physical nature can either attract or repel. The role of hydrophobicity in adhesion has received attention[147] and is considered to play a part in pathogenesis.[13] At the microbe–skin interface, the two hydrophobic surfaces would seem to be naturally repellent; a variety of physical conditions, however, may alter the forces between two surfaces. These include surface tension at the interface, which is dependent on the viscosity of the intercellular material, changes in the electrostatic charge on either of the cell surfaces or the matrix between cells, and alterations on the cell surfaces that would change the hydrophobicity, which could be brought about by either of the above-mentioned conditions. The bacterial cell surface is relatively easy to study as compared to the skin surface, which is a poorly defined mixture of degraded proteinaceous–lipid material bathed in a complex solution with electrically charged ions. Under these circumstances, the relative forces of attraction and repulsion are difficult to define. In other simpler systems, physical factors have been studied and conditions defined which may have some relevance in adherence of microorganisms to skin. The surface properties of *Candida albicans* and their relation to aggregation and adhesion have received the most attention.[148, 149] Hydrophobicity is generally considered to be a major factor in adherence to inert surfaces,[150] and buccal cells,[151] and has been shown to be temperature dependent.[152] In addition, electrical surface charge[148] and elemental surface composition[149] play a part in adherence and may also affect hydrophobicity. There is also evidence that the combination of hydrophobicity and surface tension at different interfaces, liquid–liquid, and liquid–solid, alter adhesive properties.[153] The production of an emulsifier by *Candida albicans* in vitro has also been described[154] and may be important in colonizing skin by solubilizing the lipid surface. Production of biosurfactants by phytopathogenic coryneforms has been described[155] and has been considered in adhesion to epithelial cells.[156] The forces between surfaces are obviously complex and this issue raises many questions, even when examined under defined in vitro conditions.[157, 158] It is important, however, to consider the potential of these factors at the skin–microbe interface.

The presence of fimbriae in microorganisms is of importance for attachment and pathogenicity. The importance of fimbriae (pili) in the attachment of *Neisseria gonorrhoeae* to epithelial cells of the cervix and vagina has been well documented.[159] Similarly, uropathogenic *Escherichia coli* colonize the uro-genital tract by means of fimbriae.[160] Thus far, the presence of fimbriae in microorganisms colonizing the skin has received little attention, although fibrillae have been described in *Streptococcus pyogenes* as contributing to attachment to epithelial cells, and adherence was also found to be related to a decrease in hydrophobicity.[161] Although this area of research is largely specu-lative at present, the question is raised whether Gram-positive colonization of acetone-treated skin[162] might actually be due to the removal of inhibitory lipids or to an alteration of the hydrophobic surface of the skin, thus permitting adherence. The efficacy of detergent scrubs in removing bacteria from skin[80] tends to support this hypothesis.

Light

Light derived from the sun is necessary for sustaining life on this planet. Living organisms convert solar energy to chemical bonds, thus providing the necessary energy for biosynthetic processes. The sun has been worshipped by man as religious deity from the preChristian era throughout the world, by North American and Mexican Indians, by the Hindus and by the Babylonians in ancient Persia, as well as in ancient Greece. This widespread worship of the sun suggests that it provides life-sustaining properties: the sun is a major source of heat; it is also responsible for the production of vitamin D in the skin, which is linked to the prevention of disease; it can be used for therapy, as in psoriasis; and it is responsible for the degradation of bilirubin in the skin.[163] Interestingly, in recent years, most research on the effects of light on skin has focused on the harmful aspects of light, such as sunburn and cancer. Although a great deal of information has been gathered on the effects of light on the skin, very little is understood of these effects, either direct or indirect, in relation to bacteria living on or in the skin, or of the role of light in skin disease of microbial aetiology.

Radiation from the sun is divided on the basis of wavelength into ultraviolet, visible and near infrared. These are portrayed diagrammatically in Fig. 3.4. Visible light has wavelengths between 400 and 700 nm and is responsible for vision by absorption on the retina. Radiation of these wavelengths is not known to be harmful. The ultraviolet spectrum has been further divided into types described as UVA, UVB and UVC in decreasing order of wavelength. The wavelengths of UVA are from 320 to 400 nm; UVA is referred to as long-wave or near ultraviolet because of its proximity to visible light. It has also

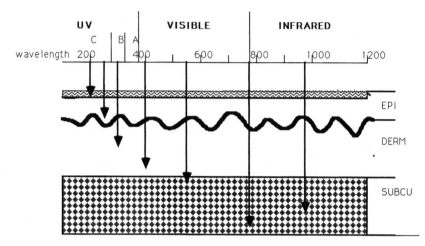

Fig. 3.4. Penetration of different wavelengths of light into human skin (*adapted from*:
Diffey BL. Optical properties of skin: measurement of erythema. In: Marks RM,
Barton SP, Edwards C, eds. The physical nature of skin. Lancaster: MTP Press; 1988:
180).

been called 'blacklight' for its ability to cause substances to fluoresce in the
dark. Radiation from UVA causes erythema and stimulates melanin, but is not
as harmful as UVB, which has wavelengths between 290 and 320 nm, is
responsible for sunburn, and considered to be a significant factor in skin
cancer. UVC (200–290 nm) is known as 'short-wave' or 'far' radiation
because it is farthest from the visible spectrum. It is filtered out by the ozone
layer and does not reach the earth's surface but experimentally causes
erythema of the skin and kills unicellular organisms.

It has long been known that UVB is lethal to microorganisms in vitro,[164, 165]
and although many studies have been done of the effects of UVB on skin, none
has examined these effects on the skin microflora. Faergemann and Larkö[166]
compared the effects of UVB and UVA in vitro on the killing of microorganisms commonly found on skin: *Candida albicans*, *Malassezia furfur*,
Staphylococcus epidermidis and *S. aureus*. Using UVB and irradiation doses
from 250 to 900 mJ/cm^2, *M. furfur* and *C. albicans* were killed. Only at
900 mJ/cm^2 was *S. epidermidis* killed and *S. aureus* inhibited, but total killing
was not achieved. Using UVA, *M. furfur* was found to be the most sensitive,
although a small proportion of cells survived. Wikler and colleagues[167] studied
the effects of UVA on the ultrastructure of *Malassezia*. They found killing with
UVA at 50 mJ/cm^2 but no significant killing with UVB until 900 mJ/cm^2.
They suggested that these findings could explain the curative effects of sunlight
on seborrheic dermatitis.

While there is good evidence that light can affect skin microorganisms in vitro, it has not been possible to demonstrate any real changes in vivo. Gerber and co-workers[168] studies the effects of sunbathing on microbial flora of the skin in 9 frequent sunbathers and 10 comparable volunteers who denied sunbathing. No differences in overall populations were observed when sun-exposed and non-exposed areas were compared, but sunbathers had a higher proportion of carotenoid-pigmented bacteria than non-sunbathers. The usual wide individual variations in total populations were found, which make interpretation of the data difficult; a larger number of subjects may be needed in order to draw meaningful conclusions. It is difficult to compare precisely in vitro exposure to UVA and UVB with in vivo exposure to sunlight because the amount of UV light in sunlight is variable and difficult to measure.

Photosensitization of bacteria by long-wave ultraviolet light has been recognized for some time; it involves a variety of chemicals as sensitizing agents.[169] The group of compounds that have excited the greatest interest are the furocoumarins of plant origin, in particular, 8-methoxypsoralen, which is widely used for treatment of psoriasis and vitiligo. Scherwitz and colleagues[170] described ultrastructural changes in *C. albicans* exposed to 8-methoxypsoralen and UV light at 365 nm. Damage was seen in both the cytoplasm, involving mitochondria, and the cell wall. The site of damage may vary between organisms and wavelengths; Fujita and Suzuki[171] described the induction of prophages and mutation in *Escherichia coli* with UV wavelengths of 320–340 nm, indicating damage to DNA. Daniels used the photosensitivity of *C. albicans* as a test for identifying photosensitizing agents.[172] *Candida albicans* is streaked on a plate and the compounds to be tested are spotted on the surface. The plates are grown under blacklight and zones of inhibition of growth and sensitizing compounds are evident. Mitchell suggested that, as a large number of plants in nature are potential photosensitizers, micro-organisms on the skin may themselves act as sensitizers and have toxic effects on other members of the microflora.[173] He found that *M. furfur* inhibits *S. aureus*, *S. epidermidis*, *E. coli* and *Corynebacterium minutissimum*. Extracts from *Pseudomonas aeruginosa* and *Propionibacterium acnes* were also found to be toxic. Faergemann and Larkö made similar experiments with comparable findings.[174] Their further studies showed phototoxicity of *Streptococcus viridans* to the same organisms.[175] These observations have implications on the effects of light on the microecology of the skin. Mitchell questions whether the predilection of corynebacteria responsible for trichomycosis axillaris and erythrasma for dark sites is a result of photosensitivity of these organisms in light-exposed areas.[173]

An attempt has been made to show an effect of photosensitization on the microflora of normal skin in the study of psoriatics undergoing psoralen (P)

UVA treatment.[176] The result were not remarkable, but a slight decrease in *P. acnes* populations correlated with skin lipid levels at the beginning of the study, and this was not the case after PUVA treatment.

Whether photosensitization of microorganisms on skin can have a beneficial effect in preventing diseases of microbiological aetiology is still questionable. Experimental infections of *Trichophyton mentagrophytes* in guinea-pigs were shown to respond to treatment with 8-methoxypsoralen and blacklight.[177] Seborrheic dermatitis, currently believed to be caused by *M. furfur* has responded to treatment with PUVA and other wavelengths in the UVA range.[178] Although it is popularly believed that light is beneficial to acne, clinical studies[179,180] using UVA and UVB and 8-methoxypsoralen did not support the view that photosensitization was helpful.

In considering the effects of light on skin, one must not ignore the possibility of indirect effects. Light may induce changes in the skin that can indirectly affect microbial life. One of the best described sunlight-mediated events is the photosynthesis of previtamin D_3 and its inhibitory effect on *Mycobacterium tuberculosis*.[181] While this may be the reason why *M. tuberculosis* causes skin infections only infrequently, other non-tuberculous *Mycobacterium* spp. are well-recognized skin pathogens, many of which produce carotenoid pigments that may have evolved as a protective mechanism against the lethal effect of ultraviolet light. When these various aspects of light are considered, it is obvious that a great deal is yet to be learned of the effects of light on the microbial ecosystem of the skin.

Conclusion

In summary, recent knowledge of the organization of the skin structure and its biophysical properties has provided a greater understanding of the factors, and the interaction between them, that are necessary for establishment of the microbial ecosystem. By the same token, it is possible to see what changes or alterations are necessary in these physical properties to provide the opportunity for microorganisms to overcome the barrier properties of skin and initiate infection. Unfortunately, microbiologists in recent years have been seduced by technological advances in biochemistry and have tended to overlook the role of physical factors in the microbial colonization and invasion of skin.

References

1 Evans CA. Persistent individual differences in bacterial flora of the skin of the forehead: numbers of propionibacteria. J Invest Dermatol 1975; 64: 42–46.

2 Evans CA, Strom MS. Eight year persistence of individual differences in the bacterial flora of the forehead. J Invest Dermatol 1982; 79: 51–52.

3 Marples MJ. The ecology of human skin. Springfield, IL: Thomas; 1965.

4 Noble WC, Pitcher DG. Microbial ecology of human skin. Advances in microbial ecology 1976; 2: 245–89.

5 Noble WC. Microbiology of Human Skin. 2nd ed. London: Lloyd-Luke; 1981.

6 Maibach HI, Hildick-Smith G. Skin bacteria and their role in infection. New York: McGraw-Hill; 1965.

7 Maibach HI, Aly R. Skin microbiology: relevance to clinical infection. New York: Springer-Verlag; 1981.

8 Haustein UF. Bacterial skin flora, host defence and skin infections. Dermatol Monatsschr 1989; 175: 665–80.

9 Roth RR, James WD. Microbiology of the skin: resident flora, ecology, infection. J Am Acad Dermatol 1989; 20: 367–90.

10 Parrish JA. Responses of skin to visible and ultraviolet light. In: Goldsmith LA, ed. Biochemistry and physiology of the skin. New York: Oxford University Press; 1983: 3–63.

11 Edwards C. The electrical properties of the skin In: Marks RM, Barton SP, Edwards C, eds. The physical nature of skin. Boston: MTP Press; 1988: 209–13.

12 Lévêque JL, Rasseneur L. Mechanical properties of stratum corneum: influence of water and lipids. In: Marks RM, Barton SP, Edwards C, eds. The physical nature of skin. Boston: MTP Press; 1988: 155–64.

13 Absalom DR. The role of bacterial hydrophobicity in infection: bacterial adhesion and phagocytic ingestion. Adv Microbiol Ecol 1986; 9: 355–93.

14 Montagna W, Parakaal PF. The structure and function of skin. New York: Academic Press; 1974.

15 Holbrook KA, Wolff K. Structure and Development of Skin. In: Fitzpatrick TB, Eisen AZ, Wolff K, Freedberg IM, Austen KF, eds. Dermatology in general medicine. 3rd ed. New York: McGraw-Hill; 1987: 93–130.

16 Woodcock-Mitchell J, Eichner R, Nelson WG, Sun TT. Immunolocalization of keratin polypeptides in human epidermis using monoclonal antibodies. J Cell Biol 1982; 95: 580–88.

17 Sun TT, Eichner R, Nelson WG, Tseng SCG, Weiss RA, Jarvinen M, Woodcock-Mitchell J. Keratin classes: molecular markers for different types of epithelial differentiation. J Invest Dermatol 1983; 81: 109–15S.

18 Rheinwald JA, Green H. Epidermal growth factor and multiplication of human epidermal cells. Nature Lond 1977; 265: 421–24.

19 Milstone LM, Edelson RL, eds. Endocrine, metabolic and immunologic functions of keratinocytes. Ann NY Acad Sci 1988; 548: 1–3.

20 Odland GP, Holbrook K. The lamellar granules of epidermis. Curr Prob Dermatol 1987; 9: 29–49.

21 Elias PM, Feingold KR. Lipid related barrier and gradients in the epidermis. Ann NY Acad Sci 1985; 458: 4–17.

22 Miller SJ, Aly R, Shinefield HR, Elias P. In vitro and in vivo antistaphylococcal activity of human stratum corneum lipids. Arch Dermatol 1988; 124: 209–15.

23 Sengel P. Role of extracellular matrix with development of skin and cutaneous

appendages. In: Lash JW, Saven L, eds. Developmental mechanisms: normal and abnormal. Progr Clin Biol Res 1985; 171: 123–35.

24 Robertshaw D. Biology of apocrine sweat glands. In: Goldsmith LA, ed. Biochemistry and physiology of the skin. Oxford University Press: New York; 1983: 209.

25 Jackman PJH. Body odour – the role of skin bacteria. Sem Dermatol 1982; 1: 143–48.

26 Leyden JJ, Zeng XN, McGinley K, Lawley HJ, Preti G. Characterization of pungent axillary odors. J Invest Dermatol 1990; 94: 549.

27 Ezoe K, Katsumata M. Immunohistochemical study of lysozyme in human apocrine glands. J Dermatol 1990; 17: 159–63.

28 Strauss JS. Sebaceous glands. In: Fitzpatrick TB, Eisen AZ, Wolff K, Freedberg IM, Austen KF, eds. Dermatology in general medicine. New York: McGraw-Hill; 1987: 666–84.

29 Cunliffe WJ. Acne. Chicago/London: Martin Dunitz/Yearbook Medical; 1989.

30 Ito M. Biological roles of the innermost cell layer of the outer root sheath in human anagen hair follicle: further electron microsopic study. Arch Dermatol Res 1989; 281: 254–59.

31 Kloos WE, Musselwhite MS. Distribution and persistence of *Staphylococcus* and *Micrococcus* species and other anerobic bacteria on human skin. Appl Microbiol 1975; 30: 381–95.

32 Pitcher DG. Corynebacterium and related genera of the normal human skin. Hautzart 1981; 32 (suppl V): 273–75.

33 McGinley KJ, Webster GF, Leyden JJ. Regional variations of cutaneous propionibacteria. Appl Environ Microbiol 1978; 35: 62–66.

34 Leeming JP, Notman FH. Improved methods for isolation and enumeration of *Malassezia furfur*. J Clin Microbiol 1987; 25: 2017–19.

35 Price PB. The bacteriology of the normal skin: a new quantitative test applied to a study of the bacterial flora and disinfection action of mechanical cleansing. J Infect Dis 1938; 63: 301–18.

36 Röckl H, Müeller E. Beitrag fur Lokolization der mikroben der Haut. Arch Klin Exp Dermatol 1959; 209: 13–23.

37 Updegraff DM. A cultural method of quantitatively studying microorganisms on skin. J Invest Dermatol 1964; 43: 129–37.

38 Montes LF, Wilborn WH. Location of bacterial skin flora. Br J Dermatol 1969; 81 (Suppl 1): 23–26.

39 Somerville DA, Noble WC. Microcolony size of microbes on human skin. J Med Microbiol 1973; 6: 323–28.

40 Holt RJ. Aerobic bacterial counts of human skin after bathing. J Med Microbiol 1971; 4: 319–27.

41 McBride ME, Duncan WC, Knox JM. Correlations between epithelial cells and bacterial populations in bacteriological skin samples. Brit J Dermatol 1978; 99: 537–43.

42 Hölzle E, Plewig G, Ledoller A. Corneocyte exfoliative cytology: A model to study normal and diseased stratum corneum. In: Marks R, Plewig G, eds. Skin models. Berlin: Springer Verlag; 1986: 181–90.

43 Taylor D, Whatling C, Kearney JN, Matthews B, Holland KT. The effect of bacterial products on human fibroblast and keratinocyte detachment. Br J Dermatol 1990; 122: 23–28.

44 Montes LF, McBride ME, Johnson WP, Owens DW, Knox JM. Ultrastructural study of host–bacteria relationship in erythrasma. J Bacteriol 1965; 90: 1489–92.

45 Jahn H, Nielsen EH, Elberg JJ, Bierring F, Ronne M, Brandrup F. Ultrastructure of psoriatic epidermis. APMIS 1988; 96: 723–31.

46 Marples RR, Heaton CL, Kligman AM. *Staphylococcus aureus* in psoriasis. Arch Dermatol 1973; 107: 568–70.

47 David TJ, Cambridge GC. Bacterial infection and atopic eczema. Arch Dis Child 1986; 61: 20–23.

48 White MI, Noble WC. *Staphylococcus aureus* in atopic dermatitis. Clin Exp Dermatol 1986; 11: 34–40.

49 Dahl MV. *Staphylococcus aureus* and atopic dermatitis. Arch Dermatol 1983; 119: 840–46.

50 Kearney JN, Harnby D, Gowland G, Holland KT. Follicular distribution and abundance of resident bacteria on human skin. J Gen Microbiol 1984; 130: 797–801.

51 Leeming JP, Holland KT, Cunliffe WJ. The microbial ecology of pilosebaceous units isolated from human skin. J Gen Microbiol 1984; 130: 803–07.

52 Brown E, Wenzel RP, Hendley JO. Exploration of the microbial anatomy of normal skin by using plasmid profiles of coagulase negative staphylococci. J Infect Dis 1989; 160: 644–50.

53 Knutson D. Ultrastructural observations in acne vulgaris: the normal sebaceous follicle and acne lesions. J Invest Dermatol 1974; 62: 288–307.

54 Duncan WC. Bacterial folliculitis. In: Demis JD, ed. Clinical dermatology, vol 3 (16–5). Philadelphia: Lippincott; 1988: 1–3.

55 Bäck O, Faergemann J, Hörnqvist R. Pityrosporum folliculitis: a common disease of young and middle-age. J Am Acad Dermatol 1985; 12: 56–61.

56 Fulton JE, McGinley K, Leyden JJ, Marples R. Gram negative folliculitis, recognition and treatment. Arch Dermatol 1968; 98: 349–53.

57 Duncan WC, McBride ME, Knox JM. Experimentally induced cutaneous infections in man. In: Maibach HI, Aly R, eds. Skin microbiology relevance to clinical infection. New York: Springer-Verlag; 1981: 220–30.

58 Hill MK, Goodfield MJD, Rodgers FG, Crowley JL, Saihan EM. Skin surface electron microscopy in *Pityrosporum* folliculitis. Arch Dermatol 1990; 126: 1071–74.

59 Williams M, Cunliffe WJ, Gould D. Pilosebaceous duct physiology: I effect of hydration on pilo-sebaceous duct orifice. Br J Dermatol 1974; 90: 631–35.

60 Ratnam S, Hogan K, March SB, Butler RW. Whirlpool-associated folliculitis caused by *Pseudomonas aeruginosa*: report of an outbreak and review. J Clin Microbiol 1986; 23: 655–59.

61 Bibel DJ, Lovell DJ. Skin flora maps: a tool in the study of cutaneous ecology. J Invest Dermatol 1976; 66: 265–69.

62 McGinley KJ, Webster G, Ruggieri MR, Leyden JJ. Regional variations in density of cutaneous propionibacteria: correlation of *Propionibacterium acnes* populations with sebaceous secretion. J Clin Microbiol 1980; 12: 672–75.

63 Leyden JJ, McGinley KJ, Nordstrom KM, Webster GF. Skin microflora. J Invest Dermatol 1987; 88 (Suppl 3): 65–72.

64 Jackman PJH, Noble WC. Normal axillary microflora in various populations. Clin Exp Dermatol 1983; 8: 259–68.

65 Noble WC, Hope YM, Midgley G, Moore MK, Patel S, Virani Z, Lison E. Toe webs as a source of gram negative bacilli. J Hosp Infect 1986; 8: 248–56.

66 Kates SG, Nordstrom KM, McGinley KJ, Leyden JJ. Microbial ecology of interdigital infections of toe web spaces. J Am Acad Dermatol 1990; 22: 578–82.

67 Shuster S. The aetiology of dandruff and the mode of action of therapeutic agents. Brit J Dermatol 1984; 111: 235–42.

68 Marchionini A, Pascher G, Röckl H. Der pH-wert der Hautoberfläche und seine bedeutung im rahmen der Bakterienabwehr. New York: Excerpta Medica; 1963: 396–402.

69 Anderson DS. Acid–base balance of the skin. Br J Dermatol 1951; 63: 283–96.

70 Arbenz H. Untersuchungen uber die pH-luerte der normalen Hautoberfläche. Dermatologica 1952; 105: 333–42.

71 Beare JM, Cheeseman EA, Gailey AAH, Neill DW, Merrett JD. The effect of age on the pH of the skin surface in the first week of life. Br J Dermatol 1960; 72: 62–66.

72 Behrendt H, Green M. Patterns of skin pH from birth through adolescence. Springfield, IL: Thomas; 1971.

73 Sato K, Kang WH, Jaga K, Sato T. Biology of sweat glands and their disorders: I normal sweat gland function. J Am Acad Dermatol 1989; 20: 537–63.

74 Usher B. Human sweat as culture medium for bacteria; preliminary report. Arch Dermatol Syphol 1928; 18: 276–80.

75 Marchionini A, Hausknecht W. Saeuremantel der Haut und Bakterienabwehr Die regionaere Verschiedenheit der Wassenstaffionen-Konzentration der Hautaberfläeche. Klin Wochnschr 1938; 17: 663–66.

76 Noble WC. Observations on the surface flora of the skin and on skin pH. Br J Dermatol 1968; 80: 279–81.

77 Arnold L. Relationship between certain physico-chemical changes in the cornified layer and the endogenous bacterial flora of the skin. J Invest Dermatol 1942; 5: 207–23.

78 Korting HC, Kober M, Mueller M, Braun-Falco O. Influence of repeated washings with soap and synthetic detergents on pH and resident flora of the skin of forehead and forearm. Acta Dermatol Venereol Stockh 1987; 67: 41–47.

79 Korting HC, Hübner K, Greiner K, Hamm G, Braun-Falco O. Differences in skin pH and bacterial microflora due to long-term application of synthetic detergent preparations of pH 5.5 and pH 7.0. Acta Dermatol Venereol Stockh 1990; 70: 429–57.

80 Williamson P, Kligman AM: A new method for the quantitative investigation of cutaneous bacteria. J Invest Dermatol 1965; 45: 498–503.

81 Bayer ME, Sloyer JL. The electrophoretic mobility of gram negative and gram positive bacteria. J Gen Microbiol 1990; 136: 867–74.

82 Richmond DV, Fisher DJ. The electrophoretic mobility of microorganisms. Adv Microbiol Physiol 1973; 9: 1–29.

83 Hartman AA. Effect of occlusion on resident flora skin moisture and skin pH. Arch Dermatol 1983; 275: 251–54.

84 Marples RR. The effect of hydration on bacterial flora of the skin. In: Maibach HI, Hildick-Smith G, eds. Skin bacteria and their role in infection. New York: McGraw-Hill; 1965: 33–42.

85 Aly R, Shirley C, Cunico B, Maibach H. Effect of prolonged occlusion on the

microbial flora, pH, carbon dioxide and transepidermal water loss on human skin. J Invest Dermatol 1978; 71: 378–81.

86 Marshall J, Leeming JP, Holland KT. The cutaneous microbiology of normal human feet. J Appl Bacteriol 1987; 62: 139–46.

87 Marshall J, Holland KT, Gribbon EM. A comparative study of the cutaneous microflora of normal feet with low and high levels of odour. J Appl Bacteriol 1988; 65: 61–68.

88 Newrick PG, O'Brien IAD, Smart A, Corrall RJM, Speller DCE. Impaired sweating in the diabetic neuropathic foot and its influence on skin flora. Diabetes Research 1989; 12: 173–76.

89 Nielsen PG. Skin pH on soles in patients with hereditary palmoplantar keratoderma and pathogenicity of dermatophytes. Mykosen 1985; 28: 310–12.

90 Meevootisom V, Niederpruem DJ. Control of exocellular proteases in dermatophytes and especially *Trichophyton rubrum*. Sabouraudia 1979; 17: 91–106.

91 Tsuboi R, Ko IJ, Takamori K, Ogawa H. Isolation of a keratinolytic proteinase from *Trichophyton mentagrophytes* with enzymatic activity at acidic pH. Infect Immun 1989; 57: 3479–88.

92 El-Maghrabi EA, Dixon DM, Burnett JW. Characterization of *Candida albicans* epidermolytic proteases and their role in yeast-cell adherence to keratinocytes. Clin Exp Dermatol 1990; 15: 183–91.

93 Todd JK, Todd BH, Franco-Buff A, Smith CM, Lawellin DW. Influence of focal growth conditions on the pathogenesis of toxic shock syndrome. J Infect Dis 1987; 155: 673–81.

94 Scheuplein RJ. Mechanisms of temperature regulation in the skin. In: Medicine. Fitzpatrick TB, Eisen AZ, Wolff K, Freedberg TM, Austen KF, eds. Dermatology in general medicine. New York: McGraw-Hill; 1987: 347–67.

95 Leithead CS, Linn AR. Heat stress and heat disorders. Philadelphia: FA Davies; 1964.

96 Benzinger TH. Peripheral cold reception and central warm reception, sensory mechanisms of behavior and autonomic thermostasis. In: Hardy JD, ed. Physiological and behavioral temperature regulation. Springfield, IL: Thomas; 1968: 831–55.

97 Hardy JD. Body temperature regulation. In: Mountcastle VB, ed. Medical physiology, vol 2. St Louis: CV Mosby; 1980: 1417–33.

98 Roddie IC. Circulation to skin and adipose tissue. In: Shepherd JT, Abboud FM, eds. Handbook of physiology, sec. 2, vol III. Bethesda, MD: American Physiological Society; 1983: 285–317.

99 Ladell WSS. Terrestrial animals in humid heat: Man. In: Dill, D. B., ed. Handbook of physiology. Sec. 4: adaptation to the environment. Washington, DC: American Physiological Society; 1964: 625–59.

100 Rippon JW. Medical mycology. 3rd ed. Philadelphia: WB Saunders; 1988: 304–05.

101 Somers HM, Good RL. Mycobacterium. In: Lennette EH, Balows A, Hausler WJ, Shadomy JH, eds. Manual of clinical microbiology. 4th ed. Bethesda, MD: Amer Soc Microbiol; 1985: 218.

102 McBride ME, Rudolph AH, Tschen JA, Brown BA, Wallace RJ, Cernoch P, Davis J. Diagnostic and therapeutic considerations for cutaneous *Mycobacterium haemophilum*. Arch Dermatol 1991; 127: 276.

103 Polla B. Heat (shock) and the skin. Dermatologica 1990; 180: 113–17.

104 Lindquist C, Craig EA. The heat shock proteins. Ann Rev Genet 1988; 22: 631–77.

105 Pelham H. Heat shock proteins: coming in from the cold. Nature 1988; 332: 776–77.

106 Young D, Lathigra R, Hendrix R, Sweetson D, Young R. Stress proteins are immune targets in leprosy and tuberculosis. Proc Natl Acad Sci USA 1988; 85: 4267–70.

107 Quoronfleh MW, Streips UN, Wilkinson BJ. Basic features of the staphylococcal heat shock response. Antonie van Leeuwenhoek 1990; 58: 79–86.

108 Blank IH. Factors which influence the water content of the stratum corneum. J Invest Dermatol 1952; 18: 433–40.

109 Middleton JD. The mechanism of water binding in the stratum corneum. Br J Dermatol 1968; 80: 437–50.

110 Grubauer G, Feingold KR, Harris RM, Elias PM. Lipid content and lipid type as determinants of the epidermal barrier. J Lipid Res 1989; 30: 89–96.

111 Grubauer G, Elias PM, Feingold KR. Transepidermal water loss: the signal for recovery of barrier structure and function. J Lipid Res 1989; 30: 323–33.

112 Elsner P, Maibach HI. The effect of prolonged drying on transepidermal water loss, capacitance and pH of human volar and forearm skin. Acta Dermatol Venereol Stockh 1990; 70: 105–09.

113 Willis I. The effects of prolonged water exposure on human skin. J Invest Dermatol 1973; 60: 166–71.

114 Bibel DJ, LeBrun JR. Changes in cutaneous flora after wet occlusion. Can J Microbiol 1975; 21: 496–500.

115 Duncan WC, McBride ME, Knox JM. Bacterial flora: the role of environmental factors. J Invest Dermatol 1969; 52: 479–84.

116 Stender IM, Blichman C, Serup J. Effects of oil and water baths on the hydration state of the epidermis. Clin Exper Dermatol 1990; 15: 206–09.

117 Pankurst R. The use of thermal baths in the treatment of skin disease in old time Ethiopia. Int J Dermatol 1990; 29: 451–56.

118 Sanderson PH, Sloper JC. Skin disease in the British Army in S.E. Asia: I influence of environment on skin disease. Br J Dermatol 1956; 65: 252–64.

119 Allen AM, Taplin D, Lowy JA. Skin infection in Vietnam. Military Med. 1972; 137: 295–301.

120 Hope YM, Clayton YM, Hay RJ, Noble WC, Elder-Smith JG. Foot infection in coal miners: a reassessment. Br J Dermatol 1985; 112: 405–13.

121 Davis JA, Leyden JJ, Grove GL, Rauner WJ. Comparison of disposable diaper with fluff absorbent and fluff plus absorbent polymers: effects on skin hydration, skin pH, and diaper dermatitis. Ped Dermatol 1989; 6: 102–08.

122 Sarkany I, Taplin D, Blank H. The etiology and treatment of erythrasma. J Invest Dermatol 1961; 37: 283–89.

123 Crissey JT, Rebell GC, Laskas JJ. Studies on the causative organism of trichomycosis axillaris. J Invest Dermatol 1952; 19: 187–97.

124 McBride ME, Freeman RG, Knox JM. The bacteriology of trichomycosis axillaris. Brit J Dermatol 1968; 80: 509–13.

125 Savin JA, Somerville DA, Noble WC. The bacterial flora of trichomycosis axillaris. J Med Microbiol 1970; 3: 352–56.

126 Shelley WB, Miller MA. Electron microscopy, histochemistry, and

microbiology of bacterial adhesion in trichomycosis axillaris. J Am Acad Dermatol 1984; 10: 1005–14.

127 White SW, Smith J. Trichomycosis pubis. Arch Dermatol 1979; 115: 444–45.

128 Daniel CR. Paronychia. Dermatologic Clinics 1985; 3: 461–64.

129 Farm G. Paronychia...an occupational disease. Contact Dermatol 1990, 22: 116–17.

130 Lapière M, Nusgens BV, Pierard GE. The architectural organization and function of the macromolecules in the dermis. In: Marks RM, Barton SP, Edwards C, eds. The physical nature of the skin. Boston: MTP Press; 1988: 163–76.

131 Marks RM. Mechanical properties of skin. In: Goldsmith LA, ed. Biochemistry and physiology of the skin. Oxford: Oxford University Press; 1983: 1237–53.

132 Cua AB, Wilhelm KP, Maibach HI. Elastic properties of human skin: relation to age, sex, and anatomical region. Arch Dermatol Res 1990; 282: 283–86.

133 Lévêque JL, Rasseneur L. Mechanical properties of stratum corneum: influence of water and lipids. In: Marks RM, Barton SP, Edwards C, eds. The physical nature of the skin. Boston; MTP Press; 1988: 155–61.

134 Somerville DA. A quantitative study of erythrasma lesions. Br J Dermatol 1972; 87: 130–37.

135 Zimmerer RE, Lawson KD, Calvert CJ. The effects of wearing diapers on skin. Ped Dermatol 1986; 3: 95–101.

136 Wimberley PD, Pedersen KG, Thode J, Fogh-Andersen N, Sorensen AM, Sigguurd-Anderson O. Transcutaneous and capillary pCO_2 and pO_2 measurements in healthy adults. Clin Chem 1983; 29: 1471–73.

137 Grønlund J. Evaluation of factors affecting relationship between transcutaneous pO_2 and probe temperature. J Appl Physiol 1985; 59: 1117–27.

138 Hansen TN, Sonoda Y, McIlroy M. Transfer of oxygen, nitrogen, and carbon dioxide through normal adult human skin. J Appl Physiol 1980; 49: 438–43.

139 King RD, Dillarou CL, Greenberg JH, Jeppsen JC, Jaeger JS. Identification of carbon dioxide as a dermatophyte inhibitory factor produced by *Candida albicans*. Can J Microbiol 1976; 22: 1725.

140 Evans CA, Mattern KL. The aerobic growth of *Propionibacterium acnes* in primary cultures from skin. J Invest Dermatol 1979; 72: 103–06.

141 Costerton JW, Cheny XJ, Greesey GG, Ladd TA, Nickel JC, Dasgupta M, Marrie T. Bacterial biofilms in nature and disease. Ann Rev Microbiol 1987; 41: 435–64.

142 Hamilton WA. Biofilms: Microbial interactions and metabolic activities. In: Fletcher M, Gray TRG, Jares JG, eds. Ecology of microbial communities. Cambridge: Cambridge University Press; 1987: 361–85.

143 Berardesca E, Maibach HI. Skin occlusion: treatment or drug-like device? Skin Pharmacol 1988; 1: 207–15.

144 Bibel DJ, Aly R, Shinefield HR. Importance of the keratinized epithelial cell in bacterial adherence. J Invest Dermatol 1982; 79: 250–53.

145 Cole GW, Silverberg NL. The adherence of *Staphylococcus aureus* to human corneocytes. Arch Dermatol 1986; 122: 166–69.

146 Kinsman OS. Attachment to the host as a preliminary to infection. Sem Dermatol 1982; 1: 127–36.

147 Rosenberg M, Kjellenberg S. Hydrophobic interactions: role in bacterial adhesion. Adv Microbiol Ecol 1986; 9: 353–93.

148 Kihn JC, Masy CL, Mestdagh MM. Yeast flocculation: competition between nonspecific repulsion and specific bonding in cell adhesion. Can J Microbiol 1988; 34: 773–78.

149 Mozes N, Leonard AJ, Rouxhet PG. On the relations between elemental surface composition of yeasts and bacteria and their charge and hydrophobicity. Biochim Biophys Acta 1988; 945: 324–34.

150 Klotz SA, Drutz DJ, Zajic JE. Factors governing adherence of Candida species to plastic surfaces. Infect Immun 1985; 50: 97–101.

151 Macura AB. Hydrophobicity of *Candida albicans* related to their adherence to mucosal epithelial cells. Zentrlbl Bakteriol Mikrobiol Hyg Serv A 1987; 266: 491–96.

152 Hazen BW, Hazen KC. Dynamic expression of cell surface hydrophobicity during initial yeast cell growth and before germ tube formation of *Candida albicans*. Infect Immun 1988; 56: 2521–25.

153 Klotz SA. Surface active properties of *Candida albicans*. Appl Environ Microbiol 1989; 55: 2119–22.

154 Klotz SA. A bioemulsifier produced by *Candida albicans* enhances yeast adherence to intestinal cells. J Infect Dis 1988; 158: 636–39.

155 Akit J, Cooper DG, Manninen KL, Zajic JE. Investigation of potential biosurfactant production among phytopathogenic corynebacteria and related soil microbes. Curr Microbiol 1981; 6: 145–50.

156 Rosenberg E, Gottlieb A, Rosenberg M. Inhibition of bacterial adherence to hydrocarbons and epithelial cells by emulsion. Infect Immun 1983; 39: 1024–28.

157 Pashley RM, McGuiggan PM, Ninham BW. Attractive forces between uncharged hydrophobic surfaces: Direct measurements in aqueous solutions. Science 1985; 229: 1088–89.

158 Israelachvili JN, McGuiggan PM. Forces between surfaces in liquids. 1988; 241: 795–800.

159 Swanson I, Kraus SJ, Gotschlich EC. Studies on gonococcus infection. I Pili and zones of adhesion: their relation to gonococcal growth patterns. J Exp Med 1971; 134: 886–906.

160 Nowicki B, Hölthofer H, Saraneva T, Rhen M, Väisänen-Rhen V, and Korhonen TK. Localization of adhesion sites for P-fimbriated and for 075X-positive *Escherichia coli* in the human kidney. Microb Pathog 1986; 1: 169–180.

161 Ravdonikas LE, Rye M, Grabovskaya KB, Totolian AA. Adherence to epithelial cells and ultrastructure of fosfomycin-resistant mutants of Group A streptococci. Folia Microbiol Praha [Czechoslovakia] 1988; 33: 513–19.

162 Aly R, Maibach HI. Survival of pathogenic organisms on human skin. J Invest Dermatol 1972; 58: 205–10.

163 Parrish JA, Rosen CF, Grange RW. Therapeutic uses of light. Ann NY Acad Science 1985; 453: 354–64.

164 Zelle MR, Hollaender A. Effects of radiation on bacteria. In: A. Hollaender, ed. Radiation biology. New York: McGraw-Hill; 1955: 365–400.

165 Sharp DG. The lethal action of short ultraviolet rays on several common pathogenic bacteria. J Bacteriol 1939; 37: 447–60.

166 Faergemann J, Larkö O. The effect of UV-light on human skin microorganisms. Acta Dermatol Venereol Stockh 1987; 67: 69–72.

167 Wikler JR, Janssen N, Bruynzeel DP, Nieboer C. The effect of UV-light on

Pityrosporum yeasts: ultrastructural changes and inhibition of growth. Acta Dermatol Venereol Stockh 1990; 70: 69–71.

168 Gerber D, Matthews-Roth M, Fahlund C, Hummel D, Rosnor B. Effect of frequent sun exposure on bacterial colonization of the skin. Int J Dermatol 1979; 18: 571–74.

169 Oginsky EL, Green GS, Griffith DG, Fowlks WL. Lethal photosensitization of bacteria with 8-methoxypsoralen to long wavelength ultraviolet radiation. J Bacteriol 1959; 78: 821–33.

170 Scherwitz C, Rassner G, Martin R. Effects of 8-methoxypsoralen plus 365 nm UVA light on *Candida albicans* cells. Arch Dermatol Res; 1978; 263: 47–58.

171 Fujita H, Suzuki K. Effect of near-UV light on *Escherichia coli* in the presence of 8-methoxypsoralen: wavelength dependency of killing induction of prophage, and mutation. J Bacteriol 1978; 135: 345–62.

172 Daniels F. A simple microbiological method for demonstrating phototoxic compounds. J Invest Dermatol 1965; 44: 259–62.

173 Mitchell JC. Cutaneous flora and microfloral phototoxicity. Contact Dermatitis. 1982; 8: 75–76.

174 Faergemann J, Larkö O. Phototoxicity of skin microorganisms tested with a new model. Arch Dermatol Res 1988; 280: 168–70.

175 Faergemann J, Larkö O. The phototoxic inhibitory effect and phototoxic killing effect of microorganisms. Photodermatology 1990; 7: 35–37.

176 Weissman A, Noble WC. Photochemotherapy of psoriasis: effects on bacteria and surface lipids in uninvolved skin. Br J Dermatol 1980; 102: 185–93.

177 Oberste-Lehn H, Plempel M. Zur Wirkung von. 8-Methoxypsoralen (8-MOP) und Blacklight auf Mikoorganismen *in vitro* und den Ablauf der experimentellen Meerschweinchen-Trichophytie. Dermatologica 1977; 154: 193–202.

178 Salo VO, Lassus A, Juvakoski T, Kanerva L, Lauwaranta J. Behandlung der Dermatitis atopica und der Dermatitis seborrhoica mit selecktiver UV-Phototherapie and PUVA. Dermatol Monatsschr 1983; 169: 371–75.

179 Mills OH, Kligman AM. Ultraviolet phototherapy and photochemotherapy of acne vulgaris. Arch Dermatol. 1978; 114: 221–23.

180 Parish JA, Strauss J, Fleming TS, Fitzpatrick TB. Oral methoxsalen photochemotherapy for acne vulgaris. Arch Dermatol 1978; 114: 1241–42.

181 Crowle AJ, Ross EJ. Comparative abilities of various metabolites of vitamin D to protect cultured human macrophages against tubercle bacilli. J Leuk Biol 1990; 47: 545–50.

4

Coryneform bacteria

J. J. LEYDEN & K. J. McGINLEY

Coryneform bacteria include both aerobic and anaerobic, non-acid fast, non-branching, pleomorphic, Gram-positive rods that do not form spores. Because of their similarity to the diphtheria bacillus, these organisms were formerly referred to as 'diphtheroids'. They are commonly arrayed in palisades giving the appearance of Chinese lettering; cells vary from short, coccobacilli to long, bacillary forms and may be rod-shaped or club-shaped. Coryneform is thus a designation of a large, ill-defined group of bacteria. The diverse genera that have been included with the coryneforms include *Actinomyces*, *Arachnia*, *Arcanobacterium*, *Arthobacter*, *Bacterionema*, *Bifidobacterium*, *Brevibacterium*, *Cellulomonas*, *Corynebacterium*, *Eyrsipelothrix*, *Eubacterium*, *Kurthia*, *Listeria*, *Mycobacterium*, *Nocardia*, *Oerskovia*, *Propionibacterium*, *Rhodococcus* and *Rothia*.[1,2]

Classification

In the past, coryneforms found on humans were assumed to belong to the genus 'corynebacterium'. Attempts were made to construct taxonomic classifications through the use of various biochemical tests. During the past 20 years, important advances in methods for classifying bacteria have been developed, many of which have been applied to coryneforms.[2-15] While this has led to clarification of their taxonomy, much further work is needed to establish agreed-upon species and their role in skin and systemic infections.

The early work of Somerville[16] provided a classification scheme based on a battery of biochemical tests as well as other properties such as fluorescence under ultraviolet light, lipid requirement (lipophilia) and lipolysis. Other schemes, such as those of Evans[17] and Marples[18], also used biochemical variables. In early studies of skin coryneforms, lipid dependency was a major feature of identification schemes.[19-21] More recently, McGinley and co-workers[22] found that a major attribute of many coryneforms on skin was a

102

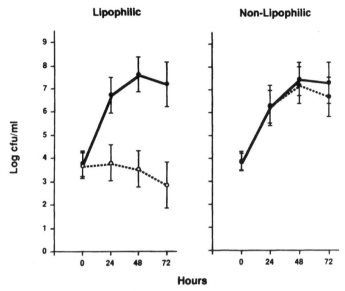

Fig. 4.1. Growth curves (cfu, colony-forming units) for aerobic coryneforms. Small-colony, lipophilic coryneforms demonstrate a lipid nutritional requirement for growth and expansion of an inoculum. Large-colony coryneforms do not require lipid for growth (after McGinley and coworkers[21]).

strict nutritional requirement for lipid (Fig. 4.1). Like Smith,[21] McGinley and colleagues found that all coryneforms which showed enhanced growth in the presence of lipid (lipolysis) were lipid dependent. Others, such as Somerville,[16] reported lipophilia for many cutaneous coryneforms but only rarely found lipid dependence. These differences may reflect variations in the media used by various investigators or the distinction between survival, proliferation and continued expansion of an inoculum on lipid-depleted media. Somerville,[16] for example, used solid media in which lipids were depleted by solvent extraction. Others used charcoal inactivation or solvent extraction of broth media.[19-22] McGinley and colleagues[22] determined growth curve characteristics over time (Fig. 4.1); Somerville used agar streak plates and determined the presence or absence of visible colonies. It is clear, however, that coryneforms found on skin can be divided into those whose growth is dependent on and enhanced by lipid and those whose growth is not. These were formerly referred to as 'lipophilic' and 'non-lipophilic diphtheroids' or small-colony and large-colony diphther-oids.[16, 18, 21, 23]

More recent identification of cell-wall components, including amino acids, sugars, fatty acids and mycolic acids, has been extremely useful for clarifying coryneform taxonomy. Furthermore, DNA base composition, the isoprenoid quinones and the cytochromes have been useful in defining genera. DNA–

DNA hybridization studies have been of value in indicating that organisms previously ascribed to different genera were similar enough to be a single species. Hybridization studies between DNA and rRNA have provided estimates of the more distant relationships between genera in view of the fact that genes which specify rRNA sequences have evolved more slowly than the overall genome. Most agree that cell-wall analysis is one of the most important criteria. In defining coryneform genera, Pitcher[14] studied more than a thousand isolates of coryneforms from human skin. He reported that about 60 per cent had cell-wall constituents consisting of *meso*-diaminopimelic acid (*meso*-DAP), arabinose as the major sugar, and mycolic acids with chain lengths of approximately 30 carbons. Twenty per cent had *meso*-DAP, galactose and no mycolic acids. The cell-wall characteristics of the former are now recognized to be that of *Corynebacterium* spp. while the latter is that of *Brevibacterium* spp.

The genus *Corynebacterium* is now characterized by the presence of *meso*-DAP, arabinogalactan in the cell wall, short-chain (C_{22}–C_{36}) mycolic acids, dihydrogenated menaquinones with eight or nine isoprene units or both, and a DNA base composition within the range of 51–63 mol per cent $G + C$. Other prominent features include straight to curved rods, sometimes showing club-shaped forms, a tendency to form palisades or Chinese characters formation, Gram positivity, metachromatic granules, non-motility and catalase-positivity.[24]

While substantial advances have been made in the taxonomy of this diverse group of organisms, much work is still required before clinical laboratories can routinely identify coryneform isolates.

Corynebacterium spp.

Corynebacterium diphtheriae is not an inhabitant of normal skin, though it may be recovered from intact skin under epidemic conditions. This organism is more commonly found on mucous membranes.[25–27] Strains of *C. diphtheriae* have been divided into gravis, intermedius and mitis types on the basis of physiological, morphological, and molecular characteristics. Its pathogenic properties depend on the ability to produce toxins.[24, 28]

Corynebacterium minutissimum is recognized as a valid species.[29] This organism is a non-lipid dependent, large-colony coryneform, which produces white and grey colonies. Other than the lack of lipid dependency, there is no characteristic that clearly distinguishes *C. minutissimum* from the lipid-dependent coryneforms found in human skin. This organism does not reduce nitrate, is urease negative, and does not digest gelatin. Production of acid from

Table 4.1. *Taxonomic characteristics of cutaneous aerobic coryneforms*

Characteristics	C. jeikeium	Group CD2	Group CLC	C. minutissimum	C. xerosis	B. epidermidis
DNA G+C (mol%)	59/61	ND	ND	56/59	55/59	63/64
Cell wall						
m-DAP	+	+	+	+	+	+
Arabinose	+	+	+	+	+	−
Mycolic acids	+	+	+	+	+	−
Fatty acids	S	S	S	S	S	B
Lipid requirement	+	+	+	−	−	−
Biochemical test						
Phosphatase	+	+	ND	+	−	ND
Gelatinase	−	−	−	−	−	+
Urease	−	+	−	−	−	+
Acid from						
Glucose	+	−	−	+	+	−
Galactose	+	−	−	ND	+	ND

S, straight chain; **B**, branched; ND, not done.

maltose is not seen with *C. minutissimum* and is variable for lipid-dependent coryneforms.

Corynebacterium xerosis is a recognized species found on human skin and grows as a large-colony coryneform. This organism is catalase positive, urease negative, reduces nitrate, ferments sugars and produces white-grey, pale yellow and tan colonies. It has short-chain mycolic acids and long-chain fatty acids.[3,4,24]

Cutaneous lipophilic corynebacteria (group CLC)

It has long been recognized that many cutaneous coryneforms isolated from human skin show enhanced growth on media supplemented with lipids. As described above, lipid dependency was a major feature of previous identification schemes for coryneform bacteria. McGinley and coworkers[22] suggested that lipid-dependent coryneforms may represent a single species (*C. lipophilicus*), based on cell-wall fatty acid, mycolic acid, a strict nutritional requirement for lipid, and negative responses to glucose and urea (our unpublished observations) (Table 4.1). Lipid-dependent coryneforms are major constituents of the cutaneous flora, particularly in the nose, axillae, perineum and foot. (Tables 4.2, 4.3). These coryneforms differ significantly from other species recovered from skin and perhaps deserve to be classified as a separate species.

C. jeikeium *CDC group JK*

In 1979, Riley and colleagues[30] from the Centers for Disease Control (CDC) characterized 95 coryneforms isolated from clinical specimens and reported multiple antibiotic resistance as a dominant characteristic. These coryneform bacteria came to be called group JK. These multiple-antibiotic resistant coryneforms have become recognized as important causes of systemic infection, particularly in immunocompromised individuals. The definition of multiple-antibiotic resistant coryneforms described by the CDC and called group JK has been officially accepted by the International Committee on Systematic Bacteriology as *Corynebacterium jeikeium*. Such organisms are catalase positive, produce acid from glucose, and are negative in a variety of biochemical tests in which other coryneforms produce positive reactions.[30,31] Antimicrobial resistance has been a key feature in identification and many surveys have used media with multiple antibiotics as the primary means of identification. However, there are other coryneforms that show multiple antibiotic resistance, such as group D2, which are biochemically distinct in that these are urease positive and do not produce acid from glucose. We have recently demonstrated multiple antibiotic resistance in cutaneous lipophilic

Table 4.2. *Prevalence and density of cutaneous lipophilic corynebacterium from 50 young healthy adults*

Site	Prevalence (%)	Density[a]
Scalp	27	4.62 ± 1.13
Forehead	16	4.21 ± 1.26
Nose	92	5.23 ± 1.07
Axilla	66	4.66 ± 1.48
Forearm	10	2.14 ± 1.14
Perineum	100	3.62 ± 1.87
Calf	15	3.62 ± 1.87
Toe interspace	98	6.22 ± 1.50

[a] Log mean and standard deviation when present: (1) per cm^2 (scalp, forehead, forearm, calf, axilla, perineum); (2) per 2-ml swab (nose, toe).

corynebacteria. The taxonomist defines *C. jeikeium* on the basis of a DNA base composition between 58–61 mol per cent $G + C$, mycolic acids of carbon length C_{32}–C_{36} and greater than 60 per cent homology of both DNA and cell-wall protein with National Collection of Type Cultures (NCTC) type strain NCTC 11913.[32] This definition includes a number of strains resistant to penicillin but susceptible to many other antimicrobial agents.[33] Thus, there currently is a nosological problem in that the clinical microbiologist and the taxonomist include some organisms in the 'JK' group that were not part of the initial clinical definition. McGowan[33] raises the spectre of having to distinguish 'JK' from 'JK-like' organisms in hospital cross-infection, as the organisms of clinical consequence seem to be those resistant to multiple antimicrobials. There clearly is need for a rapid, easily performed definitive test for identification of *C. jeikeium*. Towards that end, Moore and coworkers[34] have employed rocket and rocket–line immunoelectrophoresis and immunoblotting techniques. They demonstrated that rocket immunoelectrophoresis clearly distinguished *C. jeikeium* from other coryneforms and that immunoblotting was sufficiently sensitive to distinguish within *C. jeikeium* strains and thus serve as an epidemiological tool.

Pitcher and colleagues[35] analysed multiresistant *C. jeikeium* strains isolated over a 1-year period in a surgical unit with regard to their plasmid content and the use of rRNA to probe restriction fragment length polymorphism (RFLP). Seven of 12 strains showed similar RFLP profiles, consistent with their being related epidemiologically. Kerry-Williams and Noble[36] reported that 23 of 39 *C. jeikeium* isolates had plasmids that were grouped according to restriction fragment patterns and concluded that the plasmid analysis provided strong

Table 4.3. *Prevalence (number) and density of lipid-dependent corynebacterium from 30 young healthy adult males*[a]

	Group CLC[b]		C. jeikeium		Group D2	
	Prevalence	Density	Prevalence	Density	Prevalence	Density
Anterior nares	9	5.38 ± 0.62	15	6.18 ± 0.92	0	0
Axilla	5	3.66 ± 1.94	7	4.40 ± 1.21	8	4.28 ± 1.49
Perineum	18	6.74 ± 1.36	5	6.65 ± 1.64	0	0
Toe interspace	18	7.53 ± 1.62	3	7.74 ± 2.70	0	0

[a] Log mean density and standard deviation when present: (1) per cm^2 (axilla, perineum); (2) per 2-ml swab (anterior nares, toe interspace).

[b] CLC, cutaneous lipophilic corynebacterium.

evidence for the strains having a common origin, thus suggesting person-to-person transmission. Another study that also used plasmid profiling concluded that patient-to-patient transmission did not occur,[37] as only 2 of 27 isolates from a cancer ward were found to harbour the same plasmid. Chromosomal analysis showed that prolonged colonization with a single strain occurred. Strains from two clusters of infection had distinctive patterns, making nosocomial transmission unlikely.

Studies have now shown that the prevalence of skin colonization with *C. jeikeium* is highest in patients with malignancies or other severely immuno-compromising disorders. Rates range from 40 to 82 per cent compared with 13 to 73 per cent in immunologically normal individuals.[31] As the perineum is the primary site of *C. jeikeium* colonization in most studies, it has been postulated that antibiotic-resistant strains may originate in the gastrointestinal tract and then spread to the skin.[31]

CDC corynebacteria group D2

Coryneform group D2, occasionally referred to as '*C. urealyticum*', is strongly positive for urease activity, does not produce acid from glucose and frequently is resistant to many antibiotics.[38] This organism thus resembles *C. jeikeium*, except for its urease activity and inability to acidify glucose. This organism has been associated primarily with urinary tract infections and, on occasion, with other infections such as pneumonitis. Like *C. jeikeium*, these organisms have been found to be highly resistant to multiple antibiotics but have been uniformly sensitive to vancomycin and the quinolones, and often are sensitive to erythromycin and tetracyclines.[39, 40]

Marples[18] reported that urease-positive coryneforms were occasionally recovered from the skin. In a recent survey of healthy individuals we found urease-positive, glucose-negative lipophilic coryneforms in the axilla in eight individuals but not in the anterior nares, perineum or toe-web space (see Table 4.3). Soriano[41] also reported recovery of group D2 from the skin of patients with urinary tract infection.

Corynebacterium amycolatum

As described by Collins and coworkers,[42] six coryneforms recovered from human skin demonstrated cell-wall arabinose and galactose, *meso*-DAP with a $G+C$ ratio of 61 mol per cent but no mycolic acids. These investigators proposed the species *C. amycolatum*, referring to the absence of cell-wall mycolic acids. How frequently and in what body areas this organism can be found on human skin will have to be determined.

Dermabacter hominis

Four strains isolated from the forearm of healthy adults were Gram-positive, non-spore forming, rod-shaped bacteria that had biochemical and chemical characteristics distinct from all taxa described to date. Cell-wall analysis showed *meso*-DAP and no mycolic acids. The principal menaquinone was MK-9, with MK-8 and MK-7 also present. These organisms were proposed as a new genus *Dermabacter*, and named *Dermabacter hominis*.[43]

Brevibacterium spp.

It is now recognized that some large-colony coryneforms isolated from skin, and formerly assumed to be *Corynebacterium* spp., differ in their cell-wall composition and DNA base-pair composition and belong to *Brevibacterium* spp. *Brevibacterium* strains have the following characteristics: catalase positive, DNAase, gelatinase, phosphatase, rod to coccus morphogenesis, sensitive to lysozyme, negative for starch hydrolysis, acid fastness, methyl red reaction, production of methanethiol from L-methionine, acetoin production, indole production, sulphatase, presence of *meso*-DAP, and absence of arabinose and cell-wall mycolic acids. *Brevibacterium epidermidis* has been suggested for the species found in human skin.[44]

Carriage of aerobic coryneforms on human skin

Pitcher,[14] in an extensive study of more than 1000 isolates of aerobic coryneforms from human skin, found that 60 per cent were *Corynebacterium* and 20 per cent were *Brevibacterium*. Using a modification of the scheme of Noble,[45] we have identified the species of coryneforms found on the skin of two cohorts of healthy individuals (Tables 4.2–4.4). Cutaneous lipophilic coryne-bacteria were found in the greatest frequency and number in the wet body areas such as the anterior nares, axilla, perineum and toe-web space. They were far less prevalent in the extremities, face and scalp. These organisms have a strict nutritional requirement for lipid (Fig. 4.1), and are glucose and urease negative. Their cell walls contain *meso*-DAP, arabinose and short-chain mycolic acids. *C. jeikeium*, glucose-positive, urease-negative, lipid-dependent coryneforms, were recovered from the anterior nares in 50 per cent of individuals, from the axilla in 23 per cent, from the perineum in 17 per cent and from the toe-web space in 10 per cent (Table 4.3). Only two of these strains were resistant to multiple antibiotics. In another study,[46] utilizing antibiotic resistance as a primary character, we found multiple-resistant coryneforms to be most prevalent on the perineum in a group of cancer patients (Table 4.5). It

Table 4.4. *Prevalence and density of non-lipid dependent coryneforms from 30 young healthy adult males*[a]

Site	C. minutissimum		C. xerosis		B. epidermidis	
	Prevalence	Density	Prevalence	Density	Prevalence	Density
Oily						
Scalp	7	3.62	0	0	0	0
Forehead	10	2.21	0	0	0	0
Cheek	7	1.59	0	0	0	0
Wet						
Anterior nares	27	6.12	7	2.39	0	0
Axilla	17	5.10	7	3.19	0	0
Perineum	63	7.36	47	6.66	40	6.28
Toe interspace	53	6.51	20	6.53	40	6.16

[a] Per cent prevalence and log mean density when present: (1) per cm^2 (scalp, forehead, cheek, axilla, perineum); (2) per 2-ml swab (anterior nares, toe interspace).

Table 4.5. *Isolation of* C. jeikeium

	Hospitalized patients (n = 43)		Healthy adults (n = 80)	
	Prevalence (%)	Density[a] (log_{10})	Prevalence (%)	Density (log_{10})
Nose	34.8	4.80	0	0
Axilla	48.8	4.67	0	0
Perineum	69.7	5.94	15.0	3.76
Toe interspace	67.4	5.95	6.3	4.27

[a] Density when found.
Based on Larson and coworkers.[46]

now appears that those strains may represent a variety of species with antibiotic resistance, that is, *C. jeikeium* and cutaneous lipophilic coryne-bacteria (Table 4.6).

CDC group D2 (lipid dependent, glucose negative, urease positive) were found in the axilla of 27 per cent of subjects but not on other body areas.

The common lipid-dependent coryneform is found in varying densities at various body sites (see Tables 4.2, 4.3). While the density of this organism might be thought to correlate with areas rich in sebaceous glands, the primary ecological factor seems to be the presence of water as the toe-web space, perineum and axilla have the highest levels of this organism even though they

Table 4.6. *Antibiotic-resistant lipid-dependent corynebacterium from 30 young healthy adult males*[a]

| | Group CLC | | C. jeikeium | | Group D2 | |
	Prevalence	Density	Prevalence	Density	Prevalence	Density
Anterior nares	0	0	1	7.32	0	0
Axilla	1	2.96	0	0	0	0
Perineum	11	3.70 ± 1.36	1	4.96	0	0
Toe interspace	6	7.71 ± 2.3	1	4.65	0	0

[a] Numerical prevalence, log mean density and standard deviation when present: (1) per cm^2 (axilla, perineum); (2) per 2-ml swab (anterior nares, toe interspace).

are not 'sebaceous-rich' areas. Presumably there is enough lipid available from the exfoliating, degrading portion of the stratum corneum.

Anaerobic coryneforms

Anaerobic coryneforms recovered from human skin fall into the genus *Propionibacterium* and include the species *P. acnes*, *P. granulosum* and *P. avidum*. Confusion as to the taxonomy of these bacteria dates back to the beginning of the century when the term 'Bacillus acnes'[47] was used. Subsequently, these bacteria were classified as corynebacterium until Johnson and Cummins[48] showed that the proper genus was *Propionibacterium*, on the basis of cell-wall composition, DNA–DNA homology and base-pair composition. Marples and McGinley[49] and Cummins[8] showed that *P. acnes* and *P. avidum* were each composed of two serotypes and that these serotypes were distinct with reference to cell-wall sugar and biochemical tests. The difference in serotype and species is also reflected in bacteriophage susceptibility.[50]

Anaerobic coryneforms from skin can be classified as *P. acnes* if they are catalase positive, produce indole and/or reduce nitrate, liquify gelatin, produce only a small zone of lysis in milk agar and are lysed by *P. acnes* phage (ATCC 29399B). *Propionibacterium granulosum* is catalase positive but negative for the other characters, while *P. avidum* is catalase positive, gelatinase positive, produces large zones of caseinolysis in milk agar, and is negative for the other tests (Table 4.7).[51]

Carriage of propionibacteria

Propionibacterium acnes is the most numerous anaerobic coryneform recovered from human skin (Table 4.8). In general, *P. acnes* is most prevalent,

Table 4.7. *Taxonomic characteristics of cutaneous propionibacteria*

Characteristics	P. acnes		P. avidum		P. granulosum
	Biovar I	Biovar II	Biovar I	Biovar II	
DNA, G+C mol%	57/60		62/63		62/64
DAP isomer	L-	L- or *meso*	L-	L- or *meso*	L-
Sugars	Galactose Glucose Mannose	Glucose Mannose	Galactose Glucose Mannose	Glucose Mannose	Galactose Mannose
Biochemical tests					
Catalase	+	+	+	+	+
Asculin hydrolysis	–	–	+	+	–
Indole production	+	+	–	–	–
Nitrate reductase	+	+	–	–	–
β-haemolysis	v	v	+	+	–
Gelatin liquefaction	+	+	++	++	–
Litmus milk agar	+	+	++	++	–
Fermentation of					
Glucose	+	+	+	+	+
Sorbitol	+	–	–	–	–
Sucrose	–	–	+	+	+
Maltose	–	–	+	+	+

v, variable.

Table 4.8. *Prevalence (per cent) and density of propionibacteria from 50 young healthy adults*[a]

Site	P. acnes		P. granulosum		P. avidum	
	Prevalence	Density	Prevalence	Density	Prevalence	Density
Scalp	100	5.34	29	4.25	0	0
Forehead	100	5.70	26	4.07	0	0
Ear	72	4.61	32	3.17	0	0
Alae nasi	100	5.95	85	4.86	9	4.14
Dry						
Arm	56	2.27	12	2.90	0	0
Leg	38	1.63	0	0	0	0
Wet						
Nares	79	4.48	18	3.36	26	4.07
Axilla	47	3.81	6	3.67	32	3.82
Perineum	62	3.89	9	3.65	44	3.41
Rectum	56	4.14	6	2.77	41	4.36

[a] Log mean when present: (1) per cm^2 (scalp, forehead, arm, leg, axilla, perineum); (2) per 2-ml swab (ear, nares, rectum); (3) per 0.1 mg of wet weight (alae nasi squeezings). Based on McGinley.[51]

Table 4.9. *Propionibacteria*[a] *in relation to age and sex*

Age (years)	n	Males	n	Females	p value
0–10	38	1.53 (0.21)	54	1.14 (0.17)	NS
11–20	42	2.02 (0.37)	44	1.88 (0.32)	NS
21–30	58	5.82 (0.20)	22	4.55 (0.49)	0.01
31–80	87	5.63 (0.18)	17	4.64 (0.51)	0.05

[a] Values derived from 362 subjects, expressed as log/per cm^2 and standard error of the mean.
From Leyden and colleagues.[52]

and found in the greatest numbers in body areas rich in sebaceous glands, while *P. avidum* is more common in areas rich in eccrine sweat glands.[51] Significant age-associated differences are seen in the number of *Propionibacterium* in areas rich in sebaceous glands (Table 4.9). Moreover, the density of *Propionibacterium* correlates well with the total amount of lipid excreted on to the skin surface. A direct correlation also exists between the amount of triglycerides and free fatty acids; the latter are hydrolysed by propionibacteria from sebaceous gland triglycerides.

There are significant variations in the density of propionibacteria for various body areas (Table 4.8). The highest numbers are found in areas richest in sebaceous glands but significant levels are also found in areas where sebaceous glands are relatively sparse.

References

1 Keddie RM. What do we mean by coryneform bacteria? In: Bousfield I, Callely A, eds. Coryneform bacteria. London: Academic Press; 1978: 1–12.
2 Goodfellow M, Minnikin DE. Introduction to the coryneform bacteria. In: Starr M, Stolp H, Truper H, Balows A, Schlegel H, eds. The prokaryotes: a handbook on habitats, isolation and identification of bacteria. Berlin: Springer-Verlag; 1981: 1811–26.
3 Athalye M, Noble WC, Mallet AI, Minnikin DE. Gas chromatography-mass spectrometry of mycolic acids as a tool in the identification of medically important coryneform bacteria. J Gen Microbiol 1984; 130: 513–19.
4 Athalye M, Noble WC, Minnikin DE. Analysis of cellular fatty acids by gas chromatography as a tool in the identification of medically important coryneform bacteria. J Appl Bacteriol 1985; 58: 507–12.
5 Collins MD, Goodfellow M, Minnikin DE. Fatty acid composition of some mycolic acid-containing coryneform bacteria. J Gen Microbiol 1982; 128: 2503–09.
6 Corina DL, Sesardic D. Profile analysis of total mycolic acids from skin corynebacteria and from named *Corynebacterium* strains by gas–liquid chromatography and gas–liquid chromatography/mass spectrometry. J Gen Microbiol 1980; 116: 61–68.
7 Crombach WHU. DNA base ratios and DNA hybridization studies of coryneform bacteria, mycobacteria and nocardiae. In: Bousfield I, Callely A, eds. Coryneform bacteria. London: Academic Press; 1978: 161–79.
8 Cummins CS. Identification of *Propionibacterium acnes* and related organisms by precipitin tests with trichloroacetic acid extracts. J Clin Microbiol 1975; 2: 104–10.
9 Grasmick AE, Bruckner DA. Comparison of rapid identification method and conventional substrates for identification of *Corynebacterium* group JK isolates. J Clin Microbiol 1987; 25: 1111–12.
10 Gross CS, Ferguson DA, Cummins CS. Electrophoretic protein patterns and enzyme mobilities in anaerobic coryneforms. Appl Environ Microbiol 1978; 35: 1102–09.
11 Jackman PJH. Classification of *Corynebacterium* species from axillary skin by numerical analysis of electrophoretic protein patterns. J Med Microbiol 1982; 15: 485–92.
12 Jackman PJH, Pelczynska S. Characterization of *Corynebacterium* group JK by whole-cell protein patterns. J Gen Microbiol 1986; 132: 1911–15.
13 Johnson JL, Cummins CS. Cell wall composition and deoxyribonucleic acid similarities among the anaerobic coryneforms, classical propionibacteria, and strains of *Arachnia propionica*. J Bacteriol 1972: 109: 1047–66.
14 Pitcher DG. Rapid identification of cell wall components as a guide to the classification of aerobic coryneform bacteria from human skin. J Med Microbiol 1977; 10: 439–45.

15 Pitcher DG. Aerobic cutaneous coryneforms: recent taxonomic findings. Br J Dermatol 1978; 98: 363–70.

16 Somerville DA. A taxonomic scheme for aerobic diphtheroids from human skin. J Med Microbiol 1973; 6: 215–24.

17 Evans NM. The classification of aerobic diphtheroids from human skin. Br J Dermatol 1968; 80: 81–83.

18 Marples RR. Diphtheroids of normal human skin. Br J Dermatol 1969; 81 (Suppl I): 47–54.

19 Ward MK. Effect of Tween 80 on certain strains of *C. diphtheriae*. Proc Soc Exp Biol Med 1948; 67: 527–28.

20 Pollock MR, Wainwright SD, Manson EED. The presence of oleic acid-requiring diphtheroids on human skin. J Pathol Bacteriol 1949; 61: 274–76.

21 Smith RF. Characterization of human cutaneous lipophilic diphtheroids. J Gen Microbiol 1969; 55: 433–43.

22 McGinley KJ, Labows JN, Zechman JM, Nordstrom KM, Webster GF, Leyden JJ. Analysis of cellular components, biochemical reactions, and habitat of human cutaneous lipophilic diphtheroids. J Invest Dermatol 1985; 85: 374–77.

23 Leyden JJ, Nordstrom KM, McGinley K. Cutaneous microbiology. In: Goldsmith L, ed. Biochemistry and physiology of the skin. Oxford: Oxford University Press; 1991. [In press].

24 Jones D, Collins MD. Irregular, nonsporing Gram-positive rods. In: Sneath P, Mair N, Sharpe M, eds. Bergey's manual of systematic bacteriology, vol. 2. Baltimore: Williams & Wilkins; 1986: 1261–310.

25 Belsey MA. Isolation of *Corynebacterium diphtheriae* in the environment of skin carriers. Am J Epidemiol 1970; 91: 294.

26 Belsey MA, LeBlanc DR. Skin infections and the epidemiology of diphtheria: acquisition and persistence of *C. diphtheriae* infection. Am J Epidemiol 1975; 102: 179–84.

27 Cockcroft WH, Boyko WJ, Allen DE. Cutaneous infection due to *Corynebacterium diphtheriae*. Can Med Assoc J 1973; 108: 329.

28 Coyle MB, Groman NB, Russell JQ, Harnisch JP, Rabin M. The molecular epidemiology of three biotypes of *Corynebacterium diphtheriae* in the Seattle outbreak, 1972–1982. J Infect Dis 1989; 159: 670–79.

29 Collins MD, Jones D. *Corynebacterium minutissimum* sp. nov., nom. rev. Int J Syst Bacteriol 1983: 33: 870–71.

30 Riley PS, Hollis DG, Utter GB, Weaver RE, Baker CN. Characterization and identification of 95 diphtheroid (group JK) cultures isolated from clinical specimens. J Clin Microbiol 1979; 9: 418–24.

31 McGinley KJ, Labows JN, Zechman JM, Nordstrom KM, Webster GF, Leyden JJ. Pathogenic JK group corynebacteria and their similarity to human cutaneous lipophilic diphtheroids. J Infect Dis 1985; 152: 801–06.

32 Jackman PJH, Pitcher DG, Pelczynska S, Borman P. Classification of corynebacteria associated with endocarditis (group JK) as *Corynebacterium jeikeium* sp. nov. Syst Appl Microbiol 1987; 9: 83–90.

33 McGowan JJ. JK coryneforms: a continuing problem for hospital infection control. J Hosp Infect 1988; 11 (Suppl A): 358–66.

34 Moore MK, Chaudhry S, Noble WC. Antigenic cross-reactivity among isolates of group JK corynebacteria. J Hosp Infect 1990; 16: 123–32.

35 Pitcher D, Johnson A, Allerberger F, Woodford N, George R. An

investigation of nosocomial infection with *Corynebacterium jeikeium* in surgical patients using a ribosomal RNA gene probe. Eur J Clin Micro Infect Dis 1990; 9: 643–48.

36 Kerry-Williams SM, Noble WC. Plasmids in group JK coryneform bacteria isolated in a single hospital. J Hyg 1986; 97: 255–63.

37 Khabbaz RF, Kaper JB, Moody MR, Schimpff SC, Tenney JH. Molecular epidemiology of group JK *Corynebacterium* on a cancer ward: lack of evidence for patient-to-patient transmission. J Infect Dis 1986; 154: 95–99.

38 Soriano F, Ponte C, Santamaria M, Castilla C, Fernandez-Roblas R. *In vitro* and *in vivo* study of stone formation by *Corynebacterium* group D2 (*Corynebacterium urealyticum*). J Clin Microbiol 1986; 23: 691–94.

39 Fosse T, Carles D, Laffont C, Lefebvre J, Boquet J. Infections urinaires a *Corynebacterium* du groupe D2: epidemie hospitaliere et sensibilite aux antibiotiques. Pathol Biol 1988; 36: 742–45.

40 Marty N, Clave D, Cancet B, Henry-Ferry S, Didier J. *Corynebacterium* groupe D2 etude clinique, identification biochimique et sensibilite aux antibiotiques. Pathol Biol 1988; 36: 460–64.

41 Soriano F, Ponte C, Santamaria M, Fernandez-Roblas R. Struvite crystal formation by *Corynebacterium* group D2 in human urine and its prevention by acetohydroxamic acid. Eur Urol 1987; 13: 271–73.

42 Collins MD, Burton RA, Jones D. *Corynebacterium amycolatum* sp. nov. a new mycolic acid-less *Corynebacterium* species from human skin. FEMS Microbiol Lett 1988; 49: 349–52.

43 Jones D, Collins MD. Taxonomic studies on some human cutaneous coryneform bacteria: description of *Dermabacter hominis* gen. nov., sp. nov. FEMS Microbiol Lett 1988; 51: 51–56.

44 Collins MD, Farrow JA, Goodfellow M, Minnikin DE. *Brevibacterium casei* sp. nov. and *Brevibacterium epidermidis* sp. nov. System Appl Microbiol 1983; 4: 388–95.

45 Noble WC. Microbiology of human skin. 2nd ed. London: Lloyd-Luke; 1981.

46 Larson EL, McGinley KJ, Leyden JJ, Cooley ME, Talbot GH. Skin colonization with antibiotic-resistant (JK group) and antibiotic-sensitive lipophilic diphtheroids in hospitalized and normal adults. J Infect Dis 1986; 153: 701–06.

47 Gilchrist TC. A bacteriological and microscopical study of over 300 vesicular and pustular lesions of the skin with a research upon the etiology of acne vulgaris. John Hopkins Hosp Rep 1900; 9: 409–30.

48 Johnson JL, Cummins CS. *Corynebacterium parvum*: a synonym for *Propionibacterium acnes*? J Gen Microbiol 1974; 80: 433–42.

49 Marples RR, McGinley KJ. *Corynebacterium acnes* and other anaerobic diphtheroids from human skin. J Med Microbiol 1974; 7: 349–61.

50 Webster GF, Cummins CS. The use of bacteriophage typing to differentiate *Propionibacterium acnes* types 1 and 11. J Clin Microbiol 1978; 7: 84–90.

51 McGinley KJ, Webster GF, Leyden JJ. Regional variations of cutaneous propionibacteria. Appl Environ Microbiol 1978; 35: 62–65.

52 Leyden JJ, McGinley KJ, Mills OH, Kligman AM. Age related changes in the resident bacterial flora of the human face. J Invest Dermatol 1975; 65: 379–81.

5

Coryneforms as pathogens

J. J. LEYDEN & K. J. McGINLEY

In Chapter 4 the evolving taxonomy of the coryneform bacteria was discussed, as well as their role as members of the resident skin flora. The excellent review of Coyle and Lipsky[1] discusses the coryneforms, particularly the multiple-antibiotic resistant *Corynebacterium jeikeium* and group D2, that have been associated with systemic infections and difficult to treat urinary tract infections. *Corynebacterium xerosis* has been identified as a cause of endocarditis, septicaemia and osteomyelitis. Likewise, *C. minutissimum* has been described as a cause of septicaemia and endocarditis.

In cutaneous infections, *C. diphtheriae* is clearly involved both as a primary pathogen as well as in secondary superinfection of other cutaneous infections such as syphilis and streptococcal pyoderma. There are several cutaneous lesions from which coryneforms can be recovered and in which they are seen as playing important pathophysiological roles. These include trichomycosis axillaris, erythrasma, interdigital toe-web space infections, acne and pitted keratolysis.

Trichomycosis axillaris

Trichomycosis axillaris commonly comprises waxy, nodular coatings on the axillary hair shafts of individuals with poor hygiene. Similar lesions can arise, but less frequently, in the pubic and beard areas. Not infrequently, the waxy nodules may be red, black or yellow and will fluoresce a variety of colours under Wood's ultraviolet light.

Crissey and coworkers[2] gave the name 'C. tenuis' to the coryneforms recovered from trichomycosis axillaris. They found a number of very different colonial morphologies with varying biochemical reactions among 31 isolates studied. Subsequent studies have shown that each nodule of trichomycosis axillaris contains at least four or five groups.[3-6] It is clear that the classification

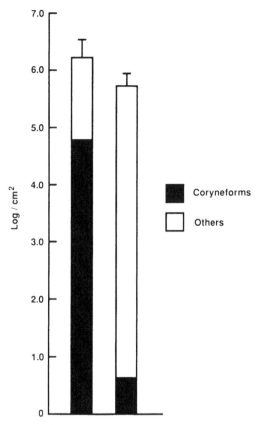

Fig. 5.1. Quantitative recovery of coryneforms in 81 subjects with intense axillary malodour (left column) and 124 subjects with absent or faint odour (right column) (after Leyden and colleagues[10]).

of the coryneforms involved in trichomycosis axillaris needs further study and that 'C. tenuis' is an invalid name that should no longer be used.

By scanning and transmission electron microscopy a continuous, irregular coating of the hair surface with bacteria is seen, the organisms being attached to neighbouring colonies by a thready material.[7] In general only the cuticular layers are involved, although the superficial portion of the cortex can be invaded in some cases; hair shafts are rarely damaged.[6,8] The origin of the waxy, amorphous material that coats the hair shaft and forms the distinctive nodules is unknown. Many have believed that the nodules are macrocolonies embedded in the mass of hair-shaft organisms. Levit[9] has proposed that the nodules are coryneform colonies that have become coated with dried apocrine sweat droplets. This theory is supported by the poor hygiene and lack of deodorant use that are commonly associated with trichomycosis axillaris – detergents physically remove coryneforms from the skin and hair, and most deodorants contain aluminium salts, which are active against coryneforms. Those who favour the theory that the nodules are embedded colonies of coryneforms are supported by the work of McBride and colleagues.[8] They found that only coryneforms isolated from affected hairs would grow on sterile hair that was inoculated in vitro. This, coupled with electron microscopic evidence of cuticular breakdown, suggests that under certain conditions the coryneforms produce keratinolytic enzymes that allow digestion of hair cuticles followed by a gradual accumulation of bacterial colonies.

Individuals with trichomycosis axillaris usually have offensive body odour. Axillary odour represents a mixture of volatile substances including fatty acids, isovaleric acid, the highly offensive steroid androstenedione and the recently identified 3-methyl-2-hexanoic acid, which is a product of bacterial action on apocrine sweat.[10, 11] Individuals with more intense, so-called apocrine odour, have an axillary flora with large numbers of aerobic coryneforms (Fig. 5.1). Seventy-five per cent of males and 25 per cent of females have heavy colonization by coryneforms, which correlates well with the finding that males have a greater tendency for axillary malodour.[12] It is not surprising that those with trichomycosis axillaris have a greater odour problem.

Trichomycosis axillaris can be simply treated by shaving or cutting infected hair shafts and instituting good hygiene practices. Topical antibiotics can be used where cutting or shaving of hair is undesirable.

Erythrasma

Erythrasma is a superficial cutaneous infection ranging from a low-grade scaling to thickly macerated areas of skin. This condition is primarily seen in intertriginous sites such as the axilla, crural areas, toe-web spaces and the submammary areas. (Table 5.1).[13–29] Most infections show a typical reddish fluorescence with Wood's light.

Sarkany and coworkers[21] isolated a coryneform from the lesions of erythrasma that could produce a red fluorescence in vitro similar to that seen in vivo. They named this coryneform *C. minutissimum*. The fluorescence is due to production of porphyrins, which fluoresce under long-wave ultraviolet light. Apparently only one colony type was characterized and sent to the National Collection of Type Cultures. Sarkany and colleagues[21] attempted experimentally to produce erythrasma by inoculating this organism under an occlusive dressing on the forearm of volunteers. A mild scaling with transient fluorescence resulted. No microbiological cultures were made from these experimental inoculations.

Table 5.1. *Incidence* (%) *of erythrasma*

No. examined	Axillae	Groins	Toe webs	Reference no.
Children				
410 (males)			17	(18)
22		5	5	(14)
Young adults				
25 (males)		36		(21)
109			23	(21)
55 (males)		9		(22)
363 (males)			18	(27)
108 (females)			6	(27)
514 (males)	3	3	16	(23)
240 (females)		2	16	(23)
Elderly adults				
308 (females)			10	(17)
Military personnel				
38 (males)			74	(16)
194 (males)			39	(16)
665 (recruits)			51	(26)
546 (discharged)			77	(26)
Institutionalized subjects				
609 (males)	5	20	29	(24)
265 (females)	1	15	41	(24)
Dermatology patients				
50 (males)	6	6		(14)
50 (females)	10			(14)
200		37		(28)
48 (males, fungus present)		25		(29)
34 (males, fungus present)		79		(29)
35 (males)	11	66	66	(19)
13 (females)	15	38	92	(19)
300			14	(13)
Coal miners				
443			4	(20)
Podiatric patients				
349			38	(15)
Diabetic subjects				
54 (males)	6	9	54	(25)
44 (females)	2	7	32	(25)
59			58	(20)

Subsequently, a number of investigators showed that fluorescent coryneforms are commonly found on normal skin. Somerville[23] cultured samples from the toe webs, axillae and perineum and found coryneforms in 42 per cent of sites. Hernandez[30] recovered *C. minutissimum* from the skin of more than a third of men with no evidence of infection, and Marples[31] found that more than 20 per cent of the normal skin flora contained fluorescent coryneforms. McBride and coworkers[32] used a series of biochemical tests in an attempt to classify 58 fluorescent coryneforms from normal skin, erythrasma and other skin lesions. Only two isolates from 25 cases of erythrasma gave identical biochemical reactions and less than half of the isolates from erythrasma gave biochemical reactions consistent with *C. minutissimum*. Somerville[33] proposed a scheme to divide fluorescent coryneforms into eight different biochemical groups. Different morphological and biochemical types of fluorescent coryneforms have been recovered from erythrasma. While there is general agreement that *C. minutissimum* plays a causative role in erythrasma, the possibility that other species are involved remains a probability. Furthermore, an important, unanswered question is: what are the factors responsible for transforming an organism frequently found on normal skin into a form that produces keratinolytic enzymes which superficially invade the stratum corneum?

Microscopically, long, thin filaments are seen in the scales recovered from erythrasma. Sarkany and colleagues[21] describe the organism in the scales as rod-like filaments with an average length of 4–7 μm, a width of 1 μm and an absence of branching. Similar appearances are seen by scanning electron microscopy. What is responsible for these morphological changes is unknown and until it is known, the pathophysiological background of erythrasma remains partially unresolved. Erythrasma may be associated with dermatophyte infection, though conflicting data have been presented. One important associated disease is diabetes mellitus.[34,35] Whether this association is the result of biochemical differences in the skin of diabetics or an impaired host response is not known. Obesity is a predisposing factor, presumably by providing larger amounts of semioccluded intertriginous areas. There also appears to be an increasing incidence with age.[23]

Erythrasma normally responds to a variety of topical or systemic antibacterial agents. Somerville and colleagues[23] also found that vigorous use of soap and water reduced the incidence of erythrasma.

Interdigital toe-web infections

Interdigital toe-web infections have been classified in the past as fungal infections, implying that dermatophytic fungi were solely responsible. How-

Table 5.2. *Coryneforms recovered from normal and macerated toe-web interspaces*[a]

Organisms	Normal (54 interspaces)		Macerated (100 interspaces)	
	Prevalence	Density	Prevalence	Density
Group CLC	100	6.5 (± 1.1)	91[b]	7.3 (± 1.0)[b]
C. jeikeium	35	4.2 (± 1.2)	58[b]	5.3 (± 1.7)[b]
B. epidermidis	39	6.0 (± 1.1)	54[b]	6.3 (± 1.5)
C. minutissimum	44	6.2 (± 1.0)	69[b]	6.7 (± 1.1)[b]
C. xerosis	6	7.0 (± 0.2)	8	6.4 (± 1.1)

[a] Per cent prevalence and log mean density when present.
[b] Statistically significant change; $p < 0.01$.
Source: Kates et al. 1990.[36]

ever, numerous and extensive studies by world authorities consistently report discrepancies between the recovery of dermatophytes and the clinical state of toe webs.[35] Fungi can be recovered from clinically normal toe spaces. Leyden and Kligman[36] proposed that interdigital toe-web infections begin with damage to the thick stratum corneum of the foot due to the keratinolytic effect of dermatophytic fungi and that subsequent overgrowth of bacteria, particularly coryneforms, produces a secondary, more symptomatic, process. The initial invasion by fungi produces superficial scaling and fissuring, and fungi can be readily recovered. Subsequent to the overgrowth of bacteria, maceration, leucokeratosis, malodour and intense symptoms develop. In some cases, overgrowth of Gram-negative bacteria, particularly *Pseudomonas* spp., results in a more severe infection. The initial scaling has been called dermatophytosis simplex while the severe infection is called dermatophytosis complex. In a more recent study,[35] a significant increase in numbers of *Brevibacterium epidermidis* and *C. minutissimum* was found in those with macerated toe-web interspaces (Table 5.2). Furthermore, there was an increase in *C. jeikeium* and a decrease in antibiotic-sensitive lipophilic coryneforms. Dermatophytes produce penicillin, which leads to ecological pressure favouring overgrowth of antibiotic-resistant coryneforms. Brevibacteria produce a variety of proteolytic enzymes, which further damage the interspace, as well as sulphur compounds, such as methanethiol, which inhibit fungi and produce malodour. The result of this ecological interaction is the transformation of a simple scaling process (dermatophytosis simplex), in which fungi are readily recovered, to a macerated, malodorous condition (dermatophytosis complex) in which fungi are recovered less frequently.

Pitted keratolysis

Pitted keratolysis is a superficial infection of the plantar surface of the foot in which small pits develop in the stratum corneum. These pits may remain discrete or coalesce to form large erosions. Most patients have associated hyperhidrosis and those with extensive erosions have considerable discomfort.

Microscopically, Gram-positive filaments and coryneform bacteria are found in the stratum corneum. Classification of these bacteria has resulted in a variety of identifications including *Dermatophilus congolensis* and *Corynebacterium* spp.[37,38] Taplin and Zaias reported reproducing pitted keratolysis by inoculating *Corynebacterium* strains on to human volunteers.[38] More recently, Nordstrom and coworkers[39,40] studied eight cases and cultured an organism identified as *Micrococcus sedentarius* on the basis of colonial morphology, micromorphology, biochemical reactions and chemical analysis of whole-cell components. *Micrococcus sedentarius* generates various thiols and thioesters that are volatile and malodorous. Patients with pitted keratolysis have severe problems with foot odour. Furthermore, pitted keratolysis was produced experimentally by applying *M. sedentarius* under occlusive dressings on the surface of the heel.

It thus appears that both unclassified *Corynebacterium* spp. and *M. sedentarius* are capable of inducing superficial pits and erosions on the foot surface. Topical antimicrobials are effective therapy.

C. diphtheriae infection

Infections due to *C. diphtheriae* may be primary, or secondary to cutaneous infections by other pathogens such as streptococci. Infection is more common in tropical and subtropical areas but epidemics have been described in temperate climates such as North America. Erosive, ulcerative lesions with thick crusts are the most common clinical findings. Over a 10-year period in Seattle, Harnisch and colleagues[41] followed diphtheria outbreaks in urban alcoholics, which were associated with poor hygiene, overcrowding, contaminated fomites, underlying skin disease, and streptococcal pyoderma. The incidence was highest in winter and spring. In an earlier report from the same group,[42] a 4-year outbreak of mainly pharyngeal cases was associated with peaks of cutaneous infection in which the majority of isolates were toxigenic. Like previous investigators,[43] they found that skin infections more frequently caused dissemination of *C. diphtheriae* than did pharyngeal infections.

Acne

Acne vulgaris is a multifactorial disease in which three areas of pathophysiological change involving sebaceous follicles have been identified. Sebaceous follicles produce puny hairs and have sebaceous glands that are much larger than those associated with terminal and vellus hair follicles. In acne there is (a) increased sebum production, (b) abnormal desquamation of follicular epithelium, which results in accumulation of large amounts of follicular corneocytes within the lumen of sebaceous follicles, and (c) proliferation of *Propionibacterium acnes* within the milieu of abnormally shed follicular cells, which leads to the production of chemoattractants and other inflammation-provoking substances.

Propionibacterium acnes was once referred to as the 'acne bacillus' or the sebobacillus by Sabouraud, who concluded that this organism played an important part in acne. Subsequently, this organism was found in the skin of young individuals who did not have acne and its role in acne was questioned. Moreover, *P. acnes* is recovered in large numbers from adults who are free of acne.[44] The paradox that a normal inhabitant of the skin can be involved in the pathogenesis of a disease seen primarily in teenagers and yet also be found in large numbers in adults free of the disease is as perplexing as why acne tends to undergo involution even in those who have never been treated. (Fig. 5.2). The answers to these questions may lie in age-associated changes in sebaceous follicles. With age, follicles tend to enlarge, and there appears to be a more substantial follicular stratum corneum (J. J. Leyden, unpublished). Conditions that may result in disease at one age may not do so at another if the microenvironment of the sebaceous follicles has changed sufficiently. Despite these paradoxes, there is agreement that antibiotic therapy, which results in a decrease of *P. acnes*, produces clinical benefit in that there is an improvement in the inflammatory lesions.

While the sequence and interaction of pathological events in acne are not entirely clear, there is agreement that the earliest pathological changes involve increased activity of sebaceous glands and abnormal desquamation of follicular epithelium, which accumulates in sebaceous follicles – the micro-comedo.[45,46] This microscopic, clinically inapparent lesion may evolve along one of two pathological pathways. If there is excessive accumulation of follicular horny material, this material becomes apparent as a small (2–3 mm) whitish impaction (closed comedo); then, as the impacted follicular material protrudes above the skin surface, it becomes visible as a 'blackhead', or open comedo. The black coloration is produced by interference with light transmission by the tightly compacted horny cells. Microcomedones, in which

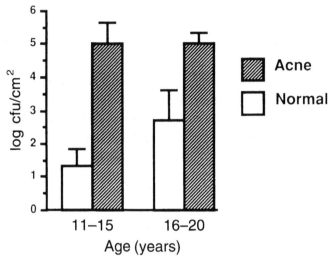

Fig. 5.2. Propionibacteria levels (cfu, colony-forming units) in teenage acne and normal subjects (after Leyden and colleagues[44]).

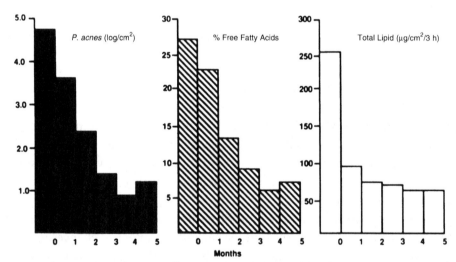

Fig. 5.3. Correlation of propionibacteria populations with sebaceous secretion during treatment with 13-*cis* retinoic acid (after Leyden and colleagues[50]).

P. acnes proliferates and generates inflammation-provoking substances, result in disruption of the follicular epithelium and progressive inflammation as the contents of the follicle are injected into the dermis. The factors responsible for determining which of the two pathways is followed in a given follicle remain to be uncovered. Follicles in which horny material accumulates and becomes clinically visible form a cocoon of horn around a central channel of sebum and *P. acnes*.[47] These follicles rarely develop into inflammatory lesions because *P. acnes* and its products are sloughed off from the dermis. Proliferation of *P. acnes* rapidly results in sufficient production of inflammation-provoking substances to produce clinical inflammation from microcomedones.

The evidence for the role of anaerobic coryneform bacteria, particularly *P. acnes*, includes the following:

1. Teenage acne patients have significantly higher densities of *P. acnes* on the skin than do age-matched controls.[48]
2. Successful suppression of *P. acnes* by systemic or topical antibiotics or 13-*cis* retinoic acid is accompanied by clinical improvement.[49,50]
3. *P. acnes* elaborates diffusible neutrophil chemotactic factors that are mostly of low molecular weight.[51,52]
4. *P. acnes* activates both the classical and the alternative pathways of complement[53-55] to produce C5-derived neutrophil chemotactic factors. Bound C3 has been reported in the tissue surrounding inflammatory acne lesions.[56,57] The activator of the alternate pathway has been identified as a cell-wall carbohydrate.[58]
5. Ingestion of *P. acnes* by neutrophils results in the release of extracellular lysosomal hydrolyases.[58] Similar release of lysosomal enzymes has been implicated in the tissue destruction in periodontal diseases and rheumatoid arthritis.
6. Intradermal injection of *P. acnes* is more inflammatory in acne patients than in controls.[59]
7. *P. acnes* antibody titres parallel the severity of inflammation in acne[60] and in vitro these titres modulate the magnitude of complement activation[54,55] and release lysosomal hydrolases.[61]
8. Patients with intensely inflammatory acne have elevated lymphocyte transformation indices to *P. acnes* antigens.[51,62]
9. *P. acnes* lipase activity on sebaceous gland triglycerides results in release of free fatty acids. Although the significance of free fatty acids has been questioned because of the minimal inflammation that develops after a single intradermal injection of amounts similar to those found in single sebaceous follicles,[63] repeated intradermal injection through ruptured follicles can reasonably be expected to contribute to the inflammatory response.
10. *P. acnes* may produce prostaglandin-like substances, which could enhance inflammation.[64]

The recent advances with 13-*cis* retinoic acid (isotretinoin) in the treatment of acne have been widely documented.[65,66] During isotretinoin therapy there are significant changes in both skin and mucous membranes, including a profound inhibition of sebum production, chapping and dryness, and resolution of the inflammation of acne.[67] Leyden and McGinley[50] showed, in a group of 10 patients treated with 1.0 mg/kg body weight/day isotretinoin, that the rates of sebum excretion were reduced by an average of 66 per cent in the first month of therapy (Fig. 5.3). Concurrently there was a fall in numbers of *P. acnes* from the pretreatment values of $10^4/cm^2$ to $10^3/cm^2$ after 1 month and to 10^2 after 5 months of therapy. On discontinuing therapy, the trend in the numbers of *P. acnes* was to recover to pretreatment levels within 2 months. As isotretinoin does not have inherent antibacterial activity, it has been concluded that the reduction in *P. acnes* is the result of decreased sebaceous gland production of lipid. Leyden and coworkers[67] further demonstrated that numbers of *P. acnes* on the face and on the trunk remained suppressed for 6 months after the discontinuation of therapy, despite the return of the rates of sebum excretion to a non-significant difference from pretreatment levels. Prolonged reduction may be an important factor in prolonged remission seen with isotretinoin therapy.

Systemic antibiotic therapy is beneficial and safe,[49] and most researchers agree that antibiotics work primarily by suppressing *P. acnes*.[68] One consequence of long-term antibiotic treatment in acne is the overgrowth of Gram-negative organisms[69, 70] in a small proportion of patients. Gram-negative bacteria overgrow in the nares, spill out on to the face, and produce pustules and nodules.

In addition to its role in acne, *P. acnes* is also a frequent opportunistic pathogen. Kaplan and Weinstein[71] reported its isolation from wound infections, osteomyelitis, and endocarditis. There are several reports of *P. acnes* meningitis,[72] and botryomycosis due to *P. acnes* has also been reported.[73] Perhaps the most significant infectious role for *P. acnes* is as a postneurosurgical pathogen.[74–77] The proximity of the scalp's reservoir of *P. acnes* to the site of incision doubtless is one source of contamination. The inability to sterilize the depths of the sebaceous follicle in preoperational preparations also prevents clearance of *P. acnes* from the site of the incision.

Coryneforms and systemic infection

C. jeikeium

First described by the Centers for Disease Control and called group JK, these aerobic coryneforms were characterized as resistant to multiple antibiotics and sensitive to vancomycin. Infections continue to be reported, mainly in patients who are immunocompromised, and particularly those with malignancies. Infections have been reported from around the world.[78–86] Newly reported clinical manifestations include pulmonary infiltrates,[87] septicaemia and cutaneous soft tissue infections in granulocytopenic patients,[81] and device-related nosocomial infection.[78, 82, 88–91]

Group D2

A case of pneumonia due to this urease-positive organism was first described in 1979,[92] but it was not until 1985 that the major pathogenic role of this organism was defined. In a series of papers,[93–96] this microorganism was associated with urinary tract infections, particularly in patients with a chronic inflammatory condition of the bladder known as alkaline encrusted cystitis. Group-D2 urinary tract infections may be hospital acquired.[93, 97] As this organism can be found on healthy skin of hospitalized patients,[98] it is possible that, after urological instrumentation, this organism gains access to the urinary tract.

There have also been a few reported non-urinary tract infections including peritonitis, endocarditis, pneumonia and bacteraemia.[92, 99–102]

C. minutissimum *and* C. xerosis

Corynebacterium minutissimum has been identified as the cause of breast abscesses,[103] bacteraemia[104] and endocarditis.[105] *Corynebacterium xerosis* has been associated with various infections of immunocompromised hosts, including endocarditis, arthritis and osteomyelitis.[106–109]

References

1 Coyle MB, Lipsky BA. Coryneform bacteria in infectious diseases: clinical and laboratory aspects. Clin Microbiol Rev 1990; 3: 227–46.
2 Crissey JT, Rebell GC, Laskas JJ. Studies on the causative organism of trichomycosis axillaris. J Invest Dermatol 1952; 19: 187–97.
3 Freeman RG, McBride ME, Knox JM. Pathogenesis of trichomycosis axillaris. Arch Dermatol 1969; 100: 90–95.
4 McBride ME, Freeman RG, Knox JM. The bacteriology of trichomycosis axillaris. Br J Dermatol 1968; 80: 509–13.
5 Savin JA, Somerville DA, Noble WC. The bacterial flora of trichomycosis axillaris. J Med Microbiol 1970; 3: 352–56.
6 Shelley WB, Miller MA. Electron microscopy, histochemistry, and microbiology of bacterial adhesion in trichomycosis axillaris. J Am Acad Dermatol 1984; 10: 1005–14.
7 Orfanos CE, Schloesser E, Mahrle G. Hair destroying growth of *Corynebacterium tenuis* in the so-called trichomycosis axillaris. Arch Dermatol 1971; 103: 632–39.
8 McBride ME, Freeman RG, Knox JM. Keratinophilic activity in species of *Corynebacterium*. Can J Microbiol 1970; 16: 1024–25.

9 Levit F. Trichomycosis axillaris: a different view. J Am Acad Dermatol 1988; 18: 778–79.

10 Leyden JJ, Zeng XN, McGinley KJ, Lawley HJ, Preti G. Characterization of pungent axillary odors. J Invest Dermatol 1990; 94: 549.

11 Labows J, Preti G, Hoelzle E, Leyden JJ. Steroid analysis of apocrine secretion. Steroids 1979; 34: 249–58.

12 Leyden JJ, McGinley KJ, Hoelzle E, Labows JN, Kligman AM. The microbiology of the human axilla and its relationship to axillary odor. J Invest Dermatol 1981; 77: 413–16.

13 Allen S, Christmas TI, McKinney W, Parr D, Oliver GF. The Auckland skin clinic tinea pedis and erythrasma study. N Z Med J 1990; 103: 391–93.

14 Burns RE, Greer JE, Mikhail G, Livingood CS. The significance of coral red fluorescence of the skin. Arch Dermatol 1967; 96: 436–40.

15 Henslee TM, Tanaka TJ, Hodson SB, Cann JE. Interdigital erythrasma. Part II: an incidence study. J Am Podiatr Med Assoc 1988; 78: 559–62.

16 Kooistra SA. Prophylaxis and control of erythrasma of the toewebs. J Invest Dermatol 1965; 45: 399–400.

17 Michalowski R, Rodziewicz H. Incidence of erythrasma in an elderly woman. Arch Dermatol 1965; 92: 396–97.

18 Munro-Ashman D, Wells RS, Clayton YM. Erythrasma in adolescence. Brit J Dermatol 1963; 75: 401–04.

19 Pitcher DG, Noble WC, Seville RH. Treatment of erythrasma with miconazole. Clin Exp Dermatol 1979; 4: 453–56.

20 Ruszczak Z, Bienias L, Proszyncka-Kuczynska W. Industrial dermatoses among the Bëthatöw brown coal miners. Med Pr 1981; 32: 365–69.

21 Sarkany I, Taplin D, Blank H. Erythrasma – common bacterial infection of the skin. J Am Med Assoc 1961; 177: 120–22.

22 Sarkany I, Taplin D, Blank H. Incidence and bacteriology of erythrasma. Arch Dermatol 1962; 85: 578–82.

23 Somerville DA. Erythrasma in normal young adults. J Med Microbiol 1970; 3: 57–64.

24 Somerville DA, Seville RH, Cunningham RC, Noble WC, Savin JA. Erythrasma in a hospital for the mentally subnormal. Br J Dermatol 1970; 82: 355–60.

25 Somerville DA, Lancaster-Smith M. The aerobic cutaneous microflora of diabetic subjects. Br J Dermatol 1973; 89: 395–400.

26 Svejgaard E, Christophersen J, Jelsdorf HM. Tinea pedis and erythrasma in Danish recruits. Clinical signs, prevalence, incidence, and correlation to atopy. J Am Acad Dermatol 1986; 14: 993–99.

27 Temple DE, Boardman CR. The incidence of erythrasma of the toewebs. Arch Dermatol 1962; 86: 518–19.

28 English MP, Turvey J. Studies in the epidemiology of tinea pedis. IX. Tinea pedis and erythrasma in new patients at a chiropody clinic. Brit Med J 1968; iv: 228–30.

29 Goto M. Ecological study of interdigital athlete's foot. Jpn J Dermatol 1970; 80: 130–42.

30 Hernandez A. Agents of dermatophytosis and other superficial mycoses. In: Mandell GL and Bennett JE, eds. Principles and practice of infectious diseases. 2nd ed. New York: Wiley Medical; 1985; 1493–98.

31 Marples RR. Diphtheroids of normal human skin. Br J Dermatol 1969; 81(Suppl I): 47–54.

32 McBride ME, Montes LF, Knox JM. The characterization of fluorescent skin diphtheroids. Can J Microbiol 1970; 16: 941–46.

33 Somerville DA. A taxonomic scheme for aerobic diphtheroids from human skin. J Med Microbiol 1973; 6: 215–24.

34 Montes LF, Dobson H, Dodge BG, Knowles WR. Erythrasma and diabetes mellitus. Arch Dermatol 1969; 99: 674–80.

35 Kates SG, Nordstrom KM, McGinley KJ, Leyden JJ. Microbial ecology of interdigital infections of toe web spaces. J Am Acad Dermatol 1990; 22: 578–82.

36 Leyden JJ, Kligman AM. Interdigital athlete's foot: the role of interaction of dermatophytes and the resident bacteria. Arch Dermatol 1978; 114: 1466–72.

37 Rubel LR. Pitted keratolysis and *Dermatophilus congolensis*. Arch Dermatol 1972; 105: 584–86.

38 Taplin D, Zaias N. Etiology of pitted keratolysis. In: Bergman Y, ed. Proceedings of the 13th International Congress of Dermatology. Princeton, NJ: Excerpta Medica; 1968: 593–95.

39 Nordstrom KM, McGinley KJ, Cappiello L, Leyden JJ. The etiology of the malodor associated with pitted keratolysis, abstracted. J Invest Dermatol 1986; 87: 159.

40 Nordstrom KM, McGinley KJ, Cappiello L, Zechman JM, Leyden JJ. Pitted keratolysis: the role of *Micrococcus sedentarius*. Arch Dermatol 1987; 23: 1320–25.

41 Harnisch JP, Tronca E, Nolan CM, Turck M, Holmes KK. Diphtheria among alcoholic urban adults. A decade of experience in Seattle. Ann Intern Med 1989; 111: 71–82.

42 Pedersen AHB, Spearman J, Tronca E, Bader M, Harnisch J. Diphtheria on Skid Road, Seattle, Washington, 1972–1975. Publ Health Reports 1977; 92: 336–42.

43 Belsey MA, LeBlanc DR. Skin infections and the epidemiology of diphtheria: acquisition and persistence of *C. diphtheriae* infection. Am J Epidemiol 1975; 102: 179–84.

44 Leyden JJ, McGinley KJ, Mills OH, Kligman AM. Age-related changes in the resident bacterial flora of the human face. J Invest Dermatol 1975; 65: 379–81.

45 Knutson DD. Ultrastructural observations in acne vulgaris: the normal sebaceous follicle and acne lesions. J Invest Dermatol 1974; 62: 288–307.

46 Leyden JJ, Shalita AR. Rational therapy for acne vulgaris: an update on topical treatment. J Amer Acad Dermatol 1986; 15: 907–16.

47 Plewig G, Kligman AM. Acne: morphogenesis and treatment. Berlin: Springer; 1975.

48 Leyden JJ, McGinley KJ, Mills OH, Kligman AM. *Propionibacterium* levels in patients with and without acne vulgaris. J Invest Dermatol 1975; 65: 382–84.

49 Leyden JJ. Systemic antibiotics for treating acne vulgaris: efficacy and safety. Arch Dermatol 1975; 111: 1630–36.

50 Leyden JJ, McGinley KJ. Effect of 13-*cis* retinoic acid on sebum production and *Propionibacterium acnes* in severe nodulo-cystic acne. Arch Dermatol Res 1982; 272: 331–37.

51 Puhvel SM, Sakamoto M. The chemoattractant properties of comedonal components. J Invest Dermatol 1978; 71: 324–29.

52 Webster GF, Leyden JJ. Characterization of serum independent polymorphonuclear leukocyte chemotactic factors produced by *Propionibacterium acnes*. Inflammation 1980; 4: 261–69.

53 Massey A, Mowbray JF, Noble WC. Complement activation by *Corynebacterium acnes*. Br J Dermatol 1978; 98: 583–84.

54 Webster GF, Leyden JJ, Norma ME, Nilsson UR. Complement activation in acne vulgaris: in vivo studies with *Propionibacterium acnes* and *Propionibacterium granulosum*. Infect Immun 1978; 22: 523–29.

55 Webster GF, Leyden JJ, Nilsson UR. Complement activation in acne vulgaris: consumption of complement of comedones. Infect Immun 1979; 261: 183–86.

56 Dahl M, McGibbon D. Complement in inflammatory acne vulgaris. Br Med J 1976; ii: 1383.

57 Dahl MGC, McGibbon DH. Complement C3 and immunoglobulin in inflammatory acne vulgaris. Br J Dermatol 1979; 101: 633–40.

58 Webster GF, Nilsson UR, McArthur WP. Activation of the alternative pathway of complement activation in human serum by *Propionibacterium acnes* (*Corynebacterium acnes*) cell fractions. Inflammation 1981; 5: 165–76.

59 Puhvel SM, Hoffman IK, Reisner RM, Sternberg TH. Dermal hypersensitivity of patients with acne vulgaris to *Corynebacterium acnes*. J Invest Dermatol 1967; 49: 154–58.

60 Puhvel SM, Barfatani M, Warnick M, Sternberg TH. Study of antibody levels to *Corynebacterium acnes*. Arch Dermatol 1964; 90: 421–27.

61 Webster GF, Leyden JJ, Tsai CG, Baehni P, McArthur WP. Polymorphonuclear leukocyte lysosomal release in response to *Propionibacterium acnes* in vitro and its enhancement by sera from inflammatory acne patients. J Invest Dermatol 1980; 74: 398–401.

62 Gowland G, Ward RM, Holland KT, Cunliffe WJ. Cellular immunity to *P. acnes* in the normal population and patients with acne vulgaris. Br J Dermatol 1978; 99: 43–49.

63 Puhvel SM, Sakamoto M. An in vivo evaluation of the inflammatory effect of purified comedonal components in human skin. J Invest Dermatol 1977; 69: 401–09.

64 Abrahamsson S, Hellgren L, Vincent J. Prostaglandin-like substances in *Propionibacterium acnes*. Experientia 1978; 34: 1446–67.

65 Peck GL, Olsen TG, Yoder FW, et al. Prolonged remission of cystic and conglobate acne with 13-*cis* retinoic acid. N Engl J Med 1979; 300: 329–33.

66 Farrell LN, Strauss JS, Stanieri AM. The treatment of severe cystic acne with 13-*cis* retinoic acid. J Am Acad Dermatol 1980; 3: 602–11.

67 Leyden JJ, McGinley KJ, Foglia AN. Qualitative and quantitative changes in cutaneous bacteria associated with systemic isotretinoin therapy for acne conglobata. J Invest Dermatol 1986; 86: 390–93.

68 Marples RR, Kligman AM. Ecological effects of oral antibiotics on the microflora of human skin. Arch Dermatol 1971; 103: 148–55.

69 Fulton JE, McGinley KJ, Leyden JJ, Marples RR. Gram negative folliculitis in acne vulgaris. Arch Dermatol 1968; 98: 349–53.

70 Leyden JJ, McGinley KJ, Mills OH, Kligman AM. Gram negative folliculitis, a complication of antibiotic therapy in acne vulgaris. Arch Dermatol 1973; 88: 533–40.

71 Kaplan K, Weinstein L. Diphtheroid infections of man. Ann Intern Med 1969; 70: 919–29.

72 Schlesinger JJ, Ross AL. *Propionibacterium acnes* meningitis in a previously normal adult. Arch Int Med 1977; 137: 921–23.

73 Schlossberg D, Keeney GE, Litton LJ, Azizhkab RG. Anaerobic botryomycosis. J Clin Microbiol 1980; 11: 184–85.

74 Beeler BA, Crowder JG, Smith JW, White A. *Propionibacterium acnes*: pathogen in central nervous system shunt infection. Am J Med 1976; 61: 935–38.

75 Everett ED, Eickhoff TC, Simon RH. Cerebrospinal fluid shunt infections with anaerobic diphtheroids (Propionibacterium spp.). J Neurosurg 1976; 44: 580–84.

76 French RS, Ziter FA, Spruance SL, Smith SB. Chronic meningitis caused by *Propionibacterium acnes*. Neurology 1974; 24: 624–28.

77 Skinner PR, Taylor AJ, Coakham H. Propionibacteria as a cause of shunt and postneurosurgical infections. J Clin Pathol 1978; 31: 1085–90.

78 Allen KD, Green HT. Infections due to a 'Group JK' corynebacterium. J Infect 1986; 13: 41–44.

79 Blom J, Heltberg O. The ultrastructure of antibiotic-susceptible and multi-resistant strains of group JK diphtheroid rods isolated from clinical specimens. Acta Pathol Microbiol Immunol Scand Sect B 1986; 94: 301–08.

80 Claeys G, Vershchraegen G, DeSmet L, Verdonk R, Claessens H. Corynebacterium JK (Johnson–Kay strain) infection of a Kuntscher-nailed tibial fracture. Clin Orthop Relat Res 1986; 202: 227–29.

81 Dan M, Somer I, Knobel B, Gutman R. Cutaneous manifestations of infection with *Corynebacterium* group JK. Rev Infect Dis 1988; 10: 1204–07.

82 Finger H, Wirsing von Koening CH, Wichmann S, Becker-Boost E, Drechsler HJ. Clinical significance of resistant corynebacteria group JK. Lancet 1983; i: 538.

83 Heltberg O, Friss-Moller A, Ersgaard H. Group JK diphtheroid bacteremia. Acta Pathol Microbiol Immunol Scand Sect B 1986; 94: 285–89.

84 Jackman PJH, Pelczynska S. Characterization of *Corynebacterium* group JK by whole-cell protein patterns. J Gen Microbiol 1986; 132: 1911–15.

85 Machka K, Balg H. In vitro activity of cipirofloxacin against group JK corynebacteria. Eur J Clin Microbiol 1984; 3: 375.

86 Telander B, Lerner R, Palmblad J, Ringertz O. *Corynebacterium* group JK in a hematological ward: infections, colonization and environmental contamination. Scand J Infect Dis 1988; 20: 55–61.

87 Waters BL. Pathology of culture-proven JK *Corynebacterium* pneumonia. Am J Clin Pathol 1989; 91: 616–19.

88 Etienne J, Barthelet M, Ninet J, Vandenesch F, Fleurette J. *Corynebacterium* group JK endocarditis after dental extraction under antibiotics. J Infect 1988; 17: 188–89.

89 Gilmour MN, Howell JA, Bibby BG. The classification of organisms termed Leptotrichia (Leptothrix) buccalis. Bacteriol Rev 1961; 25: 131–41.

90 Pierard D, Lauwers S, Mouton M, Sennesael J, Verbeelen D. Group JK corynebacterium peritonitis in a patient undergoing continuous ambulatory peritoneal dialysis. J Clin Microbiol 1983; 18: 1011–14.

91 Riebel W, Frantz N, Adelstein D, Spagnuolo PJ. *Corynebacterium* JK: a cause of nosocomial device-related infection. Rev Infect Dis 1986; 8: 42–49.

92 Jakobes NF, Perlino CA. 'Diphtheroid' pneumonia. South Med J 1979; 72: 475–76.

93 Aguado JM, Ponte C, Soriano F. Bacteriuria with a multiply resistant species of *Corynebacterium* (*Corynebacterium* group D2): an unnoticed cause of urinary tract infection. J Infect Dis 1987; 156: 144–50.

94 Bernheimer AW, Campbell BJ, Forrester LJ. Comparative toxinology of *Loxosceles reclusa* and *Corynebacterium pseudotuberculosis*. Science 1985; 228: 590–91.

95 Soriano F, Ponte C, Santamaria M, et al. *Corynebacterium* group D2 as a cause of alkaline-encrusted cystitis: report of four cases and characterization of the organisms. J Clin Microbiol 1985; 21: 788–92.

96 Soriano F, Ponte C, Santamaria M, Castilla C, Fernandez-Roblas R. In vitro and in vivo study of stone formation by *Corynebacterium* group D2 (*Corynebacterium urealyticum*). J Clin Microbiol 1986; 23: 691–94.

97 Fosse T, Carles D, Laffont C, Lefebvre J, Boquet J. Infections urinaires a *Corynebacterium* du groupe D2: epidemie hospitaliere et sensibilite aux antibiotiques. Pathol Biol 1988; 36: 742–45.

98 Soriano F, Rodriguez-Tudela JL, Fernandez-Roblas R, Aguado JM, Santamaria M. Skin colonization by *Corynebacterium* groups D2 and JK in hospitalized patients. J Clin Microbiol 1988; 26: 1878–80.

99 Van Bosterhaut B, Claeys G, Gigi J, Wauters G. Isolation of *Corynebacterium* group D2 from clinical specimens. Eur J Clin Microbiol 1987; 6: 418–19.

100 Langs JC, de Briel D. Endocardite a *Corynebacterium* du group D2, a point de depart urinaire. Med Malad Infect 1988; 5: 293–95.

101 Marshall RJ, Routh KR, MacGowan AP. *Corynebacterium* CDC group D-2 bacteraemia. J Clin Pathol 1987; 40: 813–14.

102 Marty N, Clave D, Cancet B, Henry-Ferry S, Didier J. *Corynebacterium* group D2 etude clinique, identification biochimique et sensibilite aux antibiotiques. Pathol Biol 1988; 36: 460–64.

103 Berger SA, Gorea A, Stadler J, Dan M, Zilberman M. Recurrent breast abscesses caused by *Corynebacterium minutissimum*. J Clin Microbiol 1984; 20: 1219–20.

104 Guarderas J, Karnad A, Alvarez S, Berk SL. *Corynebacterium minutissimum* bacteremia in a patient with chronic myeloid leukemia in blast crisis. Diagn Microbiol Infect Dis 1986; 5: 327–30.

105 Herschorn BJ, Brucker AJ. Embolic retinopathy due to *Corynebacterium minutissimum* endocarditis. Br J Ophthalmol 1985; 69: 29–31.

106 Lipsky BA, Goldberger AC, Tompkins LS, Plorde JJ. Infections caused by nondiphtheria corynebacteria. Rev Infect Dis 1982; 4: 1220–35.

107 Tarry DW, Carroll PJ. Summer mastitis: transmission by blood feeding flies. Vet Rec 1988; 123: 304.

108 Valenstein P, Klein A, Ballow C, Greene W. *Corynebacterium xerosis* septic arthritis. Am J Clin Pathol 1988; 89: 569–71.

109 Krish G, Beaver W, Sarubbi F, Verghese A. *Corynebacterium xerosis* as a cause of vertebral osteomyelitis. J Clin Microbiol 1989; 27: 2869–70.

6

Staphylococci on the skin

W. C. NOBLE

Taxonomy and typing

The revolution in staphylococcal taxonomy that followed the initial publications of W. E. Kloos and K-H. Schleifer (see below) has led to a much greater appreciation of the ecology of staphylococci on skin but has invalidated much earlier work. There are now 28 species and several subspecies of *Staphylococcus* (Table 6.1); subdivision within these species is possible on phenotypic or genotypic grounds and the chemistry underlying the taxonomy has been well explored.[1] The principal habitat of staphylococci is the skin and some mucous membranes of mammals and birds, though few birds and virtually no non-mammalian animals have been studied.[2]

Staphylococci are generally aerobic, Gram-positive cocci, which appear in irregular, so-called grape-like clusters under the microscope, although single and paired cells are the most common in fluid culture. They are catalase positive, have a mol per cent $G+C$ of 30–37, possess teichoic acid in the cell wall and have glycine in the interpeptide bridge of peptidoglycan, lack cytochromes c and d, and have MK6–8 as the major menaquinones. This serves to separate the staphylococci from micrococci with which they were formerly linked, as *Micrococcus* spp. have a mol per cent $G+C$ of 66–75, lack teichoic acid and glycine, possess cytochrome c and d, and have MK7(H2)–9(H2) as major quinones. *Micrococcus* and *Staphylococcus* are now regarded as very distinct genera.[3] The exceptions to aerobic growth are *S. aureus* var. *anaerobius*, a pathogen of sheep, and *S. saccharolyticus*, formerly *Peptococcus saccharolyticus*, a member of the normal human skin flora.

The basis of the current taxonomy was founded in 1975,[4] but, as much of the literature on staphylococci deals with the old taxonomies, a comment on these is not out of place. The title of S. T. Cowan's 1962 paper 'An introduction to chaos: or the classification of micrococci and staphylococci',[5] aptly described

Table 6.1. *Species of staphylococcus*

| Coagulase-positive species | Coagulase-negative species | |
	Principally of human origin	Principally of animal origin
S. aureus	*S. auricularis*	*S. caprae*
S. aureus var. *anaerobius*	*S. capitis* subssp. *capitis*	*S. carnosus*
S. delphini	*S. capitis* subssp. *ureolyticus*	*S. caseolyticus*
	S. epidermidis	*S. chromogenes*
S. hyicus[a]	*S. haemolyticus*	*S. felis*
S. intermedius	*S. hominis*	
	S. lugdunensis	
	S. saccharolyticus	*S. arlettae*[b]
	S. schleiferi	*S. equorum*[b]
	S. simulans	*S. gallinarum*[b]
	S. warneri	*S. kloosii*[b]
		S. lentus[b]
		S. sciuri[b]
	S. cohnii[b]	
	S. saprophyticus[b]	
	S. xylosus[b]	

[a] Coagulase-negative strains also occur.
[b] Novobiocin-resistant strains; these form a taxonomic group separated from the sensitive strains.

Table 6.2. *Correlation of the two classifications of the staphylococci*

Kloos and Schleifer	Baird-Parker/Marples	Agreement
S. aureus	SI	Very good
S. capitis	$SVI_3 + M3_3$	Moderate
S. cohnii	MX	Good
S. epidermidis	SII	Good
S. haemolyticus	SIV, SX, SVI, M1, M2, $M3_2$	Poor
S. hominis	SIV, SV, SVI, M1, M2, $M3_2$	Poor
S. intermedius	SI	Good[a]
S. saprophyticus	$M3_1$	Good
S. simulans	SIII, SIII maltose pos	Moderate
S. warneri	SIV, SV, SVI, M1, M2, $M3_2$	Poor
S. xylosus	M5, M6	Moderate

[a] Probably described as 'atypical *S. aureus*'.
Based on Marples.[8]

Table 6.3. *Comparison of sources of isolates identified as* S. saprophyticus (= *M3*) sensu *Baird-Parker*

Classification according to Kloos and Schleifer	Distribution (%)	
	114 strains of skin origin	72 strains of urinary tract origin
S. capitis	17.5	1.3
S. cohnii	42.0	8.6
S. haemolyticus	21.0	1.3
S. saprophyticus	12.0	76.6
S. warneri	7.0	13.0

Based on Namavar et al.[11]

the situation, but a partial, and for a decade eminently useful, classification was proposed by Baird-Parker.[6] This recognized three species, *S. aureus, S. epidermidis* and *S. saprophyticus*, each of the latter two species with four biotypes, and *Micrococcus*, also with four biotypes. *Staphylococcus epidermidis* biotype I and *S. saprophyticus* biotype III were then recognized as pathogens in catheter-associated infection and in the urinary tract, respectively. Various attempts to expand this classification, and to rectify the anomalies in it caused by a reliance on phenotypic tests, were then made.[7] Some biotypes designated as micrococci were recognized to belonging to the staphylococci. Chaos had been reduced but not eliminated. The publication of the Kloos and Schleifer scheme, based on extended phenotypic tests but later substantiated by DNA hybridization, began the evolution of the current taxonomy. An attempt at reconciling the schemes was made by Marples (Table 6.2).[8]

The initial studies on the new taxonomy[9, 10] redefined *S. epidermidis* and *S. saprophyticus*, and added descriptions of seven new species – *S. capitis, S. cohnii, S. haemolyticus, S. hominis, S. simulans, S. warneri* and *S. xylosus* – all inhabitants of normal human skin, with *S. aureus* as the only coagulase-positive species. This scheme shed light on some aspects of ecology: for example,[11] strains classified as *S. saprophyticus* in the Baird-Parker scheme had been isolated from the urinary tract but also from the skin of body and scalp. The Kloos and Schleifer scheme showed the predominance of their *S. saprophyticus* in the urine but of *S. cohnii* and *S. haemolyticus* on the skin and *S. capitis* on the scalp (Table 6.3).

New species then emerged from a consideration of habitat or pathogenic processes. Thus *S. auricularis* was identified in the human ear,[12] whilst *S.*

Table 6.4. *Host species preference in staphylococci of animal origin*

Species	Distribution (%)				
	Cattle	Goats	Pigs	Sheep	Poultry
S. chromogenes	12	1	17	0	5
S. epidermidis	29	1	0	0	2
S. gallinarum	0	0	0	0	11
S. hyicus	5	2	7	0	16
S. lentus	9	15	27	26	28
S. sciuri	3	42	22	60	9
S. xylosus	10	15	9	10	11
Other	32	24	18	4	18

Based on Devriese.[2]

Table 6.5. S. cohnii *subspp. on primate skin*

Host (Family)	Subspp.	Carriage (%)
Hominidiae (n = 40)	1	35
	2	15
Pongidae (n = 14)	2	64
Cercopithecoidea (n = 26)	2	62
New World Ceboidea (n = 16)	3	81

Based on Kloos and Wolfhohl.[22]

schleiferi and *S. lugdunensis* were found in bloodstream infections in man.[13] Attempts to discover a niche for *S. lugdunensis* on human skin have largely failed, though this remains the most probable location;[14] S. Eykyn and W. C. Noble (unpublished) have failed to find *S. lugdunensis* on the skin of 20 normal adults, although small numbers were found on the skin of newborn infants in a hospital. *S. saccharolyticus* was brought in from peptococcus and *S. caseolyticus* has been transferred from micrococcus.

Studies of animal skin flora have revealed a number of new species. *S. sciuri* and *S. lentus* were originally separated because they contained a unique cell-wall peptidoglycan.[15] Although not, in fact, confined to any one animal species, *S. caprae*, *S. chromogenes* and *S. felis* added in 1989,[16] *S. gallinarum* and *S. hyicus* do show habitat preferences (Table 6.4), whilst *S. arlettae*, *S. equorum*, *S. gallinarum*, *S. kloosii*, *S. lentus* and *S. sciuri* are, like their human-origin counterparts *S. cohnii*, *S. saprophyticus* and *S. xylosus*, novobiocin resistant.[17, 18]

The recognition of *S. aureus* as the only coagulase-positive species was also soon to be challenged, though different biovars of *S. aureus* inhabited cattle, humans and chickens. *Staphylococcus intermedius*, so called because it apparently lay between *S. aureus* and *S. epidermidis*, was recognized as an inhabitant and pathogen of dogs.[19] *S. hyicus* emerged as an inhabitant of pig and cattle skin and a pathogen of piglets,[20] whilst *S. delphini* was recovered from suppurative lesions of dolphins.[21]

There is good evidence that the species of staphylococcus have evolved together with their hosts. This is well illustrated for *S. cohnii*, where subspecies relating to humans and to Old and New World non-human primates can be distinguished (Table 6.5).[22]

A similar case can be made for divergence among the coagulase-positive species but we should be cautious that we do not overlook the possibilities of convergent evolution.[23] The chief characteristics by which we recognize the group of potential pathogens as similar – coagulase, heat-stable nuclease and possession of protein A – may be the result of selection for strains bearing these characteristics. It is worth noting that *S. aureus*, *S. intermedius* and *S. hyicus* have serologically different coagulases and nucleases.[24, 25] Protein A is found in the majority of *S. aureus* strains of human origin and in *S. hyicus* of porcine but not bovine origin, but the *S. hyicus* protein A has a different molecular weight and pI to that of *S. aureus*.[26-28] In *S. intermedius*, protein A is largely extracellular, only 4 per cent of strains producing bound protein A; in *S. aureus* of human origin, 90–95 per cent of strains produce both bound and free protein A but 50 per cent of methicillin-resistant strains produce only the extracellular form.

Subspecies recognition (typing) schemes are diverse and fairly unsatisfactory except for *S. aureus*. Typing of staphylococci has been extensively reviewed[29] and may be summarized as follows. Phage typing has proved an excellent tool for *S. aureus* of human origin, with about 70 per cent of strains typable with good discrimination. Phage sets are available for *S. aureus* of bovine and avian origin, and for *S. intermedius* and *S. hyicus*. Phage typing is less successful for the coagulase-negative staphylococci of human origin. Two sets of phages are available: those isolated by Pulverer and coworkers afford about 70 per cent typability but poor discrimination; those of Verhoef and coworkers exhibit lower levels of typability unless heat shocked but typically yield long patterns (lysis by six or more phages), making discrimination difficult.

For localized outbreaks of infection, plasmid profiles can be used. About 30 per cent of hospital strains of *S. aureus* lack plasmids but in coagulase-negative staphylococci, plasmids, especially cryptic plasmids, may be abundant (Fig. 6.1). DNA fingerprinting – the use of restriction enzymes to cut chromosomal

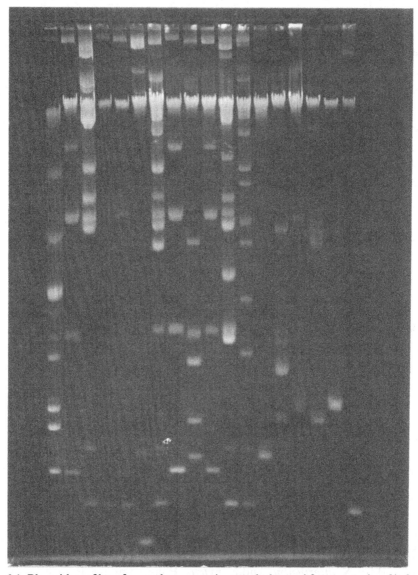

Fig. 6.1. Plasmid profiles of coagulase-negative staphylococci from a study of infection in continuous peritoneal dialysis patients.

DNA into fragments that can be resolved by electrophoresis – has limited applicability but has been used successfully in, for example, a study of methicillin-resistant *S. aureus*. Protein patterns derived by polyacrylamide gel electrophoresis of whole cell or membrane proteins will successfully separate strains to the species level and occasionally to the subspecies level.

For most epidemiological studies, especially on the coagulase-negative species, a combination of techniques is most successful. Ludlam and his colleagues,[30] in a study of skin colonization and infection of patients receiving continuous ambulatory peritoneal dialysis, found that using antibiograms gave 50 per cent discrimination with 98 per cent reproducibility; biotyping using the API STAPH system gave 26 per cent discrimination with 98 per cent reproducibility; phage typing gave 14 per cent discrimination with 100 per cent reproducibility; and plasmid profiles 48 per cent discrimination and 90 per cent reproducibility. A combination of antibiogram with plasmid profiling or with biotype plus phage each gave 95 per cent of the total discrimination possible.

Carriage

Carriage of S. aureus

The principal habitat for *S. aureus* in man is the anterior nares, with the axillae, groin and toe webs playing a lesser but still important role. The nasal carrier rate is about 30 per cent but care must be taken in interpreting rates that are higher or lower than this. Successive monthly random samples from a normal European population yielded carrier rates between 19 and 40 per cent (Table 6.6),[31] rates that technically are significantly different. There may, however, be genuine differences between different population groups. It has been suggested that nasal carriage of *S. aureus* is related to the HLA-DR type,[32] with DR3 linked to a predisposition to carriage, and DR1 and 2 linked to non-carriage. If this is so, we might expect differences between populations with differing antigenic structures. In populations of white and black children living in the same area of London, attending the same schools and having the same access to health facilities, nasal carriage was 41 per cent among 581 whites and 30 per cent among 607 blacks.[33] A family tendency to carriage has been observed in random sample studies of a population, even though the phage types recovered from different family members might differ, indicating that family carriage was not simply exposure to a common source within the home. In view of the known variance in random samples, twin studies have not assembled sufficient normals to be certain but it is agreed that identical twins have a more similar nasal flora than non-identical twins.[34, 35]

About 65 per cent of carriers in the anterior nares, the usual site of sampling, are also carriers on the turbinates and the posterior nasal space.[36] This no doubt accounts for the reappearance of an original domestic strain of *S. aureus* following temporary colonization with a 'hospital staphylococcus' as a result of inpatient exposure.[36] Other factors that affect carriage include local anatomy: 13 (65 per cent) of 20 nurses with changes due to local trauma to the nose or a deviated nasal septum were carriers compared with 55 (35 per cent) of 158 with normal nares.[37] Immune suppression (as in AIDS) is reported to

Table 6.6. *Monthly variation in carrier rate of* S. aureus *in normal respondents seen twice at an interval of 1 month*

Month	Seen first time			Seen second time		
	Total (*n*)	Carrier (%)		Total (*n*)	Carrier (%)	
		Nasal	Throat		Nasal	Throat
1964						
December	124	26	19	116	33	11
1965						
January	119	40	9	119	34	10
February	117	19	9	117	30	9
March	119	31	8	119	39	8
April	118	30	7	118	21	9
May	120	27	4	112	20	1

Taken, by kind permission of the Editor, from Noble et al.[31]

enhance nasal carrier rates, though these scarcely fall outside the limits of normal variation.[38] An immune response has been proposed to account for the loss or 'rejection' of *S. aureus* implanted in the nose.[39]

In a comparison of nasal *S. aureus* in normal individuals from 1964/65 and 1989 it was found that, although carrier rates had remained the same, there had been an increase in carriage of penicillin-resistant strains from 25 per cent to 70 per cent but that the plasmids mediating this resistance had not changed. Other relatively minor changes in antibiotic resistance pattern had also occurred: resistance to streptomycin had almost disappeared in 1989 but resistance to erythromycin and gentamicin had appeared; resistance to tetracycline had more than doubled in the 1989 sample. The balance of phage types had swung towards non-typable strains in 1989, principally away from phage group I strains (Table 6.7).[40]

Carriage in the axillae, groin and toe webs is reported at very different rates but is about 2 per cent resident carriage in the axilla with up to 7 per cent transient carriage.[41] Quantitative counts averaged about $10^4/cm^2$ in the axillae of 11 carriers over a 6-month period.[42] In the perineum or groin very diverse rates are recorded and this is due to the social difficulty in obtaining true perineal swabs. However, in skin sampling of 361 patients anaesthetized before surgery, 20 (6 per cent) appeared to carry resident and a further 25 (7 per cent) transient *S. aureus*, with no effect of age or sex.[41] Total carrier rates of about 15 per cent may therefore be expected.

Staphylococcus aureus is rare on normal skin but increasingly prevalent on

Table 6.7. *Percentage distribution of phage types of* S. aureus *in two normal populations*

Phage group	1964/65 ($n = 127$)	1989 ($n = 116$)
I	23	13
II	15.5	16.5
III	20	17
Miscellaneous	29	25
Non-typable	12.5	28

Based on Noble et al.[31] and Dancer and Noble.[59]

Table 6.8. *Skin carriage of* S. aureus *as a percentage of population studied*

Site	378 normal children	382 normal adults	98 adult diabetics[a]	46 eczema patients[b]
Forehead	6	ND	23	48
Nose	33	49	32	59
Cheek	8	ND	23	63
Chest	4	3	15	48
Axilla	1	ND	4	28
Periumbilicus	3	3	11	52
Forearm	2	3	10	63
Groin	3	6	7	41
Thigh	4	2	10	43
Shin	2	2	11	46
Toe web	1	5	5	48
Scapular area	2	2	9	46
Lumbar back	1	3	6	46

ND, not determined.
[a] All were controlled, insulin-requiring adults.
[b] The term eczema is here used loosely; if confined to patients with atopic dermatitis the rates would all have approached 100 per cent.
Based on Noble.[49]

individuals with an underlying disease such as diabetes or a skin disease such as eczema. Table 6.8 shows the results obtained by one group of workers using moistened swabs to sample an area of about 5×5 cm. If much larger areas or enrichment techniques had been used, the prevalence rates could have risen 10-fold.

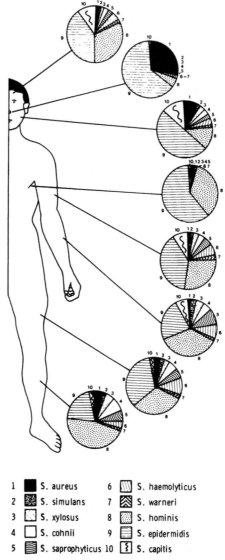

1	■	S. aureus	6		S. haemolyticus
2		S. simulans	7		S. warneri
3		S. xylosus	8		S. hominis
4		S. cohnii	9		S. epidermidis
5		S. saprophyticus	10		S. capitis

Fig. 6.2. Distribution of *Staphylococcus* spp. on different regions of the body. The mean percentages of species of total staphylococci are directly related to the shaded areas in the circles (taken, by kind permission, from Kloos and coworkers[60]).

Carriage of S. intermedius

With hindsight it seems probable that some, perhaps many, of the 'atypical' *S. aureus* occasionally recovered from carrier sites on man may strictly be species of animal origin such as *S. intermedius*. This is supported by evidence that 21 per cent of 62 human sera contained antibodies to the DNAase of *S. intermedius*, though none was positive for *S. hyicus*.[43] However, in a study of

Table 6.9. *Distribution of Staphylococcus spp. on the skin of normal adults*

Site	S. capitis	S. cohnii	S. epidermidis	S. haemolyticus	S. hominis	S. simulans	S. warneri	Other
Forehead	9.6	2.7	58.9	8.2	5.5	1.4	6.8	6.8
Nose	1.6	1.6	53.2	4.8	16.1	0.0	1.6	21
Axilla	2.0	3.9	43.1	15.7	15.7	0.0	9.8	9.8
Groin	0.0	3.6	29.7	21.4	19.0	1.2	11.9	13.1
Hip	8.2	4.9	22.9	16.4	18.0	3.3	9.8	16.4
Thigh	0.0	3.9	25.6	29.5	15.4	0.0	11.5	14.1
Toe web	4.0	1.3	30.6	13.3	8.0	13.3	10.7	10.7

Based on Marples.[46]

Table 6.10. *Isolation of* Staphylococcus *spp. from human skin in the USA and UK*

Species	Distribution (%)	
	USA	UK
S. aureus	4.6	4.4
S. capitis	4.2	10.3
S. cohnii	4.2	5.8
S. epidermidis	22.6	24.2
S. haemolyticus	11.8	10.6
S. hominis	26.9	37.5
S. saprophyticus	8.4	4.5
S. simulans	1.3	1.0
S. warneri	4.4	2.8
S. xylosus	9.9	0.0

USA: 843 isolates from Raleigh, NC and 148 from Somerville and New Brunswick, NJ.
UK: 397 isolates from east London.
Based on Kloos et al.[45]

Table 6.11. *Carriage of* Staphylococcus *spp. in relation to age*

Species	% of samples yielding species at age:			
	1 day	1 week	10–12 weeks	28–32 weeks
S. aureus	8	10	4	19
S. capitis	0	5	8	6
S. cohnii	4	10	1	4
S. epidermidis	60	80	83	90
S. haemolyticus	33	50	58	73
S. hominis	20	55	49	64
S. saprophyticus	0	0	11	8
S. simulans	0	9	4	13
S. warneri	4	4	14	5
S. xylosus	0	4	13	35

Based on Carr and Kloos.[48]

nasal carriage in veterinary college staff, only 1 of 144 persons sampled carried *S. intermedius*.[44] In skin infection in humans the organism is almost invariably typical *S. aureus*. This anomaly deserves further study.

Carriage of coagulase-negative staphylococci

The dominant species of staphyloccus on the skin is *S. epidermidis* on the face and thorax, with a lesser but still substantial role for *S. hominis*; these proportions are reversed on dry areas such as the arms and legs (Fig. 6.2).[45] More recent reports agree on the general picture but, by exploring different niches such as the toe webs or scalp, achieve slightly different distributions (Table 6.9).[46, 47] As always we should be wary of putting too much emphasis on the meaning of differences between reported studies, as these may simply reflect a geographical population difference. Studies carried out on apparently very similar populations of teenagers showed striking differences in the prevalence of *S. xylosus* and lesser differences in other species, but without altering the general pattern (Table 6.10).

The flora is built up at different rates from birth.[48] As might be anticipated, *S. epidermidis*, *S. haemolyticus* and *S. hominis* are acquired at an early stage, with the other species colonizing later (Table 6.11).

It has been suggested that organisms found on skin could be divided into three categories: 'transients', which do not multiply, 'temporary residents', contaminants that persist and multiply for a short time, and 'residents', the 'permanent' inhabitants of the skin.[49] This suggestion, an extension of Price's concept,[50] was made at a time when taxonomy of the staphylococci had not reached its present state and when typing methods for the coagulase-negative species were not available, although it could be validated for nasal *S. aureus*.[36] Because of the continuing general difficulty in readily typing large numbers of coagulase-negative staphylococci, there is relatively little information on the distribution of individual species or subspecies. However Marples[51] isolated the violagabriellae variant of *S. epidermidis* from the forehead eight times, axilla fifteen times, forearm five times, scalp once, toe webs once and anterior nares twice in 27 individuals studied. Viable counts in the axillae of 11 carriers had a mean of $3 \times 10^4/cm^2$, with a range from 8×10^2 to $2 \times 10^5/cm^2$; on the forehead the mean was 2×10^3 with a range from 3×10^0 to 4×10^4 in seven individuals. The organisms formed between 0.01 and 100 per cent of the total cocci at the sites sampled. One person sampled on three occasions yielded counts of 2600, 75800 and 790 (100, 45 and 15 per cent, respectively, of total cocci) and another 5300, 790, 290000 and 10500 (0.5, 0.6, 5.1 and 1.7 per cent of cocci). Similar studies on *S. saccharolyticus* showed that some persons carry this bacterium for long periods of time.[52] Three of 16 normal individuals studied carried *S. saccharolyticus* on the forehead over periods of at least 16, 27 and 38 months; one further person carried small numbers on one occasion only. It may be significant that the carriers were amongst those with the smallest populations of *Propionibacterium acnes*; there were no carriers of *S. saccharolyticus* amongst eight persons with *P. acnes* counts greater than $10^5/cm^2$ or the one with counts of 2×10^4 but three *S. saccharolyticus* carriers amongst the seven with *P. acnes* counts of 6×10^3 or less. *S. saccharolyticus* has also been isolated from the shoulders, back and forearm.

In a study of 17 individuals at an Antarctic base,[53] *S. capitis* was found to comprise 58 per cent of staphylococcal isolates from the scalp, and 6 of the 17 men carried their own individual clone of *S. capitis*, as determined by polyacrylamide gel electrophoresis and Western blotting, for most or all of the 42-week study, indicating that there are some essentially 'permanent' residents of the skin flora. Some individuals regularly carried a different clone on their chin to that on the scalp. In contrast, *S. haemolyticus*, *S. saprophyticus* and *S. warneri* were not recovered after the early stages of the study, suggesting that, at the sites sampled, these were temporary residents from reservoirs elsewhere.

Staphylococcus saprophyticus, *S. cohnii* and *S. xylosus* are found resident on the feet of both males and females. Before the age of puberty these species form about 5 per cent of the staphylococcal flora of the feet, with no evident difference between the sexes. At puberty the counts on females rise until they form about 45 per cent of the staphylococcal flora; in some individuals counts may rise to 90 per cent of the flora at levels of 1×10^6 colony-forming units/cm^2. The count on males remains low and rarely exceeds 5–6 per cent of the flora. In both sexes the principal species is *S. cohnii*. There is, however, an interesting change within these novobiocin-resistant staphylococcal species. Whilst the populations of *S. cohnii* remain appreciably constant after puberty, the populations of *S. saprophyticus* reach a peak at around puberty, forming about 13 per cent of the flora but declining thereafter, the counts approximately halving every 10 years until the age of 50 after which this species is rare. This corresponds well with the distribution of urinary tract infection due to *S. saprophyticus*. Whilst *S. xylosus* can be locally plentiful, it rarely exceeds $1 \times 10^4/cm^2$. As might be anticipated, there is great variation in the counts of staphylococci on the feet. The greatest numbers on healthy feet are around the toes, where counts exceed $1 \times 10^6/cm^2$, and the lowest counts are on the instep. In general, counts on males are about twice those on females.[54]

Dispersal of the skin flora

Dispersal or dissemination of the skin flora has not aroused much attention in recent years, despite its importance in postsurgical infection.[55-57] Dispersal of the skin flora takes place predominantly on skin scales or squames, and any member of the skin flora can be disseminated in this way.[57] Males disperse more than females and this is partly related to the slightly smaller squames that form the male skin and partly to the greater density of skin colonization. Males also disperse much more *S. aureus* than do females and, although perineal carriage is equal in the two sexes, males appear to shed more scales from the thigh and abdomen than do females,[58] so that dispersal of potential pathogens is related to the degree of skin contamination.

References

1 Schleifer KH, Kroppenstedt RM. Chemical and molecular classification of staphylococci. J Appl Bacteriol 1990; 69 (Symp Suppl): 9S–24S.

2 Devriese LA. Staphylococci in healthy and diseased animals. J Appl Bacteriol 1990; 69(Symp Suppl): 71S–80S.

3 Stackebrandt E, Woese CR. A phylogenetic dissection of the family Micrococcacae. Curr Microbiol 1979; 2: 317–22.

4 Kloos WE, Schleifer KH. Simplified scheme for routine identification of human *Staphylococcus* species. J Clin Microbiol 1975; 1: 82–88.

5 Cowan ST. An introduction to chaos: or the classification of micrococci and staphylococci. J Appl Bacteriol 1962; 25: 324–40.

6 Baird-Parker AC. The classification of staphylococci and micrococci from world-wide sources. J Gen Microbiol 1965; 37: 363–87.

7 Baird-Parker AC. The basis for the present classification of staphylococci and micrococci. Ann NY Acad Sci 1975; 236: 7–14.

8 Marples RR. Coagulase negative staphylococci – their classification and problems. In: Problems in the control of hospital infection. R Soc Med Int Cong Symp Ser 1980; No 23: 57–64.

9 Schleifer KH, Kloos WE. Isolation and characterization of staphylococci from human skin. I Amended description of *Staphylococcus epidermidis* and *Staphylococcus saprophyticus* and description of three new species: *Staphylococcus cohnii*, *Staphylococcus haemolyticus* and *Staphylococcus xylosus*. Int J System Bacteriol 1975; 25: 50–61.

10 Kloos WE, Schleifer KH. Isolation and characterization of staphylococci from human skin. II Description of four new species: *Staphylococcus warneri*, *Staphylococcus capitis*, *Staphylococcus hominis* and *Staphylococcus simulans*. Int J System Bacteriol 1975; 25: 62–79.

11 Namavar F. de Graaf J, McLaren DM. Taxonomy of coagulase negative staphylococci: a comparison of two widely used classification schemes. Antonie van Leeuwenhoek 1978; 44: 425–34.

12 Kloos WE, Schleifer KH. *Staphylococcus auricularis* sp.nov.: an inhabitant of the human external ear. Int J System Bacteriol 1983; 33: 9–14.

13 Freney J, Brun Y, Bes M, et al. *Staphylococcus lugdunensis* sp. nov. and *Staphylococcus schleiferi* sp.nov., two species from human clinical specimens. Int J System Bacteriol 1988; 38: 168–72.

14 Herchline TE, Ayers LW. Occurrence of *Staphylococcus lugdunensis* in consecutive clinical cultures and relationship of isolation to infection. J Clin Microbiol 1991; 29: 419–21.

15 Kloos WE, Schleifer KH, Smith RF. Characterization of *Staphylococcus sciuri* sp.nov. and its subspecies. Int J System Bacteriol 1976; 26: 22–37.

16 Igimi S, Kawamura S, Takahashi E, Mitsuoka T. *Staphylococcus felis*, a new species from clinical specimens from cats. Int J System Bacteriol 1989; 39: 373–77.

17 Schleifer KH, Kilpper-Balz R, Devriese LA. *Staphylococcus arlettae* sp.nov., *S. equorum* sp.nov. and *S. kloosii* sp.nov.: three new coagulase negative staphylococci from animals. System Appl Microbiol 1984; 5: 501–09.

18 Schleifer KH, Meyer SA, Rupprecht M. Relatedness among coagulase negative staphylococci: deoxyribonucleic acid reassociation and comparative immunological studies. Arch Microbiol 1979; 122: 93–101.

19 Hajek V. *Staphylococcus intermedius*, a new species isolated from animals. Int J System Bacteriol 1976; 26: 401–08.
Res 1977; 38: 787–92.

21 Varaldo PE, Kilpper-Balz R, Biavasco F, Satta G, Schleifer KH. *Staphylococcus delphini* sp.nov., a coagulase positive species isolated from dolphins. Int J System Bacteriol 1988; 38: 436–39.

22 Kloos WE, Wolfhohl JF. Deoxyribonucleotide sequence divergence between *Staphylococcus cohnii* sub species living on primate skin. Curr Microbiol 1983; 8: 115–21.

23 Noble WC. Systematics and the natural history of staphylococci. J Appl Bacteriol 1990; 69 (Symp Suppl): 39S–48S.

24 Igarashi H, Shingaki M, Ushida H, Fujikawa H, Terayama T. Immunological differentiation of coagulase produced by *Staphylococcus aureus*, *Staphylococcus intermedius* and *Staphylococcus hyicus* subsp. *hyicus*. Ann Rep Tokyo Met Res Lab Pub Hlth 1985; 36: 1–7.

25 Gudding R, Ness E. Identification of nuclease positive staphylococci isolated from animals. J Med Microbiol 1985; 20: 399–402.

26 Philips WE, Kloos WE. Identification of coagulase positive *Staphylococcus intermedius* and *Staphylococcus hyicus* subsp. *hyicus* isolates from veterinary clinical specimens. J Clin Microbiol 1981; 14: 671–73.

27 Muller HP, Schaeg W, Blobel H. Protein A activity of *Staphylococcus hyicus* in comparison to Protein A of *Staphylococcus aureus*. Zent Bakt 1981; 249A: 443–51.

28 Cox HU, Schmeer N, Newman SS. Protein A in *Staphylococcus intermedius* isolates from dogs and cats. Am J Vet Res 1986; 47: 1881–84.

29 Richardson JF, Noble WC, Marples RR. Species identification and epidemiological typing of the staphylococci. Soc Appl Bacteriol Microbial Identification Series; 1992: 193–219.

30 Ludlam HA, Noble WC, Marples RR, Phillips I. The evaluation of a typing scheme for coagulase negative staphylococci suitable for epidemiological studies. J Med Microbiol 1989; 30: 161–65.

31 Noble WC, Valkenburg HA, Wolters CHL. Carriage of *Staphylococcus aureus* in random samples of a normal population. J Hyg (Camb) 1967; 65: 567–73.

32 Kinsman OS, McKenna R, Noble WC. Association between histocompatibility antigens (HLA) and nasal carriage of *Staphylococcus aureus*. J Med Microbiol 1983; 16: 215–20.

33 Noble WC. Carriage of *Staphylococcus aureus* and beta haemolytic streptococci in relation to race. Acta Dermatovener (Stockh) 1974; 54: 403–05.

34 Hoeksma A, Winkler KC. The normal flora of the nose in twins. Acta Leidensia 1963; 32: 123–33.

35 Aly R, Maibach HI, Shinefield HR, Mandel AD. *Staphylococcus aureus* carriage in twins. Am J Dis Child 1974; 127: 486–88.

36 Noble WC, Williams REO, Jevons MP, Shooter RA. Some aspects of nasal carriage of staphylococci. J Clin Pathol 1964; 17: 79–83.

37 Jacobs SI, Williamson GM, Willis AT. Nasal abnormality and the carrier state of *Staphylococcus aureus*. J Clin Pathol 1961; 14: 519–21.

38 Ganesh R, Castle D, McGibbon D, Phillips I, Bradbeer C. Staphylococcal carriage and HIV infection. Lancet 1989; ii: 558.

39 Ehrenkranz NJ. Nasal rejection of experimentally inoculated *Staphylococcus aureus*: evidence for an immune reaction in man. J Immunol 1966; 96: 509–17.

40 Virani Z, Noble WC. Antibiotic resistance and plasmids in *Staphylococcus aureus* from normal populations. J Antimicrob Chemother 1992; 29: 35–39.

41 Polakoff S, Richards IDG, Parker MT, Lidwell OM. Nasal and skin carriage of *Staphylococcus aureus* by patients undergoing surgical operation. J Hyg (Camb) 1967; 65: 559–66.

42 Aly R, Maibach HI. Aerobic microbial flora of intertriginous skin. Appl Environ Microbiol 1977; 33: 97–100.

43 Hoie S, Fossum K. Antibodies to staphylococcal DNases in sera from different animal species, including humans. J Clin Microbiol 1989; 27: 2444–47.

44 Talan DA, Staatz D, Staatz A, Overturf GD. Frequency of *Staphylococcus intermedius* as nasopharyngeal flora. J Clin Microbiol 1989; 27: 2393.

45 Kloos WE, Schleifer KH, Noble WC. Estimation of character parameters in coagulase negative *Staphylococcus* species. In: Jeljaszewicz J, ed. Staphylococci and staphylococcal disease. Stuttgart: Fischer; 1976: 23–41.

46 Marples RR. The normal flora of different sites in the young adult. Curr Med Res Opin 1982; 7 (Suppl 2): 67–70.

47 Marples RR, Richardson JF, Newton FE. Staphylococci as part of the normal flora of human skin. J Appl Bacteriol 1990; 69 (Symp Suppl): 93S–99S.

48 Carr DL, Kloos WE. Temporal study of staphylococci and micrococci on normal infant skin. Appl Environ Microbiol 1977; 34: 673–80.

49 Noble WC. Microbiology of human skin. 2nd ed. London: Lloyd Luke; 1981.

50 Price PB. The bacteriology of normal skin: a new quantative test applied to a study of the bacterial flora and the disinfectant action of mechanical cleansing. J Infect Dis 1938; 63: 301–18.

51 Marples RR. Violagabrielle variant of *Staphylococcus epidermidis* on normal human skin. J Bacteriol 1969; 100: 47–50.

52 Evans CA, Mattern KL. Individual differences in the bacterial flora of the skin of the forehead: *Peptococcus saccharolyticus*. J Invest Dermatol 1978; 71: 152–53.

53 Maggs AF, Pennington TH. Temporal study of *Staphylococcus* species on the skin of human subjects in isolation and clonal analysis of *Staphylococcus capitis* by sodium dodecyl sulphate–polacrylamide gel electrophoresis. J Clin Microbiol 1989; 27: 2627–32.

54 Reuther J. Personal communication.

55 Lidwell OM. Sepsis after total hip or knee joint replacement in relation to airborne contamination. Phil Trans R Soc Lond 1983; 302: 583–92.

56 Tanner EI, Bullin J, Bullin CH, Gamble DR. An outbreak of post-operative sepsis due to a staphylococcal disperser. J Hyg (Camb) 1980; 85: 219–25.

57 Benediktsdottir E, Hambraeus A. Dispersal of non-sporeforming anaerobic bacteria from the skin. J Hyg (Camb) 1982; 88: 487–500.

58 Noble WC, Habbema JDF, van Furth R, Smith I, de Raay C. Quantitative studies on the dispersal of skin bacteria into the air. J Med Microbiol 1976; 9: 53–61.

59 Dancer SJ, Noble WC. Nasal axillary and perineal carriage of *Staphylococcus aureus* among antenatal women: identification of strains producing epidermolytic toxin. J Clin Pathol 1991; 44: 681–84.

60. Kloos WE, Musselwhite MS, Zimmerman RJ. A comparison of the distribution of *Staphylococcus* species on human and animal skin. In: Jeljaszewicz J, ed. Staphylococci and staphylococcal disease. Stuttgart: Fischer; 1976: 967.

7

Staphylococci as pathogens

W. C. NOBLE

In recent years there has been a much greater appreciation of the role of the normal skin flora in infection. The coagulase-negative staphylococci are now well-established pathogens in certain areas, whilst *Staphylococcus aureus* remains a potent pathogen, able to exhibit new antibiotic resistance patterns and to continue to infect the immunocompetent and -incompetent alike. In this chapter a brief consideration of the possible pathogenicity factors as they affect the skin will be followed by an examination of the epidemiology and aetiology of various staphylococcal infections of the skin and of the role of skin staphylococci in infection of other tissues.

With specific exceptions described below, the ability of *S. aureus* to cause infection seems to depend on the ability of the organism to produce a cocktail of enzymes or toxins that contribute to the final appearance of disease. In studies of a mouse model of infection with *S. aureus*, in which an outward sign of infection was skin necrosis due to the production of alpha toxin, it was found that strains known to produce massive amounts of alpha toxin in vitro might still prove avirulent for mice because they lacked other enzymes or toxins necessary to persist and metabolize in vivo.[1]

A list of potential pathogenicity or virulence factors is given in Table 7.1. A full description of the activity of each is beyond the scope of this chapter but this has been reviewed on several occasions.[2-4] Those that are thought to contribute directly to skin infection are described briefly below. A number of non-specific factors may also contribute to pathogenicity; these include capsules, which, by presenting a barrier between cell wall and serum, prevent efficient opsonization and hence phagocytosis. Coagulase may interfere with phagocytosis but also causes disseminated intravascular coagulation; lipase and hyaluronidase may be important in promoting the spread of staphylococci or their extracellular products in tissues.

Table 7.1. *Potential virulence factors in* S. aureus

Membrane-damaging toxins	Exoenzymes
Alpha toxin	Coagulase
Beta toxin	DNAase
Gamma toxin	Hyaluronidase
Delta toxin	Lipases
Leucocidin	Phosphatase
Epidermolytic toxins	Phospholipase
Toxic shock toxin	Proteases
Enterotoxins	Staphylokinase
Pyrogenic exotoxins	

Based on Arbuthnott and colleagues.[2]

Potential pathogenicity factors in *S. aureus*

Alpha toxin (alpha haemolysin)

Alpha toxin, which is produced by more than 90 per cent of *S. aureus* strains of human origin, is responsible for skin necrosis in experimental models because of its ability to damage blood vessels and paralyse muscle. It also impairs the response of leucocytes. Extensive dermonecrosis in rabbit or mouse skin may be due to its direct activity or to prolonged vasospasm because it increases vascular permeability. Antihistamines slow down the extravasation, suggesting that histamine and serotonin may play a part in the process. Alpha toxin may also directly affect nervous tissue and it may be that this was the cause of death in the Bundaberg disaster in which several children died after receiving vaccine contaminated with alpha toxin.[5] In experimental systems, weakly alpha-toxinogenic strains cause abscesses at the site of injection, grow relatively slowly and cause systemic infection only after 48 h. Strongly toxinogenic strains cause necrosis rather than abscess formation, grow well and invade swiftly.[2] Additional support for this role in vivo was seen in studies of mastitis in rabbits, a destructive and potentially fatal gangrenous infection that could be prevented by immunization with alphatoxoid.[6] Experimental skin infections in mice by *S. aureus* with allele replacement or transposon-inactivated alpha toxin genes showed that inactivated strains were much less virulent than intact strains, firmly establishing a role, at least in experimental systems, for alpha toxin in skin infection.[7]

Beta toxin (beta haemolysin)

Beta toxin, produced by about 10 per cent of *S. aureus* of human origin, is recognized as the hot/cold haemolysin on sheep red cells. It apparently lacks toxicity for rabbit skin, even though it is produced principally by staphylococci of animal origin.

Gamma toxin (gamma haemolysin)

Gamma toxin is a much less potent haemolysin than alpha toxin and is readily inhibited by lipids, including fatty acids. Like the other haemolysins it is lethal when injected in sufficient quantity in experimental animals.

Delta toxin (delta haemolysin)

The delta toxin gene is important because it forms part of a regulatory system for other staphylococcal toxins.[8] It is produced by more than 90 per cent of *S. aureus* of human origin and in vitro is most active as a haemolysin on horse and human erythrocytes, where it causes damage to cell membranes. Delta toxin is produced by a substantial number of coagulase-negative staphylococci, especially *S. epidermidis*, *S. saprophyticus* and *S. haemolyticus*.[9] In *S. epidermidis* the amino acid sequence of the delta toxin closely resembles that of *S. aureus*.[10] Injected into rabbit skin, delta toxin causes erythema or necrosis if very high doses are used; in human neonates, delta toxin from *S. epidermidis* has been associated with necrotizing enterocolitis.[11]

Panton–Valentine leucocidin

This is selectively toxic to polymorphonuclear leucocytes and macrophages, though other toxins that damage membranes may also act as non-specific leucocidins, and accordingly may have a role in staphylococcal disease. Panton–Valentine leucocidin is also dermonecrotic in rabbits, although antibody to the leucocidin is not protective in natural infection.

Enterotoxins

Enterotoxins are produced by many strains of *S. aureus* and by other coagulase-positive staphylococci;[12, 13] in *S. aureus* they are naturally associated with food poisoning.[14] However, Bergdoll reports that skin contact with enterotoxin in laboratory workers resulted in the development of a vesicular rash and subsequent desquamation resembling the effect of toxic shock toxin (which is also described as an enterotoxin). They are super-antigens.

Toxic shock syndrome toxin (TSST)

This toxin has been extensively investigated, cloned and sequenced. The disease was originally described in 1978 but came to prominence in 1980 when large numbers of cases were reported in menstruating women. The disease is characterized by fever, headache and confusion, with an erythematous rash resembling scarlet fever and desquamation in the later stages. The symptoms were also usually accompanied by diarrhoea, vomiting and hypotensive shock. TSST-1 is produced principally by strains of phage-group I *S. aureus*, though a strain of *S. hyicus* has also been reported to produce the toxin, as have some coagulase-negative staphylococci.[15, 16] The role of TSST-1 in disease other than the classic toxic shock syndrome can only be speculated upon.

Protein A

Protein A is a component of the cell wall of *S. aureus*, *S. intermedius* and *S. hyicus*, though these have slightly different structures (see Chapter 6). It has several interesting properties including reacting with the Fc fragment of immunoglobulin, as a result of which it has been much used as a tool in immunology. This non-specific reaction activates complement; protein A also has antiphagocytic properties and is a cytotoxigen in serum. Protein A does not penetrate the intact stratum corneum but when injected intradermally into the normal human forearm there is a biphasic reaction with an immediate weal and flare.[17] By 6 h there is induration, which persists for up to 96 h (Fig. 7.1). The initial reaction is mediated, at least in part, by release of histamine from basophils and perhaps mast cells. Between 6 and 24 h the response is predominantly by polymorphonuclear leucocytes and eosinophils, which may be responding to immune complexes. The response in normals thus resembles an immediate and delayed-type hypersensitivity, though this must actually be non-specific (protein A:Fc). A delayed-type hypersensitivity reaction can be demonstrated after immunization of the guinea-pig but not the mouse. Patients with psoriasis respond to protein A in much the same way as do normals but in patients with atopic dermatitis the response is markedly flattened (Fig. 7.1).[18] Cells rendered deficient in protein A by allele-replacement mutagenesis are slightly less virulent than their isogenic counterparts in experimental infections in mice, suggesting that protein A is a virulence factor.[7] However, it is interesting to speculate that strains which naturally have small amounts of cell-bound protein A, such as many of the methicillin-resistant *S. aureus*, may excite less local reaction and as a result are better able to colonize the host.

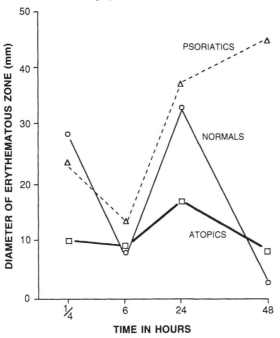

Fig. 7.1. Development of the erythematous zone resulting from intradermal injection of 5 ng protein A in patients with atopic dermatitis or psoriasis and in normals (based on White and Noble[18]).

In dogs, protein A from *S. aureus* has been shown to penetrate the skin but has not been shown to cause oedema or erythema.[19] However, prior treatment of dog skin with histamine significantly increased the penetration of protein A, suggesting that prior inflammation will facilitate penetration of many staphylococcal toxins or extracellular products.

Peptidoglycan

Peptidoglycan from the cell wall of *S. aureus* induces histamine release in human basophil leucocytes in vitro,[20] suggesting that this too could contribute to the immediate tissue response in humans and further the penetration of staphylococcal products.

Epidermolytic toxins (ET)

These are among the best-studied staphylococcal products. Two toxins are recognized: ETA, which is normally chromosomally encoded, and ETB, which is encoded on plasmid DNA. Although the amino acid sequences are only about 40 per cent similar,[21] both toxins have the same restricted host range – man, mouse, hamster and some monkeys[22, 23] – and only affect the stratum granulosum of the skin, no other epithelial tissue being involved. The mode of action seems to be destruction or disruption of desmosomes by proteolytic action, for the toxins bind to filaggrins[24] and are serine proteases.[25]

Potential pathogenicity factors in coagulase-negative staphylococci

Virulence factors in coagulase-negative staphylococci are much less well investigated than in the coagulase-positive species and the principal studies have been those on *S. epidermidis* in relation to catheter-associated or prosthetic implant infection, where the chief interest has centred around slime. Nevertheless, the various haemolysins and other toxins described above are produced by a small percentage of coagulase-negative staphylococci. Gemmel[9] records alpha toxin (2 per cent), beta toxin (2 per cent), delta toxin (13 per cent) as well as various, more generalized enzymes such as lipase (21 per cent) and gelatinase (42 per cent). The data in Gemmel's review will have been overtaken by changes in taxonomy and it would be interesting to see results from well-speciated strains. That these toxins most probably play a part in disease is also suggested in Gemmel's review, for toxins are more common in strains from infective processes (Table 7.2). However, others[26] have failed to demonstrate differences in the proportion of strains of *S. epidermidis* producing slime and extracellular enzymes from carriers or infective processes.

Slime production

The production of slime by *S. epidermidis* seems an obvious candidate as a virulence factor. Slime is implicated in the adherence of staphylococci to catheters[27-29] and is likely to interfere with phagocytosis; biofilms have been seen as of great importance in habitats as diverse as natural streams, industrial processes and the lungs in cystic fibrosis.

Slime belongs to the group of extracellular polysaccharides also known as glycocalyx or capsule: implied in the term 'slime' is a loose association with the cell wall structure whilst 'capsule' generally refers to material closely adherent to the cell. Slime is produced most abundantly when the organisms are attached to a solid surface; in studies where agar surfaces are present, slime composition may reflect to some extent the nutrient available in agar,[30] and published data on the composition of slime must be viewed in the light of this fact. Simple, defined media are now available.[31] Apart from an adhesive effect and mechanical protection, slime has other properties such as inhibiting the action of vancomycin; this may explain why this antibiotic fails to eliminate *S. epidermidis* on some occasions.[32] Early studies showed that strains of *S. epidermidis* isolated from infected patients with intravascular catheters were

Table 7.2. *Toxin production by coagulase-negative cocci*

	Positives (%)	
	Urinary tract infection	Blood, abscesses or wound infection
Alpha toxin	55	65
Delta toxin	65	50
DNAase	50	76
Gelatinase	30	64
Lipase/esterase	75	90

Based on Gemmel.[9]

Table 7.3. *Comparative pathogenicity of staphylococci*

Species	Weight retardation model			Slime production		
	n	Reduction (%)	Rank	n	Producers (%)	Rank
S. aureus	3	78	1		Not tested	
S. capitis	6	10	9	6	17	6
S. epidermidis	18	42	3	18	56	2
S. haemolyticus	10	54	2	10	20	5
S. hominis	7	19	6	7	29	4
S. lugdunensis	2	17.5	= 7	2	100	1
S. saprophyticus	5	32	4	5	0	= 7
S. simulans	3	26	5	3	0	= 7
S. warneri	6	17.5	= 7	6	50	3

Based on Gunn.[35]

more likely to produce slime than strains not isolated from patients with catheters,[33] and the relationship between slime and bacteraemia in hospitalized patients has been confirmed.[34]

Gunn,[35] in a study of comparative virulence of species of coagulase-negative staphylococci that used the model of inhibition of weight gain in the infant mouse, presented findings that might not be predicted from a consideration of disease in man. Table 7.3 shows that, although *S. aureus* was, as anticipated, the most powerful inhibitor of weight gain, *S. haemolyticus* was more inhibitory than was *S. epidermidis*. On the basis of slime production, however, the order of pathogenicity changes. Among animal staphylococci,[38] about 12 per cent of *S. hyicus* and 3 per cent of *S. chromogenes* from bovine mastitis have been found to produce slime.

Infection with *S. aureus*

Primary staphylococcal infections of the skin are chiefly boils, furuncles and other localized pustular lesions, and impetigo plus its severe manifestation, the scalded skin syndrome.

Localized infections

These occur more frequently in the first 40 years of life than later, with peaks in infection in those less than 10 years and those 30–40 years of age, the latter no doubt as a result of the presence of children in the household (Fig. 7.2). The sites of infection in those attending a general practitioner differ in nasal carriers and non-carriers (Table 7.4), with the nose as a source making a significant contribution to infections of the head and neck. In industrial injuries to the hands, however, nasal carriers are not more frequently infected than non-carriers and local contamination of the hand is more important.[37] However, in both groups, nasal and lesion strains are very frequently the same. Typical is the study from Australia in the 1960s,[38] where 65 per cent of lesion strains were the same as those carried in the nose.

In dialysis patients, the nose has long been accepted as a potent source of *S. aureus*. Haemodialysis patients studied by Rebel and coworkers[39] had principally Scribner catheter-type shunts; 10 of the 32 patients were nasal carriers and suffered 15 of the 18 shunt colonizations and five of nine infections. Others[40,41] obtained similar results and were able to relate the chance of infection to hygienic standards. In continuous ambulatory peritoneal dialysis (CAPD) patients,[42] 14 of 20 (70 per cent) nasal carriers of *S. aureus* suffered exit-site infections with their nasal strain compared with seven infections with *S. aureus* in 67 (10 per cent) non-carriers. Others have reported essentially similar results. For example, Sesso and colleagues[43] were able to distinguish between chronic carriers of *S. aureus*, yielding positive cultures on 75 per cent or more of occasions, intermittent carriers and non-carriers; 11 of the 16 chronic carriers had a total of 12 episodes of peritonitis, 4 of the 12 intermittent carriers also had peritonitis but none of the 15 non-carriers was infected with *S. aureus*.

There is a strong predominance of males infected with *S. aureus* amongst patients in general practice. Table 7.5 shows that only in lesions of the breast and axilla do females outnumber males. This male susceptibility is also seen in, for example, peritoneal dialysis, where males are much more susceptible to infection than are females,[42] and was reported for newborn infants many years previously.[44]

In experimental staphylococcal infection of man there is a direct relationship

Table 7.4. *Site distribution of* S. aureus *infections in nasal carriers and non-carriers in a single general practice*

	Distribution (%)	
Site of lesions	Nasal carriers ($n = 63$)	Non-nasal carriers ($n = 29$)
Neck and head	51	14
Eye	19	24
Axilla	3	17
Upper limb	17	14
Lower limb	6	31
Trunk	3	0

Based on Kay.[91]

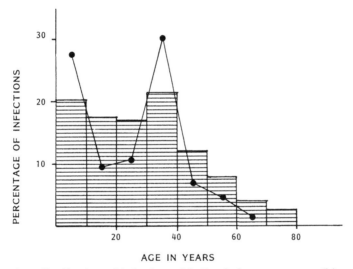

Fig. 7.2. Age distribution of infection with *Staphylococcus aureus* (histogram based on Johnson and colleagues;[38] line based on Kay[91]).

between the numbers of staphylococci applied to the skin and the likelihood that infection will occur (Fig. 7.3). This is perhaps the reason for the susceptibility of the nasal carrier to infection; the degree of contamination of the skin will be greater in carriers than in those who must aquire their staphylococci from another source.

The types of *S. aureus* causing localized infection in general practice were, historically, phage groups I and II but recently more miscellaneous or non-typable strains have been encountered. Rosdahl and coworkers in Sweden[45]

Table 7.5. *Site distribution and sex ratio of staphylococcal infection in general practice*

Site	Number of infections	M:F ratio	
Leg	374		2.1:1
Face and eyes	358	(Nose)	1:1.6
Arm	195		3.4:1
Neck	131		4.7:1
Trunk	107	(Chest and abdomen)	3.3:1
		(Breast)	1:6.25
Hand	93		4.1:1
Axilla	77		1:3.1
Toe	64		1.6:1
Anogenital area	44	(Perineum)	5.25:1
		(Genitalia)	1:2.2

Based on Johnson and colleagues.[38]

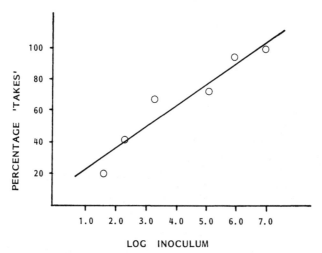

Fig. 7.3. Relationship between inoculum and experimental infection of the skin of humans with *Staphylococcus aureus* (based on Singh and coworkers[92]).

reported the following distribution: phage group 1, 13.3 per cent; II, 23.5 per cent; III, 18.5 per cent; miscellaneous, 30.5 per cent; and non-typable, 14.2 per cent. This still shows a greater predominance of phage group II than seen in normal carriers (see Chapter 6).

Table 7.6. S. aureus *and* Strep. pyogenes *in lesions of impetigo*

	Australia	UK		Sweden	Egypt
	1950s	1941	1971	1970s	1970
Number of case studies	159	190	72	200	131
Per cent with:					
S. aureus	67	81	87	86	87
Strep. pyogenes	13	47	21	25	46
Others	10.5	NR	11	2	3
Per cent of S. aureus:					
Type 80/81	18	< 3	0	10	64
Type 71	24	75	60	26	4

Some patients had both staphylococci and streptococci.
NR, not recorded.
Based on Noble.[51]

Impetigo

Impetigo is characterized by golden, stuck-on crusts or blisters (bullae); the blisters are most probably caused by small amounts of epidermolytic toxin or by the toxin in an otherwise resistant host. About three-quarters of all cases are in patients less than 20 years only with about 35 per cent less than 10 years.[46] In Europe it is chiefly a staphylococcal disease at the time of presentation to a clinician (Table 7.6), though one-third of lesions have both *Staphylococcus aureus* and *Streptococcus pyogenes*. American experience would suggest a predominantly streptococcal background, though there are signs that this may be changing.[47] In a recent series of 73 cases of impetigo from the United States, 45 (62 per cent) had *S. aureus* only, 6 (8 per cent) had streptococci only, and 14 (19 per cent) had both; the remaining eight patients had other organisms or failed to yield bacteria.[48]

In AIDS patients an extensive and atypical intertriginous form of bullous impetigo has been reported as part of AIDS-related pruritis.[49]

Scalded skin syndrome

This syndrome is the severe manifestation of epidermolytic toxin production in which the skin splits at the stratum granulosum so that the upper layers can be rubbed away by gentle sideways pressure (Nikolsky sign) in man and experimental animal models.[50] It is generally regarded as a sporadic disease with the majority of cases in children aged 0.5 to 2 years. In a collected series totalling 138 sporadic cases, 38.5 per cent of patients were less than 1 year old and 37.7 per cent between 1 and 2 years.[51] Few adult patients are reported and those chiefly in the immunosuppressed, although true cases in immunocompetent adults are known.[52] Care is needed in assessing older publications in which the term 'toxic epidermal necrolysis' was used for both diseases before the distinction was made between the staphylococcal scalded skin syndrome and drug-induced toxic epidermal necrolysis.

In recent years there have been a number of reports of outbreaks of scalded skin syndrome in newborn infants,[53-57] but it is not clear whether this reflects increased reporting or increased interest in the disease. Both scalded skin syndrome (in one incident resulting in several babies being admitted to intensive care) and the less serious pemphigus neonatorum (in one report extending to about 80 babies before and after discharge from the maternity unit) have been associated with strains bearing genes for epidermolytic toxin production. Different strains of S. aureus, including one resistant to methicillin,[58] have been responsible for each epidemic and in most cases a hospital staff member has been the apparent source or secondary cause of dissemination. In a recent survey in the United Kingdom,[59] 5 (3 per cent) of 164 S. aureus isolated from 500 normal women carried genes for epidermolytic toxin production.

Lesion colonization

Besides frank infection such as boils or impetigo, S. aureus also colonizes and aggravates lesions such as those of atopic dermatitis.[60] Some studies indicate that, when the density of S. aureus exceeds a certain level, such as $10^6/cm^2$, an exudative or impetiginized form of lesion occurs.[61, 62] There may be spread of staphylococci from these lesions such that the adjacent normal skin carries $10^2-10^3/cm^2$. Antibiotics are often used in the management of atopic dermatitis and recent studies have shown the value of topical agents in the control of bacteria, with a reduction of signs and symptoms of atopic dermatitis greater than that of hydrocortisone alone.[63] The reason for the overgrowth of S. aureus in atopic dermatitis, though much less severely or not at all in diseases such as proriasis,[64, 65] is not known. Protein A elicits a much less vigorous response in atopics than in normals or psoriatics, but this may be the result rather than a cause of colonization. Attention has recently turned to the skin lipids and there is some evidence that fatty acids which may control staphylococcal colonization are deficient in atopics (S. D. Patel and W. C. Noble, unpublished).

Infection with coagulase-negative staphylcocci

Because of the normal colonization of the skin with coagulase-negative staphylococci it has proved difficult to be sure that small localized lesions such as folliculitis are indeed caused by these organisms. An extensive infection resembling Gram-negative folliculitis but yielding an unspeciated coagulase-negative coccus has been reported,[68] but does not materially extend our knowledge of the possibility of infection due to coagulase-negative staphylococci because this would require extensive typing of resident and potentially infective isolates.

There are a number of miscellaneous infections attributed to the coagulase-negative staphylococci. These include cellulitis of the face due to *S. epidermidis* in a patient with leukaemia,[67] postoperative necrotizing fasciitis and septicaemia due to the same species,[68] two cases of cervical osteomyelitis,[69] and meningitis, also due to *S. epidermidis*.[70] Natural valve endocarditis originating in the community is increasingly recognized as due to coagulase-negative staphylococci. These, however, are the exceptions; most infections are associated with a catheter or prosthesis.[71]

Although all of the species present on human skin can be recovered from infections, all surveys[72, 73] agree in ranking *S. epidermidis* as the most frequent, followed usually by *S. hominis* and then *S. haemolyticus*, with a variable number of unidentified strains depending on the date at which the study took place. The extension of the original Kloos and Schleifer scheme (see Chapter 6) and the sequential development of commercially available kits has resulted in a reduction of the number of unspeciated strains. The best example of this is the recognition of *S. lugdunensis* as a cause of bacteraemia or septicaemia.[74]

Zierdt[75] has presented evidence that between 1 and 2 per cent of positive blood cultures are the result of contamination from skin but more interestingly he showed that *S. epidermidis* could be recovered from the blood of about 7 per cent of healthy blood donors – apparently healthy individuals have intermittent, transient, asymptomatic bacteraemia with their skin staphylococci.

The earliest infection to be recognized as regularly due to coagulase-negative staphylococci was colonization of cerebrospinal fluid shunts inserted for the relief of hydrocephalus.[76, 77] *Staphylococcus epidermidis* is responsible for about 90 per cent of these colonizations. Infection of the host may not be apparent for some time after the shunt has been inserted but many infections arise within about 2 months of surgery.[78, 79] In seven of nine such infected shunts, indistinguishable strains of *S. epidermidis* were recovered from the patient's skin at or about the time of surgery. However, other infections could not be traced to carriage at the time of surgery.

The general epidemiology of bacteraemia/septicaemia in hospital patients has been studied in 100 patients:[80] most patients were under 1 year of age or over 50 years; 73 were in intensive care units at the time of infection and mortality was 9 per cent/week. Ninety-three of the 100 had a central line or arterial catheter in place before bacteraemia and these were often of long duration. More than half of the catheters were colonized with *S. epidermidis*. Sidebottom and coworkers[81] have presented evidence that, at least in neonatal intensive-care units, the rates of infection with coagulase-negative cocci have not increased since about 1970 and represent between 26 and 70 per cent of positive blood cultures. Evidence shows that positive blood cultures represents infection and not simply contamination. Others have presented essentially similar data.[82]

In comparison with studies of dialysis patients, discussed below, few investigators seem to have sought the coagulase-negative staphylococci found in bacteraemia on the skin. Fleer and colleagues[83] have reported that 20 per cent of fluids for total parenteral nutrition are contaminated with staphylococci and attribute bloodstream infections in neonates to this source. Others[84] show the incidence of bacteraemia in granulocytopenia to have risen from 2 to 14 per cent between 1976 and 1979, but with a subsequent decrease. The source of *S. epidermidis* prior to 1977 is given as the skin but in subsequent years the respiratory and alimentary tracts are credited as the source. The adherence of *S. epidermidis* to catheter material is well established and the existence of colonies of cocci on catheter tips has been demonstrated by electron microscopy.[85, 86] Here the source of organisms is more clearly the skin, arising from the catheter entry site.

The most detailed studies of the skin origin of coagulase-negative staphylococci in infection are found in work on continuous ambulatory peritoneal dialysis (CAPD). In CAPD a 'permanent' catheter is inserted through the abdominal wall so that dialysis fluid can be introduced into and drained from the abdominal cavity every 4–8 h. In contrast to *S. aureus* infection in CAPD, the coagulase-negative cocci rarely cause exit-site infection but are responsible for a relatively mild peritonitis, usually evidenced by a 'cloudy dialysis bag' (the result of the presence of large numbers of white cells), together with mild fever and abdominal pain or tenderness. The lack of response at the exit site could result from the absence of protein A in the coagulase negatives.

Coagulase-negative staphylococci, principally *S. epidermidis*, have formed an increasing proportion of organisms causing peritonitis in CAPD patients. In one city in the United Kingdom the yearly percentages of peritonitis due to coagulase-negative staphylococci from 1983 to 1988 were 43, 45, 37, 51, 57, 53 in an annual average of 108 infections.[87] In another city the rate averaged 56 per cent of 750 infections,[88] with *S. epidermidis* causing 63 per cent of the total staphylococcal infections, followed by *S. aureus* (16 per cent), *S. haemolyticus* (6 per cent), *S. hominis* (5 per cent), *S. warneri* (4 per cent), *S. capitis* (1.4 per cent) and *S. saprophyticus* (1 per cent). Others have found esssentially similar results.

Ludlam and colleagues,[89] in a detailed study of 10 episodes of peritonitis due to coagulase-negative staphylococci, nine caused by *S. epidermidis* and one by *S. capitis*, were able to show that in six episodes the nose and/or the skin of the hand, axillae, umbilicus, exit site or groin were colonized by the infecting strain as many as 12 weeks before peritonitis, suggesting that recent acquisition of a new strain was an important factor in infection. These workers used a combination of antibiogram, biotype, phage type and plasmid profiling to distinguish between strains. Interestingly, in this series, slime production did not appear to be a pathogenicity factor since only 2 of the 10 strains produced slime in vitro. Others have been less successful in matching exit-site and peritonitis strains.[90] Perhaps differing policies in the renal units regarding prophylaxis and patient education are reflected in the different findings.

References

1 Noble WC. Virulence and the biochemical characters of staphylococci. J Pathol Bacteriol 1966; 91: 181–93.

2 Arbuthnott JP, Coleman DC, de Azevedo JS. Staphylococcal toxins in human disease. J Appl Bacteriol 1990; 69 (Symp Suppl): 101S–07S.

3 Thelestam M. Modes of membrane damaging action of staphylococcal toxins. In: Easmon CSF and Adlam C, eds. Staphylococci and staphylococcal infections, vol 2. London: Academic Press; 1983: 705–44.

4 Iandolo JJ. Genetic analysis of extracellular toxins of *Staphylococcus aureus*. Ann Rev Microbiol 1989; 43: 375–402.

5 Wadstrom T. Biological effects of cell membrane damaging toxins. In: Easmon CSF and Adlam C, eds. Staphylococci and staphylococcal infections, vol 2. London: Academic Press; 1983: 671–704.

6 Adlam C, Ward PD, McCartney AC, Arbuthnott JP, Thorley CM. Effect of immunization with highly purified alpha- and beta-toxins on staphylococcal mastitis in rabbits. Infect Immun 1977; 17: 250–56.

7 Patel AH, Nowlan P, Weavers ED, Foster T. Virulence of protein A deficient and alpha-toxin-deficient mutants of *Staphylococcus aureus* isolated by allele replacement. Infect Immun 1987; 55: 3103–10.

8 Janzon L, Arvidson S. The role of the delta lysin gene (hld) in the regulation of virulence genes by the accessory gene regulator (agr) in *Staphylococcus aureus*. EMBO J 1990; 9: 1391–99.

9 Gemmel CG. Extra-cellular toxins and enzymes of coagulase negative staphylococci. In: Easmon CFS, Adlam C, eds. Staphylococci and staphylococcal infections, vol 2. London: Academic Press; 1983: 809–27.

10 McKevitt AI, Bjornson GL, Mauracher CA, Schiefele DW. Amino acid

sequence of a deltalike toxin from *Staphylococcus epidermidis*. Infect Immun 1990; 58: 1473–75.

11 Schiefele DW, Bjornson GL, Dyer RA, Dimmick JE. Delta-like toxin produced by coagulase negative staphylococci is associated with neonatal necrotizing enterocolitis. Infect Immun 1987; 55: 2268–73.

12 Almazon J, de la Fuente R, Gomez-Lucia E, Suarez G. Enterotoxin production by strains of *Staphylococcus intermedius* and *Staphylococcus aureus* from dog infections. Zentrlbl Bakteriol Mikrobiol Hyg 1987; 264: 29–32.

13 Fukuda S, Tokuno H, Ogawa H et al. Enterotoxigenicity of *Staphylococcus intermedius* strains isolated from dogs. Zentralbl Bakteriol Mikrobiol Hyg 1984; 258: 360–67.

14 Bergdoll MS. Enterotoxins. In: Easmon CSF and Adlam C, eds. Stapylococci and staphylococcal infections, London: Academic Press; 1983: 559–98.

15 Crass BA, Bergdoll MS. Involvement of coagulase-negative staphylococci in toxic shock syndrome. J Clin Microbiol 1986; 23: 43–45.

16 Kahler RC, Boyce JM, Bergdoll MS, Lockwood WR, Taylor MR. Case report: toxic shock syndrome associated with TSST-1 producing coagulase-negative staphylococci. Amer J Med Sci 1986; 292: 310–11.

17 White MI, Noble WC. Skin response to protein A. Proc R Soc Edin 1980; 79B: 43–46.

18 White MI, Noble WC. The cutaneous reaction to staphylococcal protein A in normal subjects and patients with atopic dermatitis or psoriasis. Brit J Dermatol 1985; 113: 179–83.

19 Mason IS, Lloyd DH. Factors influencing the penetration of bacterial antigens through canine skin. In: von Tscharner C, Halliwell REW, eds. Advances in veterinary medicine, vol 1. London: Bailliere Tindall; 1990: 370–74.

20 Espersen F, Jarlov JO, Jensen C, Stahl Skov P, Norn S. *Staphylococcus aureus* peptidoglycan induces histamine release from basophil human leukocytes *in vitro*. Infect Immun 1984; 710–14.

21 Lee CY, Schmidt JJ, Johnson-Winegar AD, Spero L, Iandolo JJ. Sequence determination and composition of the exfoliative toxin A and toxin B genes from *Staphylococcus aureus*. J Bacteriol 1987; 169: 3904–09.

22 Elias PM, Fritsch P, Mittermayer H. Staphylococcal toxic epidermal necrolysis: species and tissue susceptibility and resistance. J Invest Dermatol 1976; 66: 80–89.

23 Fritsch PO, Kaaserer G, Elias PM. Action of staphylococcal epidermolysin: further observations on its species specificity. Arch Dermatol Res 1979; 264: 287–91.

24 Smith TP, Bailey CJ. Epidermolytic toxin from *Staphylococcus aureus* binds to filaggrins. FEBS Lett 1986; 194: 309–12.

25 Dancer SJ, Garratt R, Saldanha J, Jhoti H, Evans R. The epidermolytic toxins are serine proteases. FEBS Lett 1990; 268: 129–32.

26 Souto MJ, Ferreiros CM, Criado MT. Failure of phenotypic characteristics to distinguish between carrier and invasive isolates of *Staphylococcus epidermidis*. J Hosp Infect 1991; 17: 107–15.

27 Baddour LM, Smalley DL, Hill MM, Christensen GD. Proposed virulence factors among coagulase negative staphylococci isolated from two healthy populations. Can J Microbiol 1988; 34: 901–05.

28 Davenport DS, Massanari RM, Pfalkler MA, Bale MJ, Streed SA, Hierholzer WJ Jr. Usefulness of test for slime production as a marker for clinically

significant infections with coagulase-negative staphylococci. J Infect Dis 1986; 153: 332–39.

29 Diaz-Mitoma D, Harding GKM, Hoban DJ, Roberts RS, Low DE. Clinical significance of a test for slime production in ventriculoperitoneal shunt infections caused by coagulase-negative staphylococci. J Infect Dis 1987; 156: 555–60.

30 Drewny DT, Galbraith L, Wilkinson BJ, Wilkinson SG. Staphylococcal slime: a cautionary tale. J Clin Microbiol 1990; 28: 1292–96.

31 Hussain M, Hastings JGM, White PJ. A chemically defined medium for slime production by coagulase-negative staphylococci. J Med Microbiol 1991; 34: 143–47.

32 Farber BF, Kaplan MH, Clogston AG. *Staphylococcus epidermidis* extracted slime inhibits the antimicrobial action of glycopeptide antibiotics. J Infect Dis 1990; 161: 37–40.

33 Christensen GD, Simpson WA, Bisno AL, Beachey EH. Adherence of slime producing strains of *Staphylococcus epidermidis* to smooth surfaces. Infect Immun 1982; 37: 318–26.

34 Kotilainen P. Association of coagulase-negative staphylococcal slime production and adherence with the development and outcome of adult septicemias. J Clin Microbiol 1990; 28: 2779–85.

35 Gunn BA. Comparative virulence of human isolates of coagulase-negative staphylococci tested in an infant mouse weight retardation model. J Clin Microbiol 1989; 27: 507–11.

36 Watts JL, Naidu AS, Wadstrom T. Collagen binding, elastase production, and slime production associated with coagulase-negative staphylococci from bovine mammary gland infection. J Clin Microbiol 1990; 28: 580–83.

37 Williams REO, Miles AA. Infection and sepsis in industrial wounds of the hands. Med Res Coun Spec Rep Ser 1949 (No 262): 1–87.

38 Johnston A, Rountree PM, Smith K, Stanley NF, Anderson K. A survey of staphylococcal infection of the skin and subcutaneous tissue in general practices in Australia. Natl Hlth Med Res Counc Spec Rep Ser (No 10) [Canberra].

39 Rebel MH, van Furth R, Stevens P, Bosscher-Zonderman L, Noble WC. The flora of renal haemodialysis sites. J Clin Pathol 1975; 28: 29–32.

40 Kaplowitz LG, Comstock JA, Landwehr DM, Dalton HP, Mayhall CG. Prospective study of microbial colonization of the nose and skin and infection of the vascular access site in haemodialysis patients. J Clin Microbiol 1988; 26: 1257–62.

41 Yu VL, Goltz A, Wagener M, Smith PB, Rihs JD, Hanchett J, Zuravleff JJ. *Staphylococcus aureus* nasal carriage and infection in patients on haemodialysis. N Engl J Med 1986; 315: 91–96.

42 Davies SJ, Ogg CS, Cameron JS, Poston S, Noble WC. *Staphylococcus aureus* nasal carriage, exit-site infection and catheter loss in patients treated with continuous ambulatory peritoneal dialysis (CAPD). Periton Dial Internat 1989; 9: 61–64.

43 Sesso R, Draibe S, Cstelo A, Sato I, Leme I, Barbosa D, Ramos O. *Staphylococcus aureus* skin carriage and development of peritonitis in patients with continuous ambulatory peritoneal dialysis. Clin Nephrol 1989; 31: 264–68.

44 Thompson DJ, Gezon HM, Hatch TF, Rycheck RR, Rogers KD. Sex

distribution of *Staphylococcus aureus* colonization and disease in newborn infants. N Engl J Med 1963; 269: 337–41.

45 Rosdahl VT, Westh H, Jensen K. Antibiotic susceptibility and phage type patterns of *Staphylococcus aureus* isolated from patients in general practice compared to strains from hospitalized patients. Scand J Infect Dis 1990; 22: 315–20.

46 Mobacken H, Holst R, Wengstrom C, Holm SE. Epidemiological aspects of impetigo contagiosa in Western Sweden. Scand J Infect Dis 1975; 7: 39–44.

47 Barton LL, Friedman AD. Impetigo: a reassessment of etiology and therapy. Pediatr Dermatol 1987; 4: 185–88.

48 Demidovich CW, Witler RR, Ruff ME, Bass JW, Browning WC. Impetigo: current etiology and comparison of penicillin, erythromycin and cephalexin therapies. Am J Dis Child 1990; 144: 1313–15.

49 Davic M. Staphylococcal infection and the pruritis of AIDS-related complex. Arch Dermatol 1987; 123: 1599.

50 Arbuthnott JP, Kent J, Noble WC. The response of hairless mice to staphylococcal epidermolytic toxin. Br J Dermatol 1973; 88: 481–85.

51 Noble WC. Microbiology of human skin. London: Lloyd-Luke; 1981.

52 Opal SM, Johnson-Winegar AD, Cross AS. Staphylococcal scalded skin syndrome in two immunocompetent adults caused by exfoliatin-B-producing *Staphylococcus aureus*. J Clin Microbiol 1988; 26: 1283–86.

53 Dowsett EG, Petts DN, Baker SL, deSaxe MJ, Coe AE, Naidoo J, Noble WC. Analysis of an outbreak of staphylococcal scalded skin syndrome: strategies for typing 'non-typable' strains. J Hosp Infect 1984; 5: 391–97.

54 Dancer SJ, Simmons NA, Poston SM, Noble WC. Outbreak of staphylococcal scalded skin syndrome among neonates. J Infect 1988; 16: 87–103.

55 Dancer SJ, Poston SM, East J, Simmons NA, Noble WC. An outbreak of pemphigus neonatorum. J Infect 1990; 20: 73–82.

56 Curran JP, Al-Salihi FL. Neonatal staphylococcal scalded skin syndrome: massive outbreak due to an unusual phage-type. Pediatrics 1980; 66: 285–90.

57 Kaplan MH, Chmel H, Hsieh H-C, Stephens A, Brinsko V. Importance of exfoliatin A production by *Staphylococcus aureus* strains isolated from clustered epidemics of neonatal pustulosis. J Clin Microbiol 1986; 23: 83–91.

58 Richardson JF, Quoraishi AHM, Francis BJ, Marples RR. Beta-lactam negative, methicillin-resistant *Staphylococcus aureus* in a new-born nursery: report of an outbreak and laboratory investigation. J Hosp Infect 1990; 16: 109–21.

59 Dancer SJ, Noble WC. Nasal, axillary and perineal carriage of *Staphylococcus aureus* among antenatal women: identification of strains producing epidermolytic toxin. J Clin Pathol 1991; 44: 681–84.

60 Dahl MV. *Staphylococcus aureus* and atopic dermatitis. Arch Dermatol 1983; 119: 840–46.

61 Hauser C, Wuethrich B, Matter L, Wilhelm JA, Sonnabend W, Schopfer K. *Staphylococcus aureus* skin colonization in atopic dermatitis patients. Dermatologica 1985; 170: 35–39.

62 Bibel DJ, Greenberg JH, Cook JL. *Staphylococcus aureus* and the microbial ecology of atopic dermatitis. Can J Microbiol 1977; 23: 1062–68.

63 Lever R, Hadley K, Downey D, Mackie R. Staphylococcal colonization in atopic dermatitis and the effect of topical mupirocin therapy. Br J Dermatol 1988; 119: 189–98.

64 Noble WC, Savin JA. Carriage of *Staphylococcus aureus* in psoriasis. Br Med J 1968; 1: 417–19.

65 Marples RR, Heaton CL, Kligman AM. *Staphylococcus aureus* in psoriasis. Arch Dermatol 1973; 107: 568–70.

66 Lotem M, Ingber A, Filhaber A, Sandbank M. Skin infection provoked by coagulase-negative staphylococcus resembling Gram-negative folliculitis. Cutis 1988; 42: 443–44.

67 Pitlik S, Fainstein V. Cellulitis caused by *Staphylococcus epidermidis* in a patient with leukemia. Arch Dermatol 1984; 120: 1099–100.

68 Mancuso-Ungaro HR Jr. Treatment of necrotizing fasciitis caused by *Staphylococcus epidermidis*. Arch Surg 1978; 113: 288.

69 Parker MA, Tuazon CU. Cervical osteomyelitis: infection due to *Staphylococcus epidermidis* in haemodialysis patients. J Am Med Ass 1978; 240: 50–51.

70 Crowe MJ, Ward OC. *Staphylococcus epidermidis* as a cause of meningitis. Irish Med J 1977; 146: 113–15.

71 Dougherty SH. Pathobiology of infection in prosthetic devices. Rev Infect Dis 1988; 10: 1102–17.

72 Papapetropoulos M, Pappas A, Papavessiliou J, Legakis NJ. Distribution of coagulase-negative staphylococci in human infection. J Hosp Infect 1981; 2: 145–53.

73 Wantscheff AI, Kuhnen E, Brandis H. Species distribution of coagulase-negative staphylococci isolated from clinical sources. Zentralbl Bakt Hyg A 1985; 260: 41–50.

74 Freney J, Brun Y, Bes M et al. *Staphylococcus lugdunensis* sp.nov. and *Staphylococcus schleiferi* sp.nov.; two species from human clinical specimens. Int J System Bacteriol 1988; 38: 168–72.

75 Zierdt CH. Evidence for transient *Staphylococcus epidermidis* bacteremia in patients and in healthy humans. J Clin Microbiol 1983; 17: 628–30.

76 Holt RJ. The classification of staphylococci from colonized ventriculo-atrial shunts. J Clin Pathol 1969; 22: 475–82.

77 Price EH. *Staphylococcus epidermidis* infections of cerebrospinal fluid shunts. J Hosp Infect 1984; 5: 7–17.

78 Bayston R, Lari J. A study of the source of infection in colonized shunts. Develop Med Child Neurol 1974; 16 (Suppl 2): 16–22.

79 Verhoef J, Petersen PK, Williams DN, Laverdiere M, Sabath LD. Atrioventricular shunt infections and endocarditis due to *Staphylococcus epidermidis*. Zentral Bakt Hyg I Abt Orig 1978; 241: 95–100.

80 Ponce de Leon S, Wenzel RP. Hospital acquired blood stream infection with *Staphylococcus epidermidis*. Am J Med 1984; 77: 639–44.

81 Sidebotham DG, Freeman J, Platt R, Epstein MF, Goldmann DA. Fifteen-year experience with bloodstream isolates of coagulase-negative staphylococci in neonatal intensive care. J Clin Microbiol 1988; 26: 713–18.

82 Fidalgo S, Vazquez F, Mendoza MC, Perez F, Mendez FJ. Bacteremia due to *Staphylococcus epidermidis*: microbiologic, epidemiologic, clinical and prognostic features. Rev Infect Dis 1990; 12: 520–28.

83 Fleer A, Senders RC, Visser MR, Bijlmer RP, Gerards LJ, Kraaijeveld CA, Verhoef J. Septicemia due to coagulase-negative staphylococci in a neonatal intensive care unit: clinical and bacteriological features and contaminated parenteral fluids as a source of sepsis. Pediatr Infect Dis 1983; 2: 426–31.

84 Wade JC, Schimpff SC, Newman KA, Wiernik PH. *Staphylococcus epidermidis*: an increasing cause of infection in patients with granulocytopenia. Ann Int Med 1982; 97: 503–08.

85 Franson TR, Sheth NK, Roase HD, Sohnle PG. Scanning electron microscopy of bacteria adherent to intravascular catheters. J Clin Microbiol 1984; 20: 500–05.

86 Locci R, Peters G, Pulverer G. Microbial colonization of prosthetic devices. Microtopographical characteristics of intravenous catheters as detected by scanning electron microscopy. Zentralbl Bakteriol Mikrobiol Hyg I B 1981; 173: 285–92.

87 Wilcox MH, Finch RG, Burden RP, Morgan AG. Peritonitis complicating continuous ambulatory peritoneal dialysis in Nottingham 1983–88. J Med Microbiol 1991; 34: 137–41.

88 Spencer RC. Infection in continuous ambulatory peritoneal dialysis. J Med Microbiol 1988; 27: 1–9.

89 Ludlam HA, Noble WC, Marples RR, Bayston R, Phillips I. The epidemiology of peritonitis caused by coagulase negative staphylococci in continuous ambulatory peritoneal dialysis. J Med Microbiol 1989; 30: 167–74.

90 Eisenberg ES, Ambalu M, Szylagi G, Aning V, Soeiro R. Colonization of skin and development of peritonitis due to coagulase-negative staphylococci in patients undergoing peritoneal dialysis. J Infect Dis 1987; 156: 478–82.

91 Kay CR. Sepsis in the home. Br Med J 1962; 1: 1048–52.

92 Singh G, Marples RR, Kligman AM. Experimental staphylococcal infection in humans. J Invest Dermatol 1971; 57: 149–52.

8

Streptococci and the skin

M. BARNHAM

Amongst the bacteria pathogenic for man, few show such variety in clinical manifestations and epidemiology as the streptococci. *Streptococcus pyogenes* (Lancefield group A) in particular has attracted much attention over the years as one of the major human pathogens and it remains very common as a cause of skin infection throughout the world, despite the availability of antibiotics. There is an increasing appreciation of other haemolytic and non-haemolytic streptococci in clinical specimens and in disease as a result of the growing use of streptococcal identification and Lancefield grouping kits in laboratories.

Skin infection with streptococci covers a range from simple colonization to primary and secondary infections; the skin provides an important portal of entry for systemic infection by these organisms. Skin infection may be complicated by non-suppurative sequelae such as nephritis and scarlet fever; conversely, streptococcal infection at other sites in the body may lead to skin manifestations, as in rheumatic fever and acute guttate psoriasis. The following account will consider these conditions, excluding streptococcal infections of the mouth, alimentary, respiratory and genitourinary tracts or deeper structures except insofar as they are relevant to the skin.

Biology and classification of streptococci

As a group the streptococci are Gram-positive, spherical, aerobic and facultatively anaerobic bacteria arranged in chains or pairs, non-sporing, catalase negative, oxidase negative and mainly non-motile. They ferment carbohydrates with the production of lactic acid but no gas, and they fail to reduce nitrate.

Haemolysis on blood-agar culture provides a useful division of streptococci into those that are haemolytic (beta haemolytic, showing a zone of complete haemolysis) and non-haemolytic (comprising alpha haemolytic, 'greening' or 'viridans' streptococci and those with no effect on red blood cells). Haemolytic streptococci are further divided according to the carriage of polysaccharide and teichoic acid, Lancefield group antigens, a system that has proved very useful for laboratory and clinical purposes. Identification of organisms to species level usually involves more comprehensive physiological testing; standardized laboratory kits are now widely available for this purpose and for Lancefield grouping.

Table 8.1 lists the main streptococci of medical importance. The haemolytic streptococci of major concern in skin infection (particularly Lancefield groups A, C and G) are listed as pyogenic streptococci along with *S. anginosus* (formerly widely known as *S. milleri*[1,2]), an organism that produces minute colonies with variable haemolytic and Lancefield grouping properties, and the pneumococcus, which, although occasionally found in wounds or on the skin, is principally an organism of the respiratory tract. Recent studies of DNA structure showed that group C *S. equisimilis*, the large-colony group G and group L streptococci, were closely related, whereas group C *S. zooepidemicus*, an organism widely found in animals, was much more closely related to the horse pathogen *S. equi*.[3,4] Listed under the heading 'other streptococci' are the principal oral or 'viridans group' streptococci of medical significance; many other species have been described in this group and there is still disagreement over their nomenclature and classification.[5-7] As shown in the table, non-haemolytic streptococci sometimes produce Lancefield-group antigens but this has been of little value in their characterization. Some streptococcal isolates show atypical haemolytic reactions that may lead to misidentification in the laboratory;[8] haemolysis may also be influenced by the cultural conditions used, such as by the choice of basal medium, species of red blood cell and the degree of anaerobiosis.[6,9]

Faecal streptococci have now been separated on the basis of DNA analysis into a genus of their own, *Enterococcus*.[10] The four most important species of the 12 so far described in the genus[11] are shown in Table 8.1. The organisms show variable haemolysis and, in addition to carriage of the Lancefield group-D antigen, some also react with antisera to groups G or Q.[12] Enterococci form part of the normal intestinal flora and may also be found in the mouth and female genital tract; sometimes they are found on intact skin and in wounds but they are generally thought to be of little clinical significance there. However, contamination of the hands of hospital staff with enterococci may play a part in nosocomial transmission.[13] Infections with enterococci and pneumococci have been reviewed elsewhere[10,14] and will not be considered further in this account.

The strictly anaerobic cocci (including organisms of the genus *Pepto-*

Table 8.1. *Classification of the main streptococci of medical importance*

Name	Lancefield group antigens carried	Usual form of haemolysis
Pyogenic streptococci		
S. pyogenes	A	beta
S. agalactiae	B	beta
S. equisimilis	C	beta
S. zooepidemicus	C	beta
Streptococcus spp.	G	beta
Streptococcus spp.	L	beta
S. suis, type 2	R(+D)	beta
S. anginosus ('milleri')	−(F, G, A, C)	non, beta
S. pneumoniae	−	non
Other streptococci		
S. salivarius	−(K)	non
S. sanguis	−(H)	non
S. gordonii	−(H)	non
S. oralis	−	non
S. mitis	−(K, O)	non
S. mutans	−(E)	non
S. bovis	D	non
Enterococci		
E. faecalis	D	non, beta
E. faecium	D	non, beta
E. avium	D, Q	non
E. durans	D	non
'Anaerobic streptococci'		
Streptococcus spp.	−	non
Peptostreptococcus spp.	−	non

Based on Parker.[6]
The minus sign preceding some group antigens indicates 'none or variable'.

streptococcus and some of the genus *Streptococcus*) form a heterogeneous collection of bacteria, many of which are very different from the other streptococci in their metabolic characteristics.[15,16] They form part of the normal flora in the oropharynx, alimentary and genital tracts, and may be responsible for a variety of superficial and deep infections, often in association with other organisms.[17]

Typing of streptococci

Streptococci may be typed for purposes of epidemiological study, surveillance or research by a variety of means including serotyping for T, M and R surface

Table 8.2. *Serotypes of* S. pyogenes *commonly associated with skin infection*

T-typing patterns	M types
3/13/B3264	Non-typable, 33, 39, 41, 43, 52, 81; less commonly 13, 53
5/27/44	Non-typable
8/25/Imp. 19	Non-typable, 2, 25, 55, 57
14/49	Non-typable, 49, 80
15/17/19/23/47	54
Non-typable	31
4, 9, 11 or 12	Non-typable

Based on Wannamaker.[19]

Table 8.3. *Features that are mainly restricted to infection with strains within a limited range of streptococcal types*

Skin infection, throat infection
Scarlet fever
Post-streptococcal glomerulonephritis
Rheumatic fever
Invasive infections
Host specificity (man – animals)
Antibiotic resistance

antigens, bacteriocin and bacteriophage typing techniques.[6] The conventional T/M surface-antigen typing system used for *S. pyogenes* has the advantage of being widely available and well established with international standardization, although there remains a low typability for isolates from certain parts of the world.[18] Some common serotypes of skin-infecting *S. pyogenes* are shown in Table 8.2; in general these organisms have more complex T-typing patterns and 'higher number' M types than those causing respiratory tract infection, but the distinction is not entirely clear cut.[19, 20] An extended T-antigen typing system recently developed for group C and G streptococci in the United Kingdom gave 88 and 82 per cent typability, respectively, on a large collection of human isolates;[21] some of these organisms, particularly those isolated from systemic infection, also produce M proteins[22] that might be used for typing purposes. The features of streptococcal infection listed in Table 8.3 are commonly associated with strains within a restricted range of T/M types. Group B streptococci may be serotyped according to surface polysaccharide and protein antigens, and subdivided by bacteriophage typing.[23]

Recently developed techniques that might be useful for streptococcal typing include chromosomal DNA fingerprinting, which when applied to *S. pyogenes* gives patterns remarkably specific to each streptococcal M type,[24] electrophoretic analysis of whole-cell proteins and probing of restriction enzyme digests of rRNA.[25]

Natural distribution of streptococci: colonization and source of infection

Colonization and carriage in man

Haemolytic streptococci of groups A, C and G, and *S. anginosus*, are regularly found in the nasopharynx of healthy people. Carriage rates vary from time to time and according to the population studied; some reported rates are shown in Table 8.4. In closed communities with a high prevalence of streptococcal infection, nasopharyngeal carriage rates may be much higher than in open communities.[29, 30] Some patients harbouring streptococci at these sites disperse organisms in large numbers, particularly from the nose, leading to extensive contamination of the hands and clothing.[31] Streptococci carried in the respiratory tract may also be deposited on to the skin via habits such as nail biting, nose picking and the sucking of freshly inflicted wounds.[32]

The main routes of spread of the streptococci causing upper respiratory tract infection include airborne transmission from the nasopharynx, together with direct inoculation into the nose and mouth, sometimes via contamination of the skin.[33, 34] For skin infection, however, streptococcal colonization of the nasopharynx is thought to be of less epidemiological significance. The classical studies of Red Lake Indians in Minnesota, in whom streptococcal pyoderma was a common and recurring problem, showed that the nose and pharynx became colonized with the organisms on average 3 and 2 weeks, respectively, after the initial finding of streptococci on healthy skin and the development of skin lesions.[34, 35] In these and other studies of pyoderma, respiratory colonization was usually found to occur in about 25 per cent of patients.[34, 36] The conclusion drawn was that nasopharyngeal colonization was a secondary phenomenon and of little significance in the evolution of pyoderma in the individual patient.

However, upper respiratory carriage of pyoderma strains may still have some importance as a longer-term reservoir for skin contamination and as a source for the initiation of outbreaks; in a study of asymptomatic nasopharyngeal carriers applying for poultry meat-processing employment, 55 per cent of isolates of *S. pyogenes* were of T/M types with an apparent potential to cause skin infection in meat workers, as judged by typing results from contemporary infections in such workers in the United Kingdom.[28]

Haemolytic streptococci of various Lancefield groups are sometimes found on normal, healthy skin, but at non-epidemic times they are usually only

Table 8.4. *Some reported nasopharyngeal carriage rates of beta-haemolytic streptococci*

Lancefield group	Carriage rate in study (%)		
	International compilation[a]	Nigeria[b]	England[c]
A	7.0	3.0	1.5
B	0.7	0.1	0.5
C	3.9	3.6	2.0
G	3.4	6.2	1.3
F or non-groupable	1.4	—	1.1
Total (all groups)	16.3	13.0	6.5

[a] From Hare 1940: study of 3102 patients, 1935–1938.[26]
[b] From Ogunbi et al. 1978: study of 12755 school children, 1972.[27]
[c] From Barnham 1989: study of 1640 young adults, 1980–1988.[28]

present in small numbers,[26, 33, 37] Experimental inoculation of the skin with pyoderma strains of *S. pyogenes* often fails to initiate colonization or infection, a result ascribed to the bactericidal activity of unsaturated fatty acids on the skin;[33] the outcome of experiments on the growth of *S. pyogenes* from small inocula in peptone water–oleic acid broth suggested that pyoderma strains would be better able to survive on the skin than would 'throat' strains.[38] The critical inoculum size of streptococci required to initiate colonization or infection of the skin is unknown but the chances of it being achieved are more likely in endemic or outbreak conditions where the excretion of organisms from others is high. Studies in communities where pyoderma is common, as in Minnesota[34, 35] and Lagos, Nigeria,[39] showed colonization of normal skin on the wrist, ankle and back, principally with group A but also with group C and G streptococci. Rates of positive culture varied from 1.7–3.0 per cent in the African study to 37 per cent in Minnesota; in the Minnesota study there was a greater likelihood (up to 76 per cent) of subsequent pyoderma in those showing positive cultures on normal skin.[35] A study of Egyptian school-children showed colonization of the skin behind the ear with *S. pyogenes* in 14 per cent of those tested.[40] The seasonal nature of streptococcal pyoderma raises questions as yet unresolved about the possible influence of prevailing temperature and humidity on the survival and growth of streptococci on the skin.[41, 42]

The faeces provides a reservoir of haemolytic streptococci of groups B, C and G and *S. anginosus*;[26, 43, 44] this may be a source of infection for abdominal surgical wounds and perianal structures but its significance for other areas of the skin is uncertain. *S. pyogenes* was found in the faeces of 20 per cent of patients with streptococcal infections of the nasopharynx,[45] but it is rarely found in the faeces under other circumstances. Symptomless carriage of *S. pyogenes* in the perineal and perianal regions has occasionally been traced as the source of outbreaks of infection;[46] in a study of 100 children with *S. pyogenes* pharyngitis, 6 per cent were found to be anal carriers.[47] Group B streptococci commonly colonize the natal cleft and perineum from their main habitat in the rectal mucosa;[48] group G streptococci have been found on the perineal skin of 2 per cent of normal people.[37]

The normal female genital tract and the male and female urethra are commonly colonized with group B streptococci and less commonly with groups C and G, and *S. anginosus*;[49, 50] *S. pyogenes* is occasionally found in apparently normal (symptomless) patients but its presence is more usually associated with vaginal soreness and discharges.[51, 52] Babies born vaginally to mothers carrying haemolytic streptococci in the tract may become colonized at various skin sites; often this produces no illness but some babies subsequently develop local infections and in a few it is a prelude to systemic invasion.

Haemolytic streptococci of various groups will sometimes colonize areas of abnormal or damaged skin, such as in eczema and other forms of dermatitis, ulcers, burns and other wounds;[21, 53-56] The apparently healthy umbilical stump of neonates may harbour *S. pyogenes* and provide an important source for cross-infection and persistence of outbreaks in nurseries.[57]

Non-haemolytic streptococci are regularly found in large numbers in the mouth and are also commonly carried in the faeces.[44] From these reservoirs, contamination of the skin of the face and hands readily occurs, with further dispersal to other parts of the body; recovery rates exceeding 50 per cent of patients have been recorded from certain parts of the face, 30 per cent from the conjunctiva, 13–48 per cent on the hand, and 3–32 per cent on the foot.[53, 58] The generally low potential of non-haemolytic streptococci to colonize and persist after inoculation into wounds was shown in a wartime study that yielded an initial isolation rate of 15 per cent in fresh wounds, decreasing according to the length of delay before swabbing in contrast to an increasing rate for haemolytic streptococci and *Staphylococcus aureus*.[59]

Environmental and animal sources of streptococci

Most human infection with pyogenic streptococci results from autoinoculation with organisms carried on patients themselves or by direct transmission of the organisms from others by contagion or airborne droplets.[26, 33, 54] Organisms are commonly shed into the environment from sites of infection or carriage. 'Throat' strains of *S. pyogenes* are readily cultivated from contaminated clothing, bedding and fomites but they quickly lose infectivity once away from their human host; however, they may multiply if inoculated into suitable foods to produce outbreaks in those who consume them.[33] In studies during outbreaks the hardier 'pyoderma' strains are often found contaminating surfaces and equipment used by patients and, in this case, the environment may be more significant as a source of infecting organisms.[34, 38] Occasional infections with *S. pyogenes* may occur by spread from domestic pets carrying the organism[60] or transmission by contaminated wound-feeding flies, such as *Hippelates* gnats.[42]

Zoonotic streptococcal infections are uncommon in man. Examples include *S. zooepidemicus* (group C) infection, which is usually acquired by close contact with horses or by the consumption of contaminated milk or undercooked pork,[61–63] group L streptococcal infection in patients in close occupational contact with chickens or pigs,[64] and group R streptococcal infection in patients in contact with pigs or pork products.[65] Serotyping of group B, C (*S. equisimilis*) and G streptococci produces largely distinct clusters of types from human and animal sources, indicating that most human infection is with human strains and not acquired from animals.[6, 66]

Changes in the prevailing types of streptococci

The predominant serotypes of *S. pyogenes* circulating in communities change over periods of months and years. Local studies, such as those of Mayon-White and Perks in Oxfordshire, show relatively constant patterns of isolation of certain types of streptococci (endemic types), with periodic epidemics caused by other types.[67] National data show an ebb and flow of particular types over the years; in the United Kingdom, M types 6 and 49 became common in the early 1980s to be replaced by types 1 and 28 in the middle of the decade and more recently by type 4,[20] while in the United States, increases in M type 1, 3 and 18 *S. pyogenes* infection have been noticed during the 1980s.[68] No satisfactory explanation for these changes is yet available. Fluctuations in the prevalence of invasive disease, scarlet fever, rheumatic fever, nephritis and antibiotic resistance may be related at local, national and global levels to changes in the prevailing types of streptococci.[68–70] Comparable data on long-term changes in the types of non-group A streptococci in human infection are not yet available.

Streptococcal infections of the skin

Direct streptococcal infection of the skin may take a number of forms, as shown in Table 8.5. *Streptococcus pyogenes* remains the major streptococcal pathogen in these infections but non-group A streptococci also play a part and they are now more commonly recognized than before with the widespread use of modern, rapid laboratory test-kits.[71] The bacteriological assessment of skin infection needs to be made with care: a variety of haemolytic and non-haemolytic streptococci may be present on healthy intact skin or as temporary colonizers or contaminants in wounds, as discussed above; other bacteria may be present in similar manner including staphylococci, coliform and anaerobic organisms, and the production by them of substances bactericidal to streptococci may lead to displacement of the primary pathogens in infected lesions.[19, 33, 53] The various forms of streptococcal infection of the skin are described below, with a note of the organisms most commonly associated with them.

Streptococcal pyoderma

Streptococcal pyoderma is a broad term used to describe purulent infections of the skin, including the superficial form previously known as streptococcal impetigo together with localized pustular infections when caused by streptococci, such as otitis externa, angular cheilitis, paronychia and infection in tattoos and pierced ear lobes.

Superficial impetiginous lesions usually develop on traumatized, exposed areas of the skin. They start as small erythematous papules, then become vesicles and pustules, and soon develop thick, adherent, honey-coloured crusts on an enlarging erythematous base;[33, 72] lesions may be multiple and coalescent and a mild to moderate tender enlargement of local lymph nodes commonly occurs. Untreated lesions may persist for several weeks and shed large numbers of organisms before healing without a scar; in many cases they are tolerated by the patient without complaint. This form of infection is most commonly seen in young children and may be very prevalent in poor communities where patients and their families live and play together at close quarters under conditions of poor hygiene.[73-76] There is a worldwide distribution but the disease is most prevalent in tropical areas and during warm, humid seasonal conditions elsewhere.[41, 42]

Minor trauma to the skin, such as abrasions, trivial cuts and scratches, is thought to be a necessary condition to allow streptococci to initiate impetiginous infection;[19, 35, 73, 77] in patients with previous colonization of healthy skin there is a high risk of developing lesions under such conditions.[35]

Table 8.5. *Forms of direct streptococcal infection of the skin and related structures*

Pyoderma (including 'streptococcal impetigo', streptococcal paronychia, angular
  cheilitis, otitis externa, infected tattoos, etc.)
Ecthyma
Secondary infections of other rashes (including eczema and other dermatitides,
  scabies, chickenpox, etc.)
Wound infections (including ulcers, traumatic wounds, blisters, bites, burns, etc)
Lymphangitis, lymphadenitis
Cellulitis
Subcutaneous abscess
Erysipelas
Necrotizing fasciitis
Miscellaneous: omphalitis, conjunctivitis, suppurative hidradenitis

---

Bites of the skin caused by insects, scabies and lice are associated with a risk of pyoderma,[41, 73, 74] when excoriation may implant streptococci from the skin surface or from contaminated fingernails. Outbreaks of streptococcal pyoderma also occur in older children and adults grouped closely together and exposed to skin trauma, such as in rugby football teams, army units and meat-handling establishments;[32, 42, 53] these are described in more detail below.

Staphylococci and streptococci are often found either individually or mixed in cultures from pyoderma lesions and there has been controversy, not yet entirely resolved, over which is the more important pathogen.[75] Close study of patients with vesicular impetigo in Minnesota and elsewhere in the United States showed that *S. pyogenes* was first to infect, with various and sometimes changing phage types of *Staph. aureus* found in the lesions only in the later stages.[19] Other features suggesting that group A streptococci were the most important agents in this infection included the response of many patients to antibiotics active only against the streptococci, and the finding in patients with multiple lesions that streptococci were present in nearly all, but staphylococci only in some.[33, 75] However, some reports from Britain, Sweden, Egypt and Iraq have shown a higher recovery of pure *Staph. aureus* from vesicular impetigo than has been encountered in the United States.[53, 75] There is some evidence now emerging in the United States for a shift from streptococci to staphylococci as the dominant causative organisms in vesicular and crusted impetigo.[78] In contrast to the vesicular type, bullous impetigo usually yields a pure growth of *Staph. aureus*.

Studies have often shown group C and G streptococci as causative agents of pyoderma in a minority of patients[37, 39, 53, 79, 80] and sometimes they have been found in mixed culture with *Streptococcus pyogenes*;[76, 81] in certain parts of the world they have been reported as more common than *S. pyogenes* in pyoderma.[82] The lesions of angular cheilitis yield haemolytic streptococci in about 15 per cent of patients and Lancefield group B organisms are commonly found;[83] the condition sometimes occurs in outbreaks.

Ecthyma

This is a deeper and more persistent form of ulcerated pyoderma, usually showing a raised oedematous edge and a hard adherent crust.[72, 76] The lesions may be single or in groups and occur most often on exposed areas of the lower extremities. In its general epidemiological and bacteriological features, ecthyma resembles the impetiginous form of infection and the two may occur together in outbreaks.

Secondary streptococcal infection

Secondary infections of other rashes include the 'impetiginization' of scabies, dermatophytosis, eczema and other forms of dermatitis, although in some patients the organisms simply colonize the lesions without producing signs of infection.[56] Secondary infection in varicella lesions may lead to serious invasive disease,[84–86] perhaps involving a potentiation of bacterial infection by the damaging effects of virus on the host defence mechanisms.[87, 88] A chronic form of infected eczema in Jamaican children, termed 'infective dermatitis', commonly yielding beta-haemolytic streptococci or *Staph. aureus*, is associated with infection by human T-lymphotropic virus type 1.[89]

The contamination of wounds with streptococci produces variable results ranging from symptomless colonization to rapid systemic spread with minimal inflammation at the original site.[76] Factors contributing to the outcome include the extent, depth and anatomical site of the wound and the presence of devitalized tissue or foreign bodies within it. Streptococcal infection of superficial wounds, such as abrasions and minor burns, may produce a simple pyoderma, as described above, whereas infection of deeper lesions, such as ulcers, surgical incisions, accidental lacerations, the deeper burns and human or animal bites, may prove more serious. Haemolytic group A, C or G streptococcal colonization of burns may be asymptomatic in some patients but it will usually lead to a failure of skin grafting; in a few patients it may lead to serious invasive disease.[21, 55]

The factors responsible for the enhanced risk of infection with foreign bodies are still not fully understood. Experimental studies showed that much smaller inocula of *Staph. aureus* or *Strep. pyogenes* were required to initiate infection in the presence of foreign material and the severity of lesions was increased.[90,91] More recent research on foreign body-associated infection revealed decreased opsonic coating of infecting bacteria, reduced accessibility to host defences by bacterial adhesion to foreign surfaces, and deficient phagocytic bactericidal function in local polymorphonuclear leucocytes.[92]

Wound infection may occur with a variety of haemolytic streptococci, particularly those of groups A, C and G,[21] and group L streptococcal infection has been described in the wounds of chicken and pig handlers.[64] Systemic infection with group R streptococci (*S. suis*) may follow a few days after wounding of the skin in patients in contact with pigs or their meat products;[65] serological evidence of infection with this organism has been found in up to 21 per cent of those occupationally exposed to pigs but it is not known if the streptococcus can elicit signs of local wound infection.[65] There are occasional reports of serious wound infection with 'viridans group' streptococci.[86]

Streptococcal infection in the deeper wounds may lead to cellulitis, a rapidly advancing and painful deep inflammation of the skin featuring oedema and erythema; in many patients there is an associated spread of organisms into local lymphatic channels to produce ascending lymphangitis and regional lymphadenitis, and a risk that this may produce suppuration of the nodes or a rapid progression to septicaemia.[76] Subcutaneous abscess occurs as an uncommon local complication of streptococcal infection; superficial bullae have been described in patients with cellulitis and other serious forms of streptococcal skin infection.[93] Varieties of these conditions include acute perianal cellulitis, most commonly seen in children in association with streptococcal upper respiratory tract infection,[94] and pilonidal and Bartholin's gland abscesses, which are usually caused by organisms colonizing the perineum from the faeces and genital tract, including groups B and G and anaerobic streptococci, and *S. anginosus*, often in mixed infection with other organisms.

Erysipelas

This is an acute, tender, erythematous lesion with an irregular, sharply demarcated edge associated with the spread of infection in subepidermal tissues.[53,73] It occurs most commonly on the face, particularly in patients with streptococcal upper respiratory tract infection, but lesions may occur elsewhere in the body and may follow wounds and abrasions of the skin. This is a rare disease, principally of adults, and it is now mainly seen in the elderly. Due to the problems of specimen collection there may be difficulties reaching a specific bacteriological diagnosis in some patients with erysipelas but culture of blood and of aspirated fluid from the advancing edge of the lesion may prove positive.[72] The lesions may be in part due to a hypersensitivity to streptococcal products.[76] Persistent and recurrent forms of erysipelas and cellulitis sometimes occur in patients with lymphatic or vascular obstruction;[95] these lesions are usually caused by streptococci but *Haemophilus influenzae* and pneumococci account for some cases.[53]

Necrotizing fasciitis

This condition, in which acute or subacute infection spreads above the fascial planes causing thrombosis of vessels and necrosis of the dermis and subcutaneous fat, is usually caused by haemolytic or anaerobic streptococci or *Staph. aureus*.[76, 96] The disease may follow trivial or inapparent injury to the skin and present initially with cellulitis, which quickly develops a dusky discoloration, haemorrhagic bullae and underlying areas of deep necrosis. There is a risk of septicaemia and rapid death. Necrotizing fasciitis is most commonly seen in patients of older age groups, often in association with serious pre-existing medical disorders.

Other secondary and miscellaneous infections

Non-haemolytic streptococci have been isolated together with *Staph. aureus* or Gram-negative bacilli from patients with the rare condition of Meleney's postoperative progressive synergistic gangrene in which infection slowly spreads in the abdominal wall to produce necrosis and ulceration.[97] More recent study of the condition suggests that *Entamoeba histolytica* implanted into the wound from the viscera at operation may be the main microbial cause of this infection.[98]

Streptococcus pyogenes may colonize the umbilicus of neonates or older patients but in some it produces omphalitis and a persistent granuloma may form at the site;[57] in occasional patients the infection may progress to septicaemia.[73]

Miscellaneous infections associated with streptococci include ophthalmia neonatorum, in which the non-haemolytic *S. mutans* and *S. mitis* have been found more commonly than in the conjunctival sac of normal babies,[58] keratoconjunctivitis, which has been reported in patients of all ages with Lancefield group A, B and G streptococci,[99] and suppurative hidradenitis, in which *S. anginosus* and anaerobic streptococci sometimes play a part.[100]

The skin and soft tissues provide a major portal of entry for invasive haemolytic, non-haemolytic and anaerobic streptococcal infections.[86, 101] In several recent compilations of *S. pyogenes* bacteraemia these structures were the most commonly documented sources of infection; local conditions leading to invasion included impetiginous and eczematous infection, infected ulcers,

traumatic wounds, intravenous access sites and varicella lesions, cellulitis and
necrotizing fasciitis.[86, 102–104]

Epidemiological settings for outbreaks of streptococcal skin infection

Much of the global burden of streptococcal skin infection occurs among
children and their contacts under poor socioeconomic conditions of overcrowding and poor hygiene, particularly in warm and humid parts of the
world. In such communities streptococcal infection is commonly endemic,
with additional periodic widespread outbreaks caused by newly introduced
strains, and there may be a very high rate of associated complications, such as
post-streptococcal nephritis.

Even in developed parts of the world, haemolytic streptococci are still
commonly isolated from a wide range of clinical specimens.[43, 105] The
perpetuation of streptococcal infection is due to a number of factors including
the common asymptomatic carriage of organisms, the minor nature of most
infections, many untreated, and the opportunities for bacterial transmission
that exist as people work, live and play together. Outbreaks of streptococcal
skin and wound infection remain a problem in certain groups of patients and
a variety of epidemiological settings has been described in recent years,
including patients and staff on hospital wards,[53, 55] in residential schools,[30]
prisons and other detention centres, military training camps,[106] police training
centres,[107] among rugby football teams,[108] carpenters, meat handlers[28, 109, 110]
and agricultural workers.[111] When there is an adequate intake of new
susceptible patients to an institution, outbreaks may become persistent,
endemic problems.[30] Infected groups may act as reservoirs of infection,
allowing the spread of organisms to others outside the group as circumstances
permit. In patients working closely with animals there may also be opportunities for zoonotic infection with unusual haemolytic streptococci, such as *S.
zooepidemicus* (group C),[61] group L[64] and group R[65, 92], but most occupational
infections with these organisms are sporadic.

Haemolytic streptococcal cross-infection within hospitals was once a
common cause of serious illness and death. Careful clinical and epidemiological studies showed the importance of direct transmission of streptococci
on the hands of attendants by physical examinations and by unhygienic
dressing changes, indirect transmission by contaminated uniforms, instruments and airborne routes, the significance of respiratory carriers and the need
to segregate patients with active, discharging infections to prevent cross-
infection. Many workers contributed to these advances, which helped to lay

the broad foundations of modern hygienic medical and surgical practice; a particularly useful contribution to this effort was the opportunity taken by several workers to study wound infection during the two World Wars.[26, 54, 59] Despite modern arrangements, localized outbreaks of streptococcal skin and wound infection still occur within hospitals; outbreaks of postoperative *S. pyogenes* wound infection have been traced to carriers in the surgical team or other operating theatre staff;[46, 56] outbreaks in burns and plastic surgery units and in the ulcers and pressure sores of patients on geriatric medical wards have been described with groups A, C and G streptococci;[21, 55, 112, 113] 'carrier epidemics' with group B streptococci on neonatal nurseries have resulted in some local sepsis and occasional invasive infections.[48] Outbreaks tend to occur in hospital units when inadequate attention has been given to hygiene, such as during periods when there is insufficient staffing or a heavy case-load, and they often follow the inadvertent admission of an infected patient shedding large numbers of streptococci.

Streptococcal and staphylococcal skin sepsis in meat and poultry handlers has become increasingly recognized in the United Kingdom since the mid-1970s[109, 110] and there are a few reports from other parts of the world, including Norway and the United States.[114-116] Figure 8.1 gives a simplified scheme of the meat trade showing the principal occupations that have been associated with skin sepsis. In a review of 389 patients with meat-associated skin infection in North Yorkshire, 96 per cent of those with positive bacteriological cultures yielded haemolytic streptococci or *Staph. aureus*.[110] In that study there were 6 large outbreaks in chicken and turkey slaughter/processing factories and 10 outbreaks in red-meat handlers, often affecting 40–70 per cent of the workforce of the establishments; infection was seen in abattoirs, related retail butchers and pig slaughter/processing factories, and among meat inspectors, chefs and restaurateurs. The variety of skin infections seen included septic cuts and scratches, paronychia, abscess, lymphangitis and infection in pierced ear lobes and fresh tattoos. Newly employed workers suffered the highest rates of infection and spread was noted amongst the families of some workers. Studies of meat handlers have shown a clear tendency for more infection to occur in the autumn and early winter months, although prolonged outbreaks and sporadic infections may be found throughout the year;[109, 110] the seasonal increase in infection is thought to relate to the increased work done in abattoirs and processing factories at that time of year.

Injury to the skin is a major predeterminant of infection in meat and poultry handlers, as it is in other groups subject to streptococcal pyoderma. Groups of meat workers most exposed to trauma from knives, saws and sharp bones were found to have the highest rates of infection attack whereas those with low

Table 8.6. *Beta-haemolytic streptococci found in two surveys of skin infection in meat handlers*

| Lancefield group | No. of infections yielding streptococci in survey | | |
	North Yorkshire[a]	Scotland[b]	Total (%)
A	242	45	287 (87)
B	4	5	9 (2.7)
C	1	4	5 (1.5)
E	1	—	1 (0.3)
G	7	6	13 (3.9)
L	13	2	15 (4.5)
Ungroupable	1	—	1 (0.3)
Total (all groups)	269	62	331 (100)

[a] Surveys 1978–1986; [b] survey 1983–1985.
Figures in parentheses show percentage of the total streptococci found.
After Barnham and Neilson.[64]

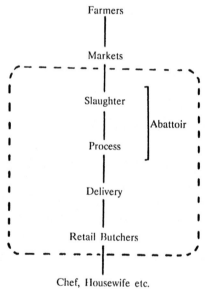

Fig. 8.1. Simplified scheme of the meat trade; the main areas in which meat-associated streptococcal sepsis has been found are marked around with a dotted line.

injury rates in the factories, such as cleaners, drivers, supervisors and office workers, were rarely affected.[32] Bone fragments might contribute to the problems of infection by contaminating the wounds of workers and acting as foreign bodies to potentiate infection.[32]

Haemolytic streptococci have been found in about two-thirds of the infected wounds of meat handlers that yield positive bacteriological cultures.[110] In extended surveys of these workers in North Yorkshire and Scotland,[64] *S. pyogenes* accounted for 87 per cent of haemolytic streptococci isolated, as shown in Table 8.6. Many different T/M types of *S. pyogenes* have now been reported from the infected lesions of meat handlers, mostly of the 'high M number' or complex T-type pattern, M-untypable profiles that are characteristic of skin infection.[20] These organisms are thought to spread from human sources person-to-person or via contaminated environmental surfaces and equipment under the conditions of work. Amongst the various non-group A streptococci isolated from the infected lesions of meat handlers, group L has been the most common, accounting in one study for 4.5 per cent of isolates (Table 8.6);[64] clinical features were similar to those associated with *S. pyogenes* and the organisms were thought to be of pathogenic significance. Group L streptococci are common in chickens and pigs, and these animals are thought to be the source of environmental contamination in the factories and infection in the meat handlers.

Skin sepsis with *S. pyogenes* is an occasional problem for teams of rugby football and American football players.[19, 53] The lesions in areas of traumatized skin are usually impetiginous in nature but more serious forms of wound infection and erysipelas sometimes occur; the infection needs to be distinguished from other forms of 'scrumpox', such as that caused by herpes simplex virus.[117] In an outbreak in a rugby team, one player suffered post-streptococcal nephritis and infection spread to affect the front-row players of at least one other team and to two girlfriends, one of whom developed salpingitis.[108]

Streptococcal pyoderma and ecthyma have been described among military servicemen, particularly when under combat conditions in tropical and subtropical ares of the world.[42, 53] Insect bites, blisters and other forms of trauma to the skin create the opportunity for infection to occur in these men; in a large outbreak amongst military trainees in south-west England, *S. pyogenes* infection developed in the scratches produced by exercising in a terrain thickly grown with gorse and thorn bushes.[106]

In outbreaks of pyoderma in prisons, detention centres, police and military training centres and school athletics teams, shared recreational equipment such as coconut matting and climbing ropes have been found to be a common cause of abrasions and burns to the skin;[106,107] during outbreaks such items are often found to be contaminated with *S. pyogenes* and they might act as an environmental source of infection.

Certain other occupational groups are subject to streptococcal skin and wound infection. Outbreaks have been observed among woodsmen and carpenters, who commonly suffer lacerations to the skin, and splinters and sawdust might act as foreign bodies to potentiate infection in their wounds. In an outbreak in a small arable farming community, infection with *S. pyogenes* occurred in the occupational wounds of farmers and in wounds acquired by their wives from household and kitchen duties.[111]

Post-streptococcal glomerulonephritis (PSGN) and skin infection

In developed countries the incidence of overt PSGN has declined markedly in recent decades, although it remains a common complication of streptococcal infections of the skin or throat in many other parts of the world. Clinical symptoms and signs develop after a latent period of usually 10–21 days after the streptococcal infection and commonly include haematuria, oedema, hypertension and a temporary reduction in urine output. There may be clusters of cases within families and other groups affected by the streptococcal infection. Laboratory findings include cultural or serological evidence of the infection, proteinuria, haematuria, reduced serum complement levels and abnormalities of renal function tests. It is a disease of variable severity and in many recorded outbreaks asymptomatic cases have outnumbered those with symptoms several-fold;[118,119] renal biopsy examination of asymptomatic children with decreased serum complement and/or abnormal urinalysis after streptococcal infection confirmed changes compatible with PSGN in a large proportion of cases.[120] In some patients the disease may progress to chronic glomerulonephritis and they may eventually require dialysis or renal transplantation.[121–124]

Nephritis occurs more readily after infection of the skin than of the throat: in a study of M-type 49 *S. pyogenes* infection on the Red Lake Indian Reservation in Minnesota, acute PSGN or unexplained haematuria developed in 24 per cent of children with pyoderma, 4.5 per cent with pharyngitis and 19 per cent of those infected with the organism at both sites.[119] Differences in the basic epidemiological features of streptococcal infections of skin and throat give rise to differences in the presentation of PSGN associated with these sites of infection: in nephritis after pyoderma, patients tend to be younger (often less than 6 years old), the sexes are equally affected (as compared with 2:1 male to female ratio after respiratory infection), there is a longer latent period (commonly 18–21 days compared with about 10 days after respiratory infection) and the seasonal peak of disease occurs typically in summer and autumn (as compared with winter and spring after respiratory infection).[19,125]

A protein believed to be a variant streptokinase enzyme with special affinity for the glomerular basement membrane – 'nephrostreptokinase' or nephritis strain-associated protein (NSAP) – is a strong contender as the pathogenic agent in glomerulonephritis developing after *S. pyogenes* infection.[126] Other candidates include endostreptosin (ESS),[123] thought to be an intracellular precursor of NSAP, and 'pre-absorbing antigen', which may be a breakdown product of NSAP.[126] Binding of nephrostreptokinase to the glomerular basement membrane may be followed by plasminogen activation, deposition of antibody and complement, and infiltration by inflammatory cells, with consequent disturbance of glomerular function; high levels of antibody to NSAP and ESS are found in patients with acute PSGN.[122,127]

Certain T/M types of *S. pyogenes* have been associated more commonly than others with PSGN, the so-called 'nephritogenic types';[128] as shown in Table 8.7, some types, such as M12 and M49, have been regularly associated with the complication whereas in others the evidence for a link has been weaker.[125] Cross-reactions have been described between epitopes of streptococcal M protein and renal glomerular basement membrane,[129,130] and conformational differences have been shown in M protein structure between nephritogenic and non-nephritogenic types;[131] however, the significance of these findings with respect to PSGN is unclear. Nephritogenicity as a character appears to be independent of the M type as such[132] but associated with certain strains within the types; some recent epidemics with classic nephritogenic serotypes of *S. pyogenes* such as M type 49 in England[20] and M type 12 in Japan[70] were not associated with increases in overt PSGN. In recent years, PSGN has also been reported to occur after infection with group C[21,133] and group G streptococci,[134] and responsible organisms of both groups have been shown to produce ESS or molecular variants of NSAP.

Seroepidemiological studies have shown that most people develop antibodies to ESS after common streptococcal infections in childhood.[122] It remains unclear whether the present low incidence of overt PSGN in developed countries is mainly due to patterns of acquired immunity in the population, perhaps with an increased proportion of subclinical disease, or to an inability of the predominant circulating strains of streptococci to produce large amounts of nephrostreptokinase.

Table 8.7. *Groups and types of haemolytic streptococci associated with post-streptococcal nephritis*

Group	Comment/species	Type
Group A[a]	Strong evidence	T12M12, M49
	Good evidence	M1, T25/Imp.19M2, M4, T25/Imp.19M55
	Reasonable evidence	T3/13/B3264M3, M25, T25/Imp.19M57, M60
	Some evidence	T5/27/44M5, T4/28M5, M6, M11, M14, M31, M52, M53, M54, M56, some non-typable strains with 'skin' T-typing patterns
Group C[b]	*S. equisimilis*	T204
	S. zooepidemicus	Several bacteriocin/bacteriophage types
Group G		Types not yet determined

[a] Based on Ferrieri.[125]
[b] See Efstratiou[21] and Barnham et al.[133]

Cutaneous manifestations of distant streptococcal infection

Table 8.8 lists a variety of rashes that may be associated with active streptococcal infection in the body, whether in the skin, wounds, throat, genital tract or at other sites. The detailed pathogenesis of these lesions remains largely unknown but a variety of mechanisms is likely to be involved, including damage from absorbed toxins, enzymes and other streptococcal products deposited in the skin, immunological reactions to these at that site or involving the deposition of circulating immune complexes in the skin vasculature, immunological cross-reactions between streptococcal and host tissue antigens, and direct damage caused by the infection in bacteraemic patients.

Scarlet fever

Scarlet fever is most commonly associated with *S. pyogenes* infection of the throat but it may also follow infection at other sites, including skin sores, burns and wounds (such as in 'surgical scarlet fever') and the genital tract (as in 'puerperal scarlet fever').[135] There is often an abrupt onset of malaise and headache with the appearance of the erythematous rash, which typically shows circumoral pallor, a 'strawberry' tongue and desquamation in convalescence.[135] The severity of the disease has varied greatly from time to time and place to place as judged by historical records; during this century there has been a great decline in complications and death due to the disease in developed

Table 8.8. *Cutaneous manifestations that may be associated with*
streptococcal infection elsewhere in the body

Scarlet fever
Rheumatic fever rashes (including papular lesions, erythema marginatum and
    subcutaneous nodules)
Urticaria and diffuse erythematous reactions
Erythema multiforme
Purpura (including petechiae and 'purpura fulminans')
Erythema nodosum
Cutaneous vasculitis
Desquamation at extremities
Peripheral gangrene (including 'auto-amputation')
Psoriasis (especially the acute guttate form)
Pityriasis alba
Skin lesions in endocarditis (including splinter haemorrhages, Osler's nodes)

countries of the world, starting before, and now perhaps reinforced by, the era of antibiotics.[136] In the United Kingdom in recent years, scarlet fever has been a mild disease, typical 'full-blown' cases have been uncommon, and there have been difficulties in reliably diagnosing the modern forms of the condition on clinical grounds alone.[137] In the United Kingdom, scarlet fever has been particularly associated with *S. pyogenes* of M types 1, 3, 4 and 6[20] and, with the increasing occurrence of M type-4 streptococci in the late 1980s, there have been increasing numbers of reports of the disease.[138]

The rash of scarlet fever is thought to result from toxicity and hypersensitivity to three antigenically distinct streptococcal pyrogenic exotoxins (SPE), termed A, B and C; a strain of *S. pyogenes* may produce one or more of these toxins but they have not been found in streptococci of other Lancefield groups.[139] Recent research on SPE-A shows its potential as a major streptococcal virulence factor. In addition to producing the scarlet fever rash it is responsible for a wide range of biological effects including enhancement of susceptibility to endotoxin shock, pyrogenicity, cytotoxicity for various tissues including the heart, depression of the clearance function of the reticulo-endothelial system, alteration of the blood–brain barrier, non-specific mitogenicity for T-cells and suppression of B-lymphocyte function.[140,141] SPE-A shows almost 50 per cent structural homology with the staphylococcal enterotoxin B, one of the main staphylococcal toxins associated with the toxic shock syndrome.[142] The gene for production of SPE-A is located on the temperate bacteriophage T12 and toxigenic conversion of *S. pyogenes* has been shown after infection with the phage.[143] SPE-C is also associated with

bacteriophage and shows structural similarity to SPE-A;[141] SPE-B has a
different structure, being secreted as a zymogen and converted to a proteinase
with functions including mitogenicity and cytotoxicity for cardiac and other
tissue cells.

Genes encoding for production of SPE-A, -B and -C have been found in 29,
100 and 50 per cent, respectively, of a recent collection of over 500 isolates of
S. pyogenes from around the world,[144] but these genes may not always be
phenotypically expressed. Isolates from patients with scarlet fever in the
United Kingdom were recently found only to produce SPE-B or -C; in
contrast 4/10 isolates saved from patients in this country before 1940 produced
SPE-A.[139,145] Scarlet fever-associated isolates in the United States gave similar
results, showing production only of SPE-B or -C,[142] but in the late 1980s,
patients with SPE A-producing *S. pyogenes* were reported again, many
featuring severe cellulitis or necrotizing fasciitis in association with marked
systemic toxicity resembling the staphylococcal toxic shock syn-
drome.[140,142,146] The serious 'toxic' form of scarlet fever seen in earlier years[135]
was perhaps due to SPE A-producing *S. pyogenes* infection and, in view of the
recent case reports, there appears to be a risk that this might become re-
established in parts of the developed world. More research is needed to
determine the significance of high-level production of SPE-B and -C by
streptococci in serious infection.[147]

A further 'septic' variety of scarlet fever was once recognized, in which the
local streptococcal infection progressed to suppuration or septicaemia with
development of foci of infection in the bones, joints or soft tissues.[135] This form
of the disease has been very rarely seen in developed countries since the
introduction of antibiotics but the recent rise in invasive M type-1 *S. pyogenes*
infections in the United Kingdom and parts of Scandinavia[20,148] has led to
reports of a few patients featuring serious invasive disease together with scarlet
fever.[149]

Many other rashes occur non-specifically in association with streptococcal
infection, including urticaria and other diffuse erythematous reactions,
erythema multiforme, erythema nodosum and, in rheumatic fever patients, a
range of papular lesions, subcutaneous nodules and erythema marginatum.[150]
Cutaneous vasculitis may occur in a variety of forms after streptococcal
infection, including the low-grade form of leucocytoclastic angiitis known as
erythema elevatum diutinum.[151] Petechial haemorrhages have been noticed in
the skin of children with streptococcal pharyngitis[152,153] and they may occur in
some patients with scarlet fever.[135] In a study of 190 children with fever and
petechiae, the most common bacterial association was with *S. pyogenes* upper
respiratory tract infection.[154] More profuse purpuric lesions, including

purpura fulminans, are sometimes seen in patients with streptococcal septicaemia and disseminated intravascular coagulation, in whom there is also a risk of peripheral gangrene and 'auto-amputation'; in convalescence from severe streptococcal infection a thick desquamation of the skin of the hands and feet may occur. Patients with streptococcal subacute bacterial endocarditis may show Osler's nodes in the fingers and toes, and splinter haemorrhages under the nails, but these signs also occur in cases of non-streptococcal background. Superficial streptococcal infections of the skin occasionally lead to pityriasis alba, a form of dermatitis in which there is a failure of affected areas to tan on exposure to sunlight.[155]

Acute guttate psoriasis

The development of acute guttate psoriasis in children and young adults, and the exacerbation of existing psoriatic lesions, is frequently preceded by haemolytic streptococcal infection of the throat.[53,156] In a study of 101 patients and controls, *S. pyogenes* was isolated from the throats of 26 per cent with acute guttate psoriasis, 14 per cent with guttate exacerbations of chronic psoriasis and 16 per cent with chronic psoriasis, but from only 7 per cent of controls;[157] serological evidence of streptococcal infection was found in two-thirds of the patients with acute guttate psoriasis. Many different T/M types of *S. pyogenes* have been isolated from such patients and streptococci of groups B, C and G have also been isolated from various sites in the body in association with the disease.[157,158] The evidence suggests that streptococci are particularly important in the aetiology of guttate psoriasis; other known triggers of the disease include some viral infections, drugs, emotional stress and physical and chemical trauma to the skin.[159] The pathogenic mechanisms involved are not yet clear; one hypothesis suggests that capillary abnormalities induced by deposited streptococcal products or hypersensivity reactions to them might trigger the rash non-specifically in susceptible patients, in the manner of the Köbner phenomenon.[53,151] Immunological cross-reactions have also been demonstrated between *S. pyogenes* and certain tissue components in human skin, and large amounts of the relevant components have been found in psoriatic lesions.[160]

Further aspects of streptococcal pathogenicity

A complex interaction of bacterial and host defence factors underlies the initiation, development and clinical manifestations of streptococcal infection. The application of modern molecular techniques has been invaluable in furthering our understanding of this, particularly in research into the surface structures and soluble products of streptococci, which are believed to contribute to their pathogenicity.

The M-protein molecule is known to be a major virulence factor of streptococci; it occurs as a double-stranded coiled-coil structure projecting from the cell surface and its functional properties include fibrinogen, fibronectin and β_2-microglobulin binding, adherence to host cells, interference with complement deposition and the conferring of resistance to phagocytosis.[130] The quantity of M protein expressed on the cell surface appears to be an important factor in pathogenesis: freshly isolated strains of group A, C and G streptococci, particularly those from invasive infections, are often rich in this substance[22] and serotypes of *S. pyogenes* such as M1, which express large quantities, are commonly associated with invasive disease.[20,148] Enhancement of M-protein expression may be a factor underlying the increased virulence observed when streptococci are rapidly passaged from host to host.[161] The binding of fibrinogen and fibronectin by streptococcal surface structures may play an important part in the attachment of organisms to wounds and clots in the first stages of colonization and infection,[162] and to foreign bodies coated with host proteins.[163]

Immunological cross-reactivities have been shown between certain streptococcal components, including M protein, and mammalian proteins in heart, kidney, brain and joint tissue,[129,130,164] but their pathological significance in relation to post-streptococcal complications remains unresolved.

Other projecting cell-surface molecules with similarities to M protein in their cell-wall attachment structure show further functions including the destruction of complement C5a, a major signal substance for the chemotactic attraction of leucocytes, and binding to the Fc portion of IgG and IgA antibodies. Immunoglobulin binding has been found in a high proportion of clinical isolates of *S. pyogenes*[165] but its role in pathogenesis remains unclear; IgG-binding activity is particularly common in pyoderma isolates while high binding of IgA has been found in a large proportion of deep-tissue isolates.[166] Other capsular and cell envelope moieties of streptococci that deter phagocytosis or are otherwise damaging to the host include hyaluronic acid, teichoic acid, lipoteichoic acid, surface polysaccharides and peptidoglycan.[167]

Some soluble products of streptococci may also contribute to the evolution of infection. Streptococcal enzymes such as nucleases, proteinases and hyaluronidases are thought to assist in the liquefaction of pus and the spread of infection in the tissues and into the lymphatic channels.[167] Streptokinase enzymes activate plasminogen to produce rapid lysis of fibrin clots. Streptolysin O damages the integrity of cholesterol-containing membranes in a variety of cells, causing a release of cytoplasmic constituents; this is thought to disrupt local phagocytic function and inhibit chemotaxis.[167] Preliminary evidence suggests that haemolytic streptococci can stimulate macrophages to produce tumour necrosis factor, a substance that plays an important part in the development of the septic shock syndrome.[168] The absorption of other particular products from the site of infection may result in certain distant manifestations of infection, such as nephritis and scarlet fever, as previously described.

Serological findings in streptococcal infection

Immunological reactions occur to many different antigens in streptococcal infection and numerous assays have been developed to detect them. Antibodies developing to streptococcal M antigens after respiratory tract or systemic infections are thought to confer immunity to challenge with the same type, and possibly other particular types, of streptococci.[19, 169, 170] M-antibody responses in streptococcal pyoderma have received much less attention and it is not known what part they might play in immunity to homotypic challenge.[19, 33] Type-specific antibody against pyoderma strains of *S. pyogenes* has been found most commonly in those patients harbouring the organism in the pharynx[171] and may depend upon the ability of the streptococcus, unusual in skin strains, to cause significant infection there. Some M proteins of skin-infecting streptococci have been found to be poorly antigenic in man and experimental animals.[172, 173]

For serological diagnosis of infection the measurement of antibodies against a number of streptococcal antigens has been used including antistreptolysin O (ASO), antideoxyribonuclease B (antiDNAase B), antihyaluronidase (using enzyme antigens from group A or groups C/G according to the antibody to be detected), antinicotinamide adenine dinucleotide glycohydrolase (anti-NADase), antistreptokinase (ASK) and antibodies to the various Lancefield-group carbohydrate antigens. The performance of multiple tests on each serum may prove useful and ideally a fourfold or greater change in titre between acute and convalescent sera should be sought. The results from single sera may prove difficult to interpret as the notional upper limits of normal for streptococcal antibodies may vary according to factors such as age, season and population group studied.[72] Early antibiotic treatment of streptococcal infection can inhibit the development of some antibody responses[173] and reduce the chances of demonstrating a rising titre.

Changes in ASO titre may be found in infection with group A, C (*S. equisimilis*) and G haemolytic streptococci but not with streptococci of other commonly encountered groups; elevation of antiDNAase B is thought to be specific for infection with *S. pyogenes*. In skin infection there is usually a brisk response in antiDNAase B[19,173,174] but feeble responses in antiNADase[33,167] and in ASO titre, the last due to an inhibitory effect of skin lipids on the enzyme.[77] In patients with post-streptococcal nephritis, marked and prolonged elevations of antibodies to the implicated streptococcal proteins NSAP and ESS have been described.[122,127]

Treatment of streptococcal infection

The rationale of antimicrobial therapy for streptococcal infections of the skin is to hasten the resolution of lesions, to reduce the risks of suppurative and non-suppurative complications and to reduce the chance of transmission of infection to others. Ideally the treatment should be highly effective in all forms of the disease, safe, cheap, brief and pleasant for the patient. The extent to which the many agents available achieve these various goals and how they compare with each other have not been fully resolved despite a long period of research and debate.[33,175]

Mechanical debridement and local disinfection of pyoderma lesions with antiseptics such as hexachlorophane or chlorhexidine give little improvement over the spontaneous resolution rate for this infection[33] but may be sufficient treatment for mild, sporadic cases.[72] Local antibiotic preparations are often prescribed for skin sepsis but many are inappropriate for streptococci, such as those containing sodium fusidate, neomycin, gentamicin, framycetin or polymyxin to which the organisms are naturally resistant, and there is a risk of sensitizing the patient to the drug or encouraging the emergence of bacterial resistance. Tetracycline is often contraindicated as a local treatment for *S. pyogenes* skin sepsis on grounds of bacterial resistance: in a large study in meat handlers, 59 per cent of skin-infecting isolates showed tetracycline resistance[28] and a review in Cambridge showed a much higher occurrence of this trait in skin- than throat-infecting streptococci.[176] The newly available topical antibiotic mupirocin has given encouraging results in the treatment of streptococcal and staphylococcal pyoderma, with comparable success rates and fewer side-effects than in control patients treated with oral erythromycin;[175,177] the agent has also been used to eradicate staphylococci from sites of carriage but resistance is now being reported amongst these organisms.[178]

Oral or injected antibiotics have generally been preferred to topical agents for the treatment of streptococcal skin infections, and penicillin and erythromycin have given high success rates;[33] in serious or invasive infections clindamycin has sometimes proved superior even to these.[179] Some isolates of viridans-group streptococci and *S. anginosus* may exhibit resistance to penicillin[180] but this character has not yet been found in *S. pyogenes*. Erythromycin resistance is currently reported in 2–5 per cent of *S. pyogenes* isolates in the United Kingdom and United States, with local increases up to 15–25 per cent, but resistance levels up to 72 per cent were reported from Japan in the 1970s;[181, 182] erythromycin resistance in Lancefield group B–G streptococci and *S. anginosus* has now been reported in 0.6–6.4 per cent of isolates.[181, 183] It remains good policy to collect specimens for bacteriological testing and to base or revise antibiotic treatment according to the susceptibility of the isolated organisms.

Haemolytic streptococci and *Staph. aureus* are often found either together or singly in septic skin lesions and it is rational to choose antibiotics active against both organisms, such as flucloxacillin, erythromycin or mupirocin, at least until bacteriological results are known. Beta-lactamase enzymes from staphylococci and other organisms greatly raise the penicillin minimum inhibitory concentration of cocultivated *S. pyogenes*;[184] however, there have been conflicting reports on the efficacy of penicillin for eradicating *S. pyogenes* from skin lesions in patients also harbouring *Staph. aureus*, most claiming that the treatment would succeed.[72, 185, 186] Flucloxacillin has enough antistreptococcal activity to give good results in the treatment of patients with mixed streptococcal and staphylococcal skin infections.[28, 109, 185]

Early antibiotic therapy of streptococcal infection is usually successful in preventing acute rheumatic fever[187] but it has proved much less effective for the prevention of glomerulonephritis. One often quoted study reported a lower rate of haematuria and acute nephritis in patients treated with penicillin for M-type 12 *Strep. pyogenes* respiratory infection than in those given placebo,[188] but others have failed to confirm this effect and no such benefit has been evident in patients treated for *S. pyogenes* skin infection.[72, 187] Early treatment may, however, reduce the chances of spread of nephritogenic streptococci to other susceptible patients.

The prophylactic administration of penicillin to susceptible patients during outbreaks of streptococcal skin infection has been found to reduce the incidence and prevalence of infection and give protection to treated individuals for several weeks.[33, 72, 113] Individuals who suffer recurrent attacks of erysipelas or other serious forms of streptococcal infection may benefit from prolonged periods of antibiotic prophylaxis.[95, 189]

General prevention of infection

The prevention of streptococcal infections of the skin is a complex topic largely beyond the scope of this review. Various relevant factors include the improvement of housing to avoid overcrowding, promotion of personal hygiene, the control of biting arthropods (such as scabies and lice, which provoke excoriation) and reduction in the risks of occupational or recreational trauma (such as exposure to sharp instruments and bone in meat-handling establishments, and abrasive coconut matting in gymnasia). A good system of surveillance and reporting of infection is helpful, particularly in settings where outbreaks of infection have been known to occur before, and prompt investigation of suspected outbreaks with early treatment of those affected should help to contain the spread of infection. Patients admitted to hospital with *S. pyogenes* infection should be nursed in isolation until at least 48 h of adequate therapy has been given to reduce the possibility of transmission to other patients.

Good teamwork and rapid dissemination of information between bacteriologist, clinicians and those with particular responsibility for public health can do much to control and reduce the burden of streptococcal skin disease.

References

1 Ball LC, Parker MT. The cultural and biochemical characters of *Streptococcus milleri* strains isolated from human sources. J Hyg Camb 1979; 82: 63–78.

2 Ruoff KL. *Streptococcus anginosus* ('*Streptococcus milleri*'): the unrecognized pathogen. Clin Microbiol Rev 1988; 1: 102–08.

3 Kilpper-Balz R, Schleifer KH. Nucleic acid hybridization and cell wall composition studies of pyogenic streptococci. FEMS Microbiol Lett 1984; 24: 355–64.

4 Farrow JAE, Collins MD. Taxonomic studies on streptococci of serological groups C, G and L and possibly related taxa. System Appl Microbiol 1984; 5: 483–93.

5 Kilian M, Mikkelsen L, Henrichsen J. Taxonomic study of viridans streptococci: description of *Streptococcus gordonii* sp. nov. and emended descriptions of *Streptococcus sanguis* (White and Niven 1946), *Streptococcus oralis* (Bridge and Sneath 1982) and *Streptococcus mitis* (Andrewes and Horder 1906). Int J System Bacteriol 1989; 39: 471–84.

6 Parker MT. Streptococcus and lactobacillus. In: Parker MT, ed. Topley and Wilson's principles of bacteriology, virology and immunity, vol. 2. London: Edward Arnold; 1983: 173–217.

7 Coykendall AL. Classification and identification of the viridans streptococci. Clin Microbiol Rev 1989; 2: 315–28.

8 Facklam RR. In: Wannamaker LW, Matsen JM, eds. Streptococci and streptococcal diseases. New York: Academic Press; 1972: 206.

9 Saunders KA, Ball LC. The influence of the composition of blood agar on beta haemolysis by *Streptococcus salivarius*. Med Lab Sci 1980; 37: 341–45.

10 Murray BE. The life and times of the Enterococcus. Clin Microbiol Rev 1990; 3: 46–65.

11 Facklam RR, Collins MD. Identification of *Enterococcus* species isolated from human infections by a conventional test scheme. J Clin Microbiol 1989; 27: 731–34.

12 Birch BR, Keaney MGL, Ganguli LA. Antibiotic susceptibility and biochemical properties of *Streptococcus faecalis* strains reacting with both D and G antisera. J Clin Pathol 1984; 37: 1289–92.

13 George RC, Uttley AHC. Susceptibility of enterococci and epidemiology of enterococcal infection in the 1980s. Epidemiol Infect 1989; 103: 403–13.

14 Gillespie SH. Aspects of pneumococcal infection including bacterial virulence, host response and vaccination. J Med Microbiol 1989; 28: 237–48.

15 Parker MT. Staphylococcus and micrococcus; the anaerobic gram-positive cocci. In: Parker MT, ed. Topley and Wilson's principles of bacteriology, virology and immunity, vol 2. London: Edward Arnold; 1983: 218–45.

16 Ezaki T, Yabuuchi E. Oligopeptidase activity of gram-positive anaerobic cocci used for rapid identification. J Gen Appl Microbiol 1985; 31: 255–65.

17 Willis AT. Anaerobic bacteriology: clinical and laboratory practice. London: Butterworths, 1977: 202–04.

18 Colman G, Efstratiou A, Gaworzewska ET. The pyogenic streptococci. PHLS Microbiol Digest 1988; 5: 5–7.

19 Wannamaker LW. Differences between streptococcal infections of the throat and of the skin. N Engl J Med 1970; 282: 23–30; 78–85.

20 Gaworzewska E, Colman G. Changes in the pattern of infection caused by *Streptococcus pyogenes*. Epidemiol Infect 1988; 100: 257–69.

21 Efstratiou A. Outbreaks of human infection caused by pyogenic streptococci of Lancefield groups C and G. J Med Microbiol 1989; 29: 207–19.

22 Jones KF, Fischetti VA. Biological and immunochemical identity of M protein on group G streptococci with M protein on group A streptococci. Infect Immun 1987; 55: 502–06.

23 Colman G. Typing methods for group B streptococci. J Med Microbiol 1984; 18: 144–46.

24 Cleary PP, Kaplan EL, Livdahl C, Skjold S. DNA fingerprints of *Streptococcus pyogenes* are M type specific. J Infect Dis 1988; 158: 1317–23.

25 Efstratiou A, Colman G, Crowley D, Pitcher D. Ribotyping of human pyogenic streptococci. In: Orefia G, ed. New perspectives on streptococci and streptococcal infections. Stuttgart: Gustav Fischer Verlag; 1992: 90–91.

26 Hare R. Sources of haemolytic streptococcal infection of wounds in war and in civil life. Lancet 1940; i: 109–12.

27 Ogunbi O, Fadahunsi HO, Ahmed I, Animashaun A, Daniel SO, Onuoha DU, Ogunbi LQO. An epidemiological study of rheumatic fever and rheumatic heart disease in Lagos. J Epidem Comm Health 1978; 32: 68–71.

28 Barnham M. A study of streptococcal skin sepsis in meat and poultry handlers. [MD thesis]. London University; 1989.

29 Colling A, Kerr I, Maxted WR, Widdowson JP. Streptococcal infection in a junior detention centre: a five-year study. J Hyg Camb 1980; 85: 331–41.

30 Leading article. Streptococci in institutions. Lancet 1981; i: 311–12.

31 Hamburger M, Green MJ. The problem of the dangerous carrier of hemolytic streptococci. J Infect Dis 1946; 79: 33–44.

32 Barnham M, Kerby J. Skin sepsis in meat handlers: observations on the causes of injury with special reference to bone. J Hyg Camb 1981; 87: 465–76.

33 Peter G, Smith AL. Group A streptococcal infections of the skin and pharynx. N Engl J Med 1977; 297; 311–17; 365–70.

34 Dudding BA, Burnett JW, Chapman SS, Wannamaker LW. The role of normal skin in the spread of streptococcal pyoderma. J Hyg Camb 1970; 68: 19–28.

35 Ferrieri P, Dajani AS, Wannamaker LW, Chapman SS. Natural history of impetigo: site sequence of acquisition and familial patterns of spread of cutaneous streptococci. J Clin Invest 1972; 51: 2851–62.

36 Barnham M, Kerby J, Skillin J. Streptococcal skin sepsis in chicken factory workers. In: Holm SE, Christensen P, eds. Basic concepts of streptococci and streptococcal diseases. Chertsey, Surrey: Reedbooks; 1982: 26–27.

37 Gaunt PN, Seal DV. Group G streptococcal infections. J Infect 1987; 15: 5–20.

38 Mortimer GE, Pinney AM, Widdowson JP. The survival of 'skin' and 'throat' streptococci in peptone water–oleic acid and their growth in simple peptone media. In: Parker MT, ed. Pathogenic streptococci. Chertsey, Surrey: Reedbooks; 1979; 120–21.

39 Ogunbi LQO, Lawal A, Lasi Q, Ogunbi O. Streptococcal pyoderma in a Lagos school population. Nigerian Med J 1974; 4: 178–80.

40 Nasr EMM, El Tayeb SHM, El Eteify GA. *Streptococcus pyogenes* as normal flora in asymptomatic children and acute glomerulonephritis. In Proceedings of the X Lancefield international symposium on streptococci and streptococcal diseases. Cologne; 1987. [In press].

41 Whittle HC, Abdullahi MT, Fakunle F, Parry EHO, Rajkovic AD. Streptococcal disease in the northern savannah of Africa. In: Haverkorn MJ, ed. Streptococcal disease and the community. Amsterdam: Excerpta Medica; 1974: 308–11.

42 Taplin D, Landsell L, Allen AM, Rodriguez R, Cortes A. Prevalence of streptococcal pyoderma in relation to climate and hygiene. Lancet 1973; i: 501–03.

43 Barnham M. The gut as a source of the haemolytic streptococci causing infection in surgery of the intestinal and biliary tracts. J Infect 1983; 6: 129–39.

44 Unsworth PF. The isolation of streptococci from human faeces. J Hyg Camb 1980; 85: 153–64.

45 Hare R, Maxted WR. The classification of haemolytic streptococci from the stools of normal pregnant women and of cases of scarlet fever by means of precipitin and biochemical tests. J Pathol Bact 1935; 41: 513–20.

46 Gryska PF, O'Dea AE. Postoperative streptococcal wound infection. JAMA 1970; 213: 1189–91.

47 Asnes RS, Vail D, Grebin B, Sprunt K. Anal carrier rate of group A beta-hemolytic streptococci in children with streptococcal pharyngitis. Pediatr 1973; 52: 438–41.

48 Parker MT. Infections with group-B streptococci. J Antimicrob Chemother 1979; 5 (Suppl A): 27–37.

49 Christensen KK, Christensen P, Flamholc L, Ripa T. Frequencies of

streptococci of groups A, B, C, D and G in urethra and cervix swab specimens from patients with suspected gonococcal infection. Acta Path Microbiol Scand 1974; 82 (Sect B): 470–74.

50 Leading article. Group G streptococci. Lancet 1984; i: 144.

51 Lewis RFM. Beta-haemolytic streptococci from the female genital tract: clinical correlates and outcome of treatment. Epidemiol Infect 1989; 102: 391–400.

52 Donald FE, Slack RCB, Colman G. Streptococcus pyogenes vulvovaginitis in children in Nottingham. Epidemiol Infect 1991; 106: 459–65.

53 Noble WC. The streptococci. In: Microbiology of human skin. London: Lloyd-Luke; 1981: 205–21.

54 Miles AA. Epidemiology of wound infection. Lancet. 1944: i: 809–14.

55 Whitby M, Sleigh JD, Reid W, McGregor I, Colman G. Streptococcal infection in a regional burns centre and a plastic surgery unit. J Hosp Infect 1984; 5: 63–69.

56 Mastro TD, Farley TA, Elliott JE, Facklam RR, Perks JR, Hadler JL, Good RC, Spika JS. An outbreak of surgical wound infections due to group A streptococcus carried on the scalp. N Engl J Med 1990; 323: 968–72.

57 Dillon HC. Group A type 12 streptococcal infection in a newborn nursery. Am J Dis Child 1966; 112: 177–84.

58 Reeder JC, Westwell AJ, Hutchinson DN. Indifferent streptococci in normal and purulent eyes of neonates. J Clin Pathol 1985; 38: 942–45.

59 Miles AA, Schwabacher H, Cunliffe AC, Ross JP, Spooner ETC, Pilcher RS, Wright J. Hospital infection of war wounds. Br Med J 1940; 2: 855–59; 895–900.

60 Roos K, Lind L, Holm SE. Beta-haemolytic streptococci group A in a cat, as a possible source of repeated tonsillitis in a family. Lancet 1988; ii: 1072.

61 Barnham M, Edwards AT. *Streptococcus zooepidemicus* infections in England, 1979–1986. In: Proceedings of the X Lancefield international symposium on streptococci and streptococcal diseases. Cologne; 1987. [In press].

62 Barnham M, Kerby J, Chandler RS, Millar MR. Group C streptococci in human infection: a study of 308 isolates with clinical correlations. Epidemiol Infect 1989; 102: 379–90.

63 Yuen KY, Seto WH, Choi CH, Ng W, Ho SW, Chau PY. *Streptococcus zooepidemicus* (Lancefield group C) septicaemia in Hong Kong. J Infect 1990; 21: 241–50.

64 Barnham M, Neilson DJ. Group L beta-haemolytic streptococcal infection in meat handlers: another streptococcal zoonosis? Epidemiol Infect 1987; 99: 257–64.

65 Robertson ID, Blackmore DK. Occupational exposure to *Streptococcus suis* type 2. Epidemiol Infect 1989; 103: 157–64.

66 Efstratiou A. The serotyping of hospital strains of streptococci belonging to Lancefield group C and group G. J Hyg Camb 1983; 90: 71–80.

67 Mayon-White RT, Perks EM. Why type streptococci? The epidemiology of group A streptococci in Oxfordshire 1976–1980. J Hyg Camb 1982; 88: 439–52.

68 Schwartz B, Facklam RR, Breiman RF. Changing epidemiology of group A streptococcal infections in the USA. Lancet 1990; 336: 1167–71.

69 Stollerman GH. Changing group A streptococci: the reappearance of streptococcal 'toxic shock'. Arch Intern Med 1988; 148: 1268–70.

70 Stollerman GH. Global changes in group A streptococcal diseases and strategies for their prevention. Adv Intern Med 1982; 27: 373–406.

71 Barnham M. Non-group-A streptococci. J Med Microbiol 1990; 33: vi–vii.

72 Wannamaker LW, Ferrieri P. Streptococcal infections updated. In: Disease-a-month. Chicago: Year Book Medical Publishers; [October] 1975: 1–40.

73 Dillon HC. Streptococcal infections of the skin and their complications: impetigo and nephritis. In: Wannamaker LW, Matsen JM, eds. Streptococci and streptococcal diseases. New York: Academic Press; 1972: 571–87.

74 Reid HFM, Birju B, Holder Y, Hospedales J, Poon-King T. Epidemic scabies in four Caribbean islands, 1981–1988. Trans R Soc Trop Med Hyg 1990; 84: 298–300.

75 Melish ME. Staphylococci, streptococci and the skin. Semin Dermatol 1982; 1: 101–09.

76 Parker MT. Streptococcal diseases. In: Smith GR, ed. Topley and Wilson's principles of bacteriology, virology and immunity, vol 3. London: Edward Arnold; 1984: 225–53.

77 Wannamaker LW, Dajani AS, Ferrieri P, Kaplan EL, Brown J. Local factors as determinants of streptococcal infection. In: Haverkorn MJ, ed. Streptococcal disease and the community. Amsterdam: Excerpta Medica; 1974: 251–57.

78 Eichenwald HF. Current abstracts: impetigo: reassessment of etiology and therapy. Pediatr Infect Dis J 1988; 7: 606.

79 Mhalu FS. Bacteriological study of superficial skin infections in Tanzanian children. E African Med J 1973; 50: 272–76.

80 Reid HFM, Bassett DCJ, Poon-King T, Zabriskie JB, Read SE. Group G streptococci in healthy school-children and in patients with glomerulonephritis in Trinidad. J Hyg Camb 1985; 94: 61–68.

81 Ferrieri P. In: Haverkorn MJ, ed. Streptococcal disease and the community. Amsterdam: Excerpta Medica; 1974: 284.

82 Belcher DW, Afoakwa SN, Osei-Tutu E, Wurupa FK, Osei L. Non-group A streptococci in Ghanaian patients with pyoderma. Lancet 1975; ii: 1032.

83 Pindberg JJ. Angular cheilitis. In: Rook A, Wilkinson DS, Ebling FJG, Champion RH, Burton JL, eds. Textbook of dermatology, vol 3. Oxford: Blackwell Scientific; 1986: 2123–24.

84 Fischbacher CM, Green ST. Varicella and life-threatening streptococcal infection. Scand J Infect Dis 1987; 19: 519–20.

85 Eichenwald HF. Current abstracts: varicella and life-threatening streptococcal infection. Pediatr Infect Dis J 1988; 7: 530.

86 Barnham M. Invasive streptococcal infections in the era before the acquired immune deficiency syndrome: a 10 years' compilation of patients with streptococcal bacteraemia in North Yorkshire. J Infect 1989; 18: 231–48.

87 Degre M. Interaction between viral and bacterial infections in the respiratory tract. Scand J Infect Dis 1986; 49 (Suppl): 140–45.

88 Rouse BT, Horohov DW. Immunosuppression in viral infections. Rev Infect Dis 1986; 8: 850–73.

89 LaGrenade L, Hanchard B, Fletcher V, Cranston B, Blattner W. Infective dermatitis of Jamaican children: a marker for HTLV-1 infection. Lancet 1990; 336: 1345–47.

90 Elek SD, Conen PE. The virulence of *Staphylococcus pyogenes* for man: a study of the problems of wound infection. Br J Exp Pathol 1957; 38: 573–86.

91 Dajani AS, Wannamaker LW. Experimental infection of the skin in the hamster simulating human impetigo: 1. natural history of the infection. J Infect Dis 1970; 122: 196–204.

92 Zimmerli W, Waldvogel FA, Vaudaux B, Nydegger UE. Pathogenesis of foreign body infection: description and characteristics of an animal model. J Infect Dis 1982; 146: 487–97.

93 Drabick JJ, Lennox JL. Group A streptococcal infections and a toxic shock-like syndrome. N Engl J Med 1989; 321: 1545.

94 Amren DP. Unusual forms of streptococcal disease. In: Wannamaker LW, Matsen JM, eds. Streptococci and streptococcal diseases. New York: Academic Press; 1972: 545–56.

95 Bitnun S. Prophylactic antibiotics in recurrent erysipelas. Lancet 1985; i: 345.

96 Barker FG, Leppard BJ, Seal DV. Streptococcal necrotising fasciitis: comparison between histological and clinical features. J Clin Pathol 1987; 40: 335–41.

97 Parker MT. Staphylococcal diseases. In: Smith GR, ed. Topley and Wilson's principles of bacteriology, virology and immunity, vol 3. London: Edward Arnold; 1984: 254–78.

98 Davson J, Jones DM, Turner L. Diagnosis of Meleney's synergistic gangrene. Br J Surg 1988; 75: 267–71.

99 Ormerod LD, Paton BG. Severe group B streptococcal eye infections in adults. J Infect 1989; 18: 29–34.

100 Roberts SOB, Highet AS. Suppurative hidradenitis. In: Rook A, Wilkinson DS, Ebling FJG, Champion RH, Burton JL, eds. Textbook of dermatology, vol 1. Oxford: Blackwell Scientific; 1986: 785–87.

101 Eykyn SJ, Gransden WR, Phillips I. The causative organisms of septicaemia and their epidemiology. J Antimicrob Chemother 1990; 25 (Suppl C): 41–58.

102 Ispahani P, Donald FE, Aveline AJD. *Streptococcus pyogenes* bacteraemia: an old enemy subdued but not defeated. J Infect 1988; 16: 37–46.

103 Yagupsky P, Gilady Y. Group A beta-hemolytic streptococcal bacteraemia in children. Pediatr Infect Dis J 1987; 6: 1036–39.

104 Francis J, Warren RE. *Streptococcus pyogenes* bacteraemia in Cambridge – a review of 67 episodes. Q J Med 1988; 68 (new series): 603–13.

105 Morris CA, Berry DM. Annual and seasonal variation in the frequency of beta-haemolytic streptococcal infections. J Clin Pathol 1985; 38: 594–95.

106 Efstratiou A, Colman G, Lightfoot NF, Cruikshank JG. Streptococcal pyoderma in a military training establishment. In: Holm SE, Christensen P, eds. Basic concepts of streptococci and streptococcal diseases. Chertsey, Surrey: Reedbooks; 1982: 23–24.

107 Barnham M, Kerby J. Pyoderma at a police training centre. PHLS Communicable Disease Report 1984: 84/35.

108 Ludlam H, Cookson B. Scrum kidney: epidemic pyoderma caused by a nephritogenic *Streptococcus pyogenes* in a rugby team. Lancet 1986; ii: 331–33.

109 Public Health Laboratory Service Working Group on Streptococcal Infection in Meat Handlers. The epidemiology and control of streptococcal sepsis in meat handlers. Environ Health 1982; 10: 256–58.

110 Barnham M, Kerby J. A profile of skin sepsis in meat handlers. J Infect 1984; 9: 43–50.

111 Barnham M. Streptococcal infection in an arable farming community. PHLS Communicable Disease Report 1983: 83/12.

112 Burnett IA, Norman P. *Streptococcus pyogenes*: an outbreak on a burns unit. J Hosp Infect 1990; 15: 173–76.

113 Allen KD, Ridgway EJ. *Streptococcus pyogenes*: an outbreak on a burns unit. J Hosp Infect 1990; 16: 178–79.

114 Tsai TF, Watson WN, Hayes PS, Facklam RR, Fraser DW. Mode of spread of group A streptococci in an abattoir outbreak of wound sepsis. In: Parker MT, ed. Pathogenic streptococci. Chertsey, Surrey: Reedbooks; 1979: 118–19.

115 Flanagan K, Kline S, Quackenbush K, Foster L. Group A, beta-hemolytic *Streptococcus* skin infections in a meat-packing plant – Oregon. Morbidity and Mortality Weekly Report 1986; 35: 629–30. [CDC, Atlanta].

116 Bjorland J, Rosef O. En epidemi med gruppe A-streptokokker ved fellesslakteriet i Oslo. Norsk Vet 1981; 93: 446.

117 Sharp JCM. Scrumpox. Communicable Diseases Scotland 1990: 90/17.

118 George JTA, McDonald JC, Payne DJH, Slade DA. Nephritis in North Yorkshire. Br Med J 1958; 2: 1381–82.

119 Anthony BF, Kaplan EL, Wannamaker LW, Briese FW, Chapman SS. Attack rates of acute nephritis after type 49 streptococcal infection of the skin and of the respiratory tract. J Clin Invest 1969; 48: 1697–704.

120 Sagel I, Treser G, Ty A, Yoshizawa N, Kleinberger H, Yuceoghi AM, Wassermann E, Lange K. Occurrence and nature of glomerular lesions after group A streptococci infections in children. Ann Intern Med 1973; 79: 492–99.

121 Lange K. The future of nephrologic research: significance and urgent problems. Clin Nephrol 1984; 21: 82–85.

122 Seligson G, Lange K, Majeed HA, Deol H, Cronin W, Bovie R. Significance of endostreptosin antibody titers in poststreptococcal glomerulonephritis. Clin Nephrol 1985; 24: 69–75.

123 Cronin W, Deol H, Azadegan A, Lange K. Endostreptosin: isolation of the probable immunogen of acute post-streptococcal glomerulonephritis. Clin Exp Immunol 1989; 76: 198–203.

124 Reid HFM, Mahabir RN, Read SE. Post streptococcal chronic glomerulonephritis: immunological profile in affected patients. In: Orefia G, ed. New perspectives on streptococci and streptococcal infections. Stuttgart: Gustav Fischer Verlag; 1992: 257–60.

125 Ferrieri P. Acute post-streptococcal glomerulonephritis and its relationship to the epidemiology of streptococcal infections. Minnesota Med 1975; 58: 598–602. [Refs p. 615].

126 Johnston KH, Zabriskie JB. Purification and partial characterization of the nephritis strain-associated protein from *Streptococcus pyogenes*, group A. J Exp Med 1986; 163: 697–712.

127 Ohkuni H, Friedman J, Van de Rijn I, Fischetti VA, Poon-King T, Zabriskie JB. Immunological studies of post-streptococcal sequelae: serological studies with an extracellular protein associated with nephritogenic streptococci. Clin Exp Immunol 1983; 54: 185–93.

128 Stollerman GH. Nephritogenic and rheumatogenic group A streptococci. J Infect Dis 1969; 120: 258–63.

129 Dale JB, Baird RW, Bronze MS, Beachey EH. Joint cross-reactive epitopes of streptococcal M proteins. In: Orefia G, ed. New perspectives on streptococci and streptococcal infections. Stuttgart: Gustav Fischer Verlag; 1992: 168–70.

130 Fischetti VA. Streptococcal M protein: molecular design and biologic behavior. Clin Microbiol Rev 1989; 2: 285–314.

131 Manjula BN, Khandke KM, Fairwell T, Relf WA, Sriprakash KS. Diagnostic patterns in the heptad periodicity of the nephritis and rheumatic fever associated Group A streptococcal M proteins. In: Orefia G, ed. New perspectives on streptococci and streptococcal infections. Stuttgart: Gustav Fischer Verlag; 1992: 171–73.

132 Treser G, Semar M, Sagel I, Ty A, Sterzel RB, Schaerf R, Lange K. Independence of the nephritogenicity of group A streptococci from their M types. Clin Exp Immunol 1971; 9: 57–62.

133 Barnham M, Cole G, Efstratiou A, Tagg JR, Skjold SA. Characterization of *Streptococcus zooepidemicus* (Lancefield group C) from human and selected animal infections. Epidemiol Infect 1987; 98: 171–82.

134 Gnann JW, Gray BM, Griffin FM, Dismukes WE. Acute glomerulonephritis following group G streptococcal infection. J Infect Dis 1987; 156: 411–12.

135 Christie AB. Streptococcal infections. In: Infectious diseases: epidemiology and clinical practice, vol 2. Edinburgh: Churchill Livingstone; 1987: 1275–99.

136 Cruikshank R. Streptococcus. In: Cruikshank R, Duguid JP, Marmion BP, Swain RHA, eds. Medical microbiology, vol 1. Edinburgh: Churchill Livingstone; 1973: 246–56.

137 Perks EM, Mayon-White RT. The incidence of scarlet fever. J Hyg Camb 1983; 91: 203–09.

138 Christie P. 30 years of scarlet fever in Scotland. Communicable Diseases Scotland. 1990: 90/10.

139 Hallas G. The production of pyrogenic exotoxins by group A streptococci. J Hyg Camb 1985; 95: 47–57.

140 Stevens DL, Tanner MH, Winship J, Swarts R, Ries KM, Schlievert PM, Kaplan E. Severe group A streptococcal infections associated with a toxic shock-like syndrome and scarlet fever toxin A. N Engl J Med 1989; 321: 1–7.

141 Watson DW. Characterisation and pathobiological properties of group-A streptococcal pyrogenic exotoxins. In: Parker MT, ed. Pathogenic streptococci. Chertsey, Surrey: Reedbooks; 1979: 62–63.

142 Cone LA, Woodard DR, Schlievert PM, Tomory GS. Clinical and bacteriologic observations of a toxic shock-like syndrome due to *Streptococcus pyogenes*. N Engl J Med 1987; 317: 146–49.

143 Weeks CR, Ferretti JJ. The gene for type A streptococcal exotoxin (erythrogenic toxin) is located on bacteriophage T12. Infect Immun 1984; 46: 531–36.

144 Yu EC, Ferretti JJ. Frequency of erythrogenic toxin gene (speA, speB and speC) among clinical isolates of group A streptococci. In: Orefia G, ed. New perspectives in streptococci and streptococcal infections. Stuttgart: Gustav Fischer Verlag; 1992: 346–47.

145 Gaworzewska ET, Hallas G. Group A streptococcal infections and a toxic shock-like syndrome. N Engl J Med 1989; 321: 1546.

146 Bartter T, Dascal A, Carroll K, Curley FJ. 'Toxic strep syndrome': a manifestation of group A streptococcal infection. Arch Intern Med 1988; 148: 1421–24.

147 Shaunak S, Gordon AM. Do streptococci cause toxic shock? Br Med J 1990; 301: 1333.

148 Leading article. Invasive streptococci. Lancet 1989; ii: 1255.

149 Shaunak S, Wendon J, Monteil M, Gordon AM. Septic scarlet fever due to *Streptococcus pyogenes* cellulitis. Q J Med 1988; 69 (new series): 921–25.

150 Vosti KL. Streptococcal diseases. In: Hoeprich PD, ed. Infectious diseases. Harperstown, MD: Harper and Row; 1977: 235–46.

151 Levene GM. Immunology of streptococcal infection. Br J Dermatol 1972; 86 (Suppl 8): 62–68.

152 Strong WB. Petechiae and streptococcal pharyngitis. Am J Dis Child 1969; 117: 156–60.

153 Leading article. Fever with purpura. Lancet 1990: 335: 889–90.

154 Baker RC, Seguin JH, Leslie N, Gilchrist MJR, Myers MG. Fever and petechiae in children. Pediatr 1989; 84: 1051–55.

155 Burton JL, Rook A, Wilkinson DS. Pityriasis alba. In: Rook A, Wilkinson DS, Ebling FJG, Champion RH, Burton JL, eds. Textbook of dermatology, vol 1. Oxford: Blackwell Scientific; 1986: 390–91.

156 Whyte HJ, Baughman RD. Acute guttate psoriasis and streptococcal infection. Arch Dermatol 1964; 89: 350–56.

157 Chalmers RJG, Whale K, Colman G. Streptococcal serotypes in patients with guttate psoriasis. Br J Dermatol 1983; 109 (Suppl 24): 44.

158 Belew PW, Wannamaker LW, Johnson D, Rosenberg EW. Beta haemolytic streptococcal types associated with psoriasis. In: Kimura Y, Kotami S, Shiokawa Y, eds. Recent advances in streptococci and streptococcal diseases. Bracknel, Berkshire: Reedbooks; 1985: 334.

159 Valdimarsson H, Baker BS, Jonsdottir I, Fry L. Psoriasis: a disease of abnormal keratinocyte proliferation induced by T lymphocytes. Immunol Today 1986; 7: 256–59.

160 Swerlick RA, Cunningham MW, Hall NK. Monoclonal antibodies cross-reactive with group A streptococci and normal and psoriatic human skin. J Invest Dermatol 1986; 87: 367–71.

161 Garrod LP. The eclipse of the haemolytic streptococcus. Br Med J 1979; 1: 1607–08.

162 Chhatwal GS, Valentin-Weigand P, Timmis KN. Bacterial infection of wounds: fibronectin-mediated adherence of group A and C streptococci to fibrin thrombi in vitro. Infect Immun 1990; 58: 3015–19.

163 Vaudaux P, Suzuki R, Valdvogel FA, Morgenthaler JJ, Nydegger UE. Foreign body infection: role of fibronectin as a ligand for the adherence of *Staphylococcus aureus*. J Infect Dis 1984; 150: 546–53.

164 Barnett LA, Cunningham MW. A new heart-cross-reactive antigen in *Streptococcus pyogenes* is not M protein. J Infect Dis 1990; 162: 875–82.

165 Lindahl G, Stenberg L. Binding of IgA and/or IgG is a common property among clinical isolates of group A streptococci. Epidemiol Infect 1990; 105: 87–93.

166 Bessen D, Fischetti VA. A human IgG receptor of group A streptococci is associated with tissue site of infection and streptococcal class. J Infect Dis 1990; 161: 747–54.

167 Ginsburg I. Streptococcal enzymes and virulence. In: Holder IA, ed. Bacterial enzymes and virulence. Boca Raton, FA: CRC Press; 1985: 121–44.

168 Cohen J, Bayston K, Tomlinson M. Do streptococci cause toxic shock? Br Med J 1990; 301: 1277–78.

169 Stollerman GH. Hypersensitivity and antibody responses in streptococcal disease. In: Wannamaker LW, Matsen JM, eds. Streptococci and streptococcal diseases. New York: Academic Press; 1972: 501–13.

170 Wiley GG, Bruno PN. The M antigens: variations and interrelationships. In:

Wannamaker LW, Matsen JM, eds. Streptococci and streptococcal diseases. New York: Academic Press; 1972: 235–49.

171 Bisno AL, Nelson KE. Type-specific opsonic antibodies in streptococcal pyoderma. Infect Immun 1974; 10: 1356–61.

172 Maxted WR. Group A streptococci: pathogenesis and immunity. In: Skinner FA, Quesnel LB, eds. Streptococci. London: Academic Press; 1978: 107–25.

173 Widdowson JP, Maxted WR, Notley CM, Pinney AM. The antibody responses in man to infection with different serotypes of group-A streptococci. J Med Microbiol 1974; 7: 483–96.

174 Kaplan EL, Anthony BF, Chapman SS, Ayoub EM, Wannamaker LW. The influence of the site of infection on the immune response to group A streptococci. J Clin Invest 1970; 49: 1405–14.

175 McLinn S. Topical mupirocin vs. systemic erythromycin treatment for pyoderma. Pediatr Infect Dis 1988; 7: 785–90.

176 Warren RE, Boissard J, Whetstone RJ. General advice about antibiotics. Lancet 1981; i: 331–32.

177 Goldfarb J, Crenshaw D, O'Horo J, Lemon E, Blumer JL. Randomized clinical trial of topical mupirocin versus oral erythromycin for impetigo. Antimicrob Ag Chemother 1988; 32: 1780–83.

178 Cookson BD. Mupirocin resistance in staphylococci. J Antimicrob Chemother 1990; 25: 497–501.

179 Fried M, Rudensky B, Golan J, Sternberg N, Isaacsohn M, Ben Hur N. Severe cellulitis caused by group A streptococcus. J Infect Dis 1990; 161: 155.

180 Phillips I, Warren C, Harrison JM, Sharples P, Ball LC, Parker MT. Antibiotic susceptibilities of streptococci from the mouth and blood of patients treated with penicillin or lincomycin and clindamycin. J Med Microbiol 1976; 9: 393–404.

181 Barnham M, Cole G. Erythromycin-resistant beta-haemolytic streptococci in North Yorkshire. J Infect 1986; 13: 200–02.

182 Phillips G, Parratt D, Orange GV, Harper I, McEwan H, Young N. Erythromycin-resistant *Streptococcus pyogenes*. J Antimicrob Chemother 1990; 25: 723–24.

183 Spencer RC, Wheat PF, Magee JT, Brown EH. Erythromycin resistance in streptococci. Lancet 1989; i: 168.

184 Brook I, Yocum P, Calhoun L. Beta-lactamase producing *Bacteroides* species recovered from children: possible clue to failure of penicillin treatment. Lancet 1981; i: 332.

185 Lowbury EJL. Streptococci in burns and plastic surgery units. J Hosp Infect 1984; 5: 339–40.

186 Whitby M, Sleigh JD, Reid W, McGregor I, Colman G. Streptococci in burns and plastic surgery units. J Hosp Infect 1985; 6: 235.

187 Gerber MA, Markowitz M. Management of streptococcal pharyngitis reconsidered. Pediatr Infect Dis 1985; 4: 518–26.

188 Stetson CA, Rammelkamp CH, Krause RM, Kohen RJ, Perry WD. Epidemic acute nephritis: studies on etiology, natural history and prevention. Medicine 1955; 34: 431–50.

189 Kremer M, Zuckerman R, Avraham Z, Raz R. Long-term antimicrobial therapy in the prevention of recurrent soft-tissue infections. J Infect 1991; 22: 37–40.

9

Other cutaneous bacteria

W. C. NOBLE

Apart from *Acinetobacter* spp. and *Micrococcus* spp., few bacteria other than coryneforms and staphylococci are found resident on skin. In this chapter are described the Gram-negative and Gram-positive bacteria regularly found on skin, together with those that contribute to well-recognized skin infection.

Gram-negative bacteria

Gram-negative bacilli are comparatively rare on normal skin, except for acinetobacter, which forms part of the normal flora in about a quarter of the population. Proteus is found on the nasal mucosa of about 5 per cent of individuals and both proteus and pseudomonas are found on the toe webs. The hands may also be temporarily colonized by a variety of bacilli. Apart from these sites the general skin surface of normal persons is sparsely colonized (Table 9.1) and the majority of organisms are probably transients or contaminants.

Acinetobacter spp.

Acinetobacter is the only genus of Gram-negative bacilli regularly found as a member of the skin flora in a significant number of individuals. About 25 per cent of normal adults carry acinetobacter in the axillae, groin, toe webs and antecubital fossa.[1] In patients with eczema the carrier rate may be higher, especially on lesions,[3] whilst in hospitalized patients with renal disease the carrier rate may exceed 50 per cent.[4] Carriage of acinetobacter is more common in the summer months,[5] probably due to increased sweating, and this is reflected in a pronounced summer maximum of endemic surgical wound infection,[6] especially in young adults. Most acinetobacter infection reported is epidemic,[1] perhaps because outbreaks command more attention than does

Table 9.1. *Total Gram-negative bacilli on skin (percentage incidence)*

	101 infants	78 children	165 adults	63 geriatrics
Forehead	7	50	18	18
Ear	6	14	5	10
Nares	16	39	21	18
Axilla	34	13	17	0
Dorsum of hand	8	35	23	18
Foot	11	38	22	12

Based on Somerville.[2]

a steady, low level of endemic disease. Skin infection by acinetobacter is rare, but cellulitis has been reported.[7,8]

Relatively recent sweeping changes in taxonomy of the acinetobacter have reduced the value of previous studies on skin carriage, which must now entail some assumptions. Most earlier work refers to one species, *Acinetobacter calcoaceticus* comprised of two varieties, *lwoffi* and *anitratus*. The former was regarded as fairly sensitive to antibiotics and the latter as frequently resistant and the cause of most hospital epidemics. In 1986, Bouvet and Grimont[9] reported a new taxonomy containing 12 genospecies, some unnamed, defined on the basis of DNA/DNA hybridization, 11 of which could be separated by phenotypic tests. This was extended to 15 groups by Tjernberg and Ursing.[10] Many strains now reported from infection seem to be referrable to *A. baumanii* but strains from normal skin are likely to be distributed amongst *A. johnsonii*, *A. lwoffi* and unnamed genospecies; however, 13 DNA groups were represented in 168 consecutive clinical isolates studied by Tjernberg and Ursing. The epidemiology and ecology of acinetobacter is in need of revision.

Many studies of epidemic spread of acinetobacters in hospital refer to temporary colonization of the skin, especially of the hands.[1] Studies on the survival of acinetobacter in experimental situations show persistence times shorter than those experienced in hospital outbreaks,[11] and it may be that the revised taxonomy will shed light on this.

Pseudomonas spp.

Pseudomonas aeruginosa is the chief pathogen among the many species of pseudomonads. When applied to normal skin, even in large numbers, disease does not occur unless the skin is hyperhydrated.[12] This is presumably why *Ps. aeruginosa* is most common in trench foot or immersion foot of soldiers, or in generalized foot infection of coal miners.[13] Much interest was generated in the late 1970s and early 1980s by the apparently new appearance of infection, described as whirlpool folliculitis or hot-tub dermatitis.[14-19] The disease was manifest as a folliculitis or pruritic skin rash in almost all individuals, with otitis media in 30–60 per cent of cases associated with swimming pools or 10–25 per cent of those associated with whirlpools or jacuzzis; mastitis appeared equally in males and females at about 10 per cent frequency. The disease was usually self-limiting but occasional severe cases occurred. Although various serotypes of *Ps. aeruginosa* were involved, 0:11 was the most common in the United States, with 0:6 and 0:9 also well represented. The risk of infection was related not only to immersion in contaminated water but to skin hydration and response to toxins produced by the organism.[19, 20] Insufficient attention to plant maintenance has been cited as a factor contributing to contamination of the water.

Other infection with *Ps. aeruginosa* includes paronychia, in which the classic green pigment pyocyanin is seen in the nail bed;[21, 22] infections of the feet or hands may also exhibit pyocyanin discoloration. The skin lesions associated with pseudomonas septicaemia range from pruritic oedematous areas through ecthyma gangrenosum, abscesses, vesicles and cellulitis to erysipelas-like infection.[23, 24] In the immunosuppressed patient with AIDS there may be a low-grade, subclinical bacteraemia, with erythematous skin nodules full of bacilli but with few neutrophils.[25]

Other *Pseudomonas* spp. reported to cause skin lesions include *Ps. cepacia* found in the macerated toe webs of swamp foot,[26] or in drug abuse.[27] *Pseudomonas paucimobilis* is found in ulcers.[28]

Other Gram-negative bacilli

Proteus spp. are found in the toe webs and, together with *Ps. aeruginosa*, *Pr. mirabilis* is considered one of the major causes of swamp foot.[29, 30] Groin carriage of *Proteeae* is correlated with urinary tract infection in the elderly.[31]

Haemophilus influenzae, usually type B, is a well-established cause of cellulitis of the face in children, especially young males,[32-34] although abscesses are also described.[35] *Pasteurella multocida* infection, which may be under-diagnosed, follows bites from animals, especially cats;[36, 37] the skin lesion may be the result of toxin production. *Aeromonas hydrophila* infection is reported in association with exposure to both fresh and salt water.[38, 39] Skin infection by various 'marine vibrios'[40-43] may be anticipated in the face of established deep-seated infection.[44] *Vibrio vulnificus* is reported as causing primary bacteraemia in 1 in 200 000 patients, a rate twice that of reported skin infection. Lesions are twice as common in males and appear as cellulitis with oedema.[45] The various

Table 9.2. *Percentage prevalence of* Neisseria *on skin*

	Infants	Children	Young adults	Geriatric adults
Nostrils	1	33	19	43
Forehead	2	25	19	25
Ear	2	4	4	3
Dorsum of hand	2	31	17	17
Nail folds	0	3	0	5
Axilla	1	5	7	8
Dorsum of foot	0	11	14	12
Toe spaces	0	10	7	5

Based on Somerville.[2]

bacteria found in water that contribute to skin infection have been reviewed,[46] but although 66 species are listed, some are clearly of skin origin and found secondarily in water. A variety of miscellaneous bacteria are reported as recovered from skin lesions, although in some instances the pathogenic role must remain in doubt. Thus legionella, which may cause a rash described as painful, non-pruritic, macular and erythematous in about 6 per cent of patients with legionellosis,[47] has also been recovered from an abscess in an immunosuppressed patient.[48] Brucella skin lesions are reported in brucellosis,[49,50] and it may be that veterinarians are especially liable to infection with these and other pathogens of animal origin such as salmonella,[51] shigella,[52] brucella[53,54] and yersinia.[55] Reports of lesions due to flavobacteria,[56] moraxella,[57] eikenella,[58,59] or serratia[60] are more difficult to assess other than, presumably, in the single original patient.

Gram-negative folliculitis is a well-established infection, which generally follows prolonged antibiotic treatment of acne vulgaris.[61-63] The causative organisms, usually *Escherichia coli* or *Pr. mirabilis*, may often also be recovered from the patient's anterior nares.

Neisseria spp.

Several species of non-pathogenic neisseria are present in the upper respiratory tract of man but, although they must frequently be deposited on the skin, they do not form part of the resident flora. Transient carriage is more frequent in the elderly (Table 9.2). However, primary cutaneous infection with *N. gonorrhoeae* has been recorded following minor trauma and genital contact,[64] whilst secondary infection following gonococcal septicaemia is well established,[65] as is a rash in meningococcal infection.[66]

Table 9.3. *Percentage of Gram-negative bacilli on the hands*

	Health care workers ($n = 255$)	Controls ($n = 104$)
Acinetobacter lwoffi	4.3	5.8
A. anitratus	3.2	10.6
Citrobacter spp.	0.4	0.0
Enterobacter spp.	17.0	40.0
Escherichia coli	0.7	0.0
Klebsiella spp.	5.0	3.0
Moraxella spp.	0.4	4.8
Proteus spp.	1.2	1.0
Pseudomonas aeruginosa	1.2	0.0
Pseudomonas spp.	0.7	1.0
Serratia spp.	5.0	8.0
Others[a]	0.8	0.0

[a] Includes *Aeromonas* spp. and unspeciated isolates.
Based on Adams and Marrie.[67]

Gram-negative flora of the hands

The hands have received special attention for the part they may play in the transmission of Gram-negative bacilli in hospital. In housewives outside hospital, the species found are chiefly those of gut origin but, in those who carry, densities average $300/cm^2$. In hospital, carrier rates may reach 90 per cent but even in nurses and physicians using antibacterial hand-washes can average about 30 per cent;[67] most had less than 1000 Gram-negative bacilli per hand, however. *Enterobacter* spp. were the most common (Table 9.3). Not all hand carriage is transient, however.[68] The same type of klebsiella, pseudomonas or enterobacter was recovered from the hands of health care or control personnel over periods of 3–6 weeks. Control subjects carried enterobacter and acinetobacter more frequently than other groups; individuals with a hand dermatitis more often carried *Ps. aeruginosa* whilst nurses carried *Klebsiella pneumoniae* more frequently than did others.

During investigations of outbreaks of hospital infection,[69] acinetobacter has been observed to colonize the hands at least temporarily.[70-72] Equally, hand colonization has been associated with the transmission of klebsiella[73,74] and citrobacter.[75] Individuals with dermatitis of the hands, which is usually ascribed to frequent hand washing, are often reported to be responsible for transmission of Gram-negative bacilli in hospital outbreaks.[71,75] *Klebsiella* spp., especially those resistant to antibiotics, survive better on fingertips than do sensitive isolates or *Ps. aeruginosa* or *E. coli*.[76,77]

Table 9.4. *Percentage distribution of Gram-negative bacilli on the toe webs in various groups*

	514 miners	100 industrial workers	100 outpatients	61 students
Acinetobacter lwoffi	18.0	8	4	1.6
A. anitratus	0.4	2	0	0.0
Alcaligenes spp.	7.4	0	0	1.6
Citrobacter spp.	1.0	3	0	0.0
Enterobacter spp.	1.6	1	1	1.6
Escherichia coli	2.3	1	1	0.0
Moraxella spp.	3.5	0	1	0.0
Proteus mirabilis	1.9	10	11	1.6
Pseudomonas aeruginosa	4.1	10	6	0.0
Pseudomonas spp. identified[a]	13.0	9	0	0.0
Pseudomonas spp. unidentified	14.4	0	0	0.0
Serratia	0.4	3	0	3.2
Other[b]	5.1	20	1	0.0

[a] Includes for miners *Ps. cepacia, Ps. diminuta, Ps. fluorescens, Ps. maltophilia, Ps. paucimobilis, Ps. putrefaciens, Ps. stutzeri, Ps. vesicularis.*
[b] Includes for miners *Achromobacter* spp., *Aeromonas* spp., *Enterobacter* spp., *Klebsiella* spp.
Based on Noble and coworkers.[78,79]

Gram-negative flora of the feet

On the feet, especially the toe webs, Gram-negative bacilli are regularly present, usually in small numbers but may also contribute to disease. In various studies in the United Kingdom the point prevalence of Gram-negative bacilli was reported as 8 per cent in normal students, 14.5 per cent in female office workers and 29 per cent in male office workers, 24 per cent in hospital outpatients with suspected tinea pedis, 41 per cent in industrial workers wearing heavy protective boots and 58 per cent in coal miners.[78,79] The species isolated are shown in Table 9.4. Most species, especially among the coal miners, are probably derived from the environment, although this point was not specifically investigated in these studies. Quantitative studies in the United States[80] report Gram-negative bacilli as minority populations in the toe webs of 10 per cent of 163 normal persons with a mean of 2.4 bacilli per web compared with over 10^5 each of staphylococci and coryneforms. The distribution was klebsiella 43 per cent, proteus 16 per cent, acinetobacter 16 per cent, enterobacter 14 per cent and escherichia 9 per cent.

'Damage to the epidermis by fungi, extreme wetness or other factors' has

Table 9.5. *Carriage of* Micrococcus *spp. in 115 adults*

	Individuals colonized (%)	Sites colonized (%)
M. luteus	90	46
M. varians	75	24
M. lylae	33	7
M. nishinomiyaensis	28	6
M. kristinae	25	6
M. roseus	15	2
M. sedentarius	13	4

Based on Kloos and Musselwhite.[5]

been described as a prerequisite for clinically apparent infection of the toe webs by Gram-negative bacilli.[81] Immersion foot, seen at its most severe in military personnel,[82,83] is an industrial hazard, although both high temperature and high humidity are necessary to bring about large skin populations.[84] Most agree that foot infection by Gram-negative bacilli is most commonly caused by *Ps. aeruginosa* and/or *Pr. mirabilis*,[29,81,85] but other *Pseudomonas* spp. such as *Ps. cepacia*[26] cause infection, whilst *Ps. putrefasciens* and *Ps. paucimobilis* may infect pre-existing lesions.[28] Infection is also caused by *Aeromonas hydrophila*.[38,39]

Studies on the treatment of foot infection in coal miners[30] show that when dermatophyte infection is suppressed by azole antifungals, lesions may remain but yield increased numbers of Gram-negative bacilli. Suppression of the bacilli by povidone iodine leads to the reappearance of dermatophytes, showing the complex ecological aspects of severe foot infection.

Gram-positive bacteria

Micrococcus spp.

The *Micrococcus* spp. were formerly considered together with the staphylococci on the grounds that both are Gram-positive cocci. However it is now considered that on taxonomic grounds, *Micrococcus* spp. are more closely related to the coryneforms than to staphylococci.[86]

There are seven species of *Micrococcus*[87] (Table 9.5) resident on human skin but those most commonly isolated are *M. luteus* and *M. varians*.[5] *Micrococcus* spp. are slower to colonize the skin of infants than are the staphylococci (Table 9.6) and may remain more common on the skin of children and adult females than adult males,[88,89] although the contrary view – that adults carry micro-

Table 9.6. *Carriage of* Micrococcus *spp. in infants in contrast*
with some staphylococci

	% of samples yielding species at infant age:			
	1 day	1 week	10–12 weeks	28–32 weeks
M. luteus	0	6	35	38
M. kristinae	3	3	8	26
M. lylae	3	0	0	18
M. varians	0	0	5	9
M. nishinomiyaensis	0	4	4	1
M. roseus	0	0	1	0
M. sedentarius	3	0	0	0
S. epidermidis	60	80	83	90
S. haemolyticus	33	50	58	73

Based on Carr and Kloos.[99]

Table 9.7. *Simplified taxonomic scheme for cutaneous mycobacteria*

Species	Pigment production		Growth at (°C)			Nitratase	Pyrazin amidase
	In dark	In light	25°	33°	45°		
Slow growers							
M. tuberculosis	−	−	−	+	−	+	+
M. ulcerans	Light lemon-yellow	Light lemon-yellow	−	+	−	−	−
M. marinum	−	Yellow	+	+	−	−	+
M. kansasii	−	Yellow	+	+	(+)	+	−
M. avium complex	−	−	+	+	+	−	+
Fast growers							
M. chelonei	Cream-buff	Cream-buff	+	+	−	−	
M. fortuitum	Buff	Buff	+	+	(+)	+	

cocci more often than do children – has also been reported,[87] whilst others
have reported about equal carriage.[90, 91] In animals, *M. varians* is the most
common species, with *M. luteus* occasionally recovered. None of the other
species has been isolated.[92]

Micrococcus spp. are not involved in skin infection (with the exception that
M. sedentarius is reported as one of the causes of pitted keratolysis)[93] and
rarely cause deep infection, although a few reports of bacteraemia have

appeared,[94-96] usually in patients at severe risk of infection. Rare infections are also reported in patients receiving peritoneal dialysis[97] and in septic arthritis.[98]

Mycobacterium spp.

Mycobacterial infection of the skin is, with the exception of lupus vulgaris and scrofula, an exogenous disease. The recovery of mycobacteria resident on skin is not reported, although some transient carriage of environmental mycobacteria must be anticipated. Even *M. smegmatis* would seem to be rare in urine,[100] for, in a survey of acid-fast bacilli in Canada, *M. smegmatis* was recovered 25 times from 1632 specimens positive for acid-fast bacilli (1107 positive for *M. tuberculosis*) in 55 254 (total) specimens screened. A simplified taxonomic scheme for cutaneous mycobacteria is shown in Table 9.7.

Mycobacterium tuberculosis infection is becoming increasingly rare in developed countries in those not affected by AIDS. Grange[101] cites evidence to show that the annual infection rate in developed countries is about 0.2 per cent and that this rate is halved every 6 years. In underdeveloped countries the annual infection rate is 2–5 per cent, with little evidence of natural decline. The risk of infection is however about 100 times greater in AIDS patients. These data relate principally to pulmonary tuberculosis. Extrapulmonary tuberculosis forms about 20 per cent of reported infection in England and Wales[102] and cutaneous infection about 1 per cent of extrapulmonary disease.

Worldwide it is estimated that there are 11 million cases of leprosy (see below) in an at-risk population of 1400 million. For tuberculosis the equivalent figures are 10–20 million new cases in 3000 million at risk.[101]

M. leprae

Recent studies have formally placed *M. leprae* amongst the mycobacteria, though this was always assumed on the basis of the Ziehl–Nielsen stain.[103] It remains true that *M. leprae* cannot be cultured in vitro and the armadillo remains a good laboratory species in which to study *M. leprae*. At least five patients are reported to have caught leprosy through hunting and handling wild armadillos,[104] and the infection is now widespread in wild armadillos in the southern United States.[105]

There are several recent reviews of leprosy and its clinical management.[106-109]

M. tuberculosis *skin infection*

This can conveniently be divided, on epidemiological grounds, into two parts: the first is scrofuloderma and lupus vulgaris and the second typified by tuberculosis verrucosa cutis. Scrofuloderma is the breakdown of tissue, characteristically via a sinus, as a result of infection of a lymph node, most frequently of the neck. In some populations it is the most prevalent form of cutaneous tuberculosis[110,111] and is a sign of current infection elsewhere. Lupus vulgaris is most frequently a manifestation of a previous infection in which bacilli are distributed about the body by haematogenous spread[112] and then lie until reactivated. In Europeans the most common site of infection is the face; the reactivating agent may be sunlight or sunburn[113-115] and organisms may be numerous.[116] In older patients, *M. bovis* may be the most common mycobacterium, as a result of former milk-borne infection,[117,118] and be of long duration.[119]

Tuberculosis verrucosa cutis or warty tubercle of the skin can be regarded, on epidemiological grounds, as inoculation of mycobacteria from the environment, though clearly this convenient distinction will not always hold true. Prosector's wart, infection usually of the hands arising from contact with necropsy material, remains the best documented example of this disease and cases are reported at regular intervals.[120-123]

In the past, exogenous infection of the skin of the legs and buttocks of children in Hong Kong was associated with playing in streets contaminated with expectorated sputum,[124] and infection of the sole of the foot in India probably had the same source.[125] Exogenous infection of the skin of the hand has been reported to follow contamination from a draining sinus on the patient's own back.[126]

M. ulcerans

Infection by *M. ulcerans* remains an epidemiological enigma. Despite the rarity of person-to-person spread, an environmental source for this organism has not been found. The appearance of lesions in a population is usually, but not always, associated with the presence of water and occurs in a belt throughout the tropics so that Northern Australia, Malaysia, New Guinea, Mexico, Bolivia and central tropical Africa are all reported as endemic zones. More recent reports include Ghana and importation into Ireland.[127,128] *Mycobacterium ulcerans* is the only member of the genus in which a toxin is implicated. The toxin is lipid soluble and causes necrosis of the subcutaneous fat.[129,130] The skin lesion progresses from a subcutaneous nodule to an ulcer with a deeply undermined edge; there is necrosis of the fatty tissue with abundant acid-fast bacilli.[131] Lesions at different stages of development may be found on the same patient.

M. marinum

The epidemiology of infection with *M. marinum* has been extensively reviewed.[132] The frequent association of this organism with some aquatic activity such as sailing, swimming or keeping tropical fish has earned the organism the names 'hobby-hazard' and 'leisure-time' pathogen. Originally associated with swimming-pool granuloma, when lesions appeared on the elbows and less often on the knees, the early reports were chiefly of epidemics involving large numbers of children. More recent outbreaks have been reported to have the same pattern.[133-135] Sporadic cases are reported in association with swimming pools and sea bathing. By their nature, cases associated with fish keeping – fish-tank granuloma – are also sporadic, and usually confined to a single patient. Lesions are usually of the back of the hands or fingers. Bacilli are very rare in these lesions and it may be more fruitful to examine the fish, if any survive.[136]

Other infections are reported in persons injured whilst fishing or boating, although a few cases appear unrelated to water.[137] Dissemination of infection is rare: one such case is reported in a renal transplant patient;[138] a second was in a 16-month-old child whose father had used the child's bath to clean out a fish tank,[139] although this more nearly resembles multiple lesions than dissemination. Deep infections, for example of the hand and wrist, also occur.[140] The name *M. marinum* was originally given to the organisms isolated from several fish in an aquarium.[141]

M. chelonei; M. fortuitum

These two fast-growing mycobacteria are usually associated with post-injection abscesses. The difficulty encountered by some workers in identifying the organism found may have resulted in some indiscriminate naming of these pathogens. Injectable materials are usually the source in epidemic outbreaks[142] but diabetics who need repeated injections may form a large part of those endemically infected.[143] For example, 13 nurses who practised injection procedures were infected at the sites of injection with *M. chelonei*, which was also found in the bottle of saline used for injections.[142] Deep infection and infection of the cornea are also reported.[144] In renal transplant patients, bacilli may be very numerous in the lesions.[145-146]

Other mycobacteria

An increasing number of other mycobacteria are reported causing skin infection, most particularly in AIDS patients. The most common are the members of the *Mycobacterium avium* complex – *M. avium*, *M. intracellulare*, *M. malmoense*, *M. haemophilum*. In about 80 per cent of cases these organisms caused a disseminated infection in the immunosuppressed,[147] but infection limited to skin and lymph nodes also occurs.[148,149] Much more rare is infection with *M. thermoresistibile*; the first skin case, or third human case, was described in 1989.[150] Inoculation mycobacterioses as a group have been reviewed by Grange and colleagues.[144] Such infections include those due to *M. szulgai*, *M. scrofulaceum* and *M. gordonae*. Infection may also follow the use of BCG.[144,151]

Other Gram-positive bacteria

Vegetative cells of clostridia are very sensitive to desiccation and it is most probably spores of *Clostridium perfringens* that are recovered in skin samples. Drewett and coworkers[152] reported that 44 of 100 patients examined carried *Cl. perfringens*, usually around the anus or natal cleft, but 24 carried in the perineum, 22 over the hip joint, 19 on the knee and 12 on the ankle. These were most probably transient organisms from the rectum. The skin is reported as a site of entry for spores in deep surgical wound infections.[153]

Bacillus spp. are recovered as part of the normal flora of the skin, but in small numbers and doubtless as a part of the transient or contaminant flora derived from the environment.[154] Apart from local skin infections in the immunodeficient,[155] only one member of the genus *B. anthracis* is a pathogen of skin, although other species are involved in food poisoning outbreaks and occasionally are reported in surgical wound infection.[156] In the Western world, 98 per cent of patients with anthrax have the cutaneous form; infection with *B. anthracis* is predominantly a disease of animals and humans are generally infected as a result of handling infected products such as hides or wool. The current status of anthrax has been well summarized at a workshop held in 1990.[157]

As with the Gram-negative bacteria, a variety of Gram-positives are reported, though relatively infrequently, as causing primary skin lesions. *Nocardia* spp. cause primary skin infection,[158,159] though more often associated with deep infection, and have been reported as contaminants on the skin of the feet.[160] *Erysipelothrix insidiosa* (*E. rhusiopathiae*) is a pathogen of fish and other animals but causes a well-established infection, erysipeloid, in man, especially where the skin is in contact with animal tissue, for example in butchers, and may lead to deep infection.[161,162] Similarly, *Listeria monocytogenes* is also reported in primary infection.[163]

Dermatophilus congolensis is a well-established and locally frequent pathogen of the skin of domestic animals (see Chapter 11), where severe infection leads to loss of weight, reduction of milk yield and even death,[164] but is a rare, probably underreported skin pathogen of man.[165] It has, however, been implicated in pitted keratolysis, where its proteolytic ability no doubt accounts for the lesions.[166,167]

Anaerobes

Apart from *Propionibacterium* spp, which are not strictly anaerobic bacteria but need to be treated as such in the laboratory, and the clostridia described above, we have been slow to appreciate that anaerobic bacteria have any real role in skin disease. Anaerobes have long been appreciated as causing deep infection.[168]

Sebaceous cysts may also contain anaerobes such as *Bacteroides* spp. and *Peptococcus* spp.[169,170] The potential for anaerobes such as fusiforms has been explored in relation to perioral dermatitis[171] and tropical ulcers.[172,173] This is an underexplored region of cutaneous microbiology.

Ulcers may contain a mixed flora of Gram-negative and Gram-positive bacteria together with anaerobes, especially in those that fail to heal.[174] The flora comprises pseudomonas, proteus, staphylococci, streptococci and bacteroides and there is little agreement on the role, if any, for the various organisms that may be present, with opposing views equally firmly held. The reader is referred to several publications,[175–182] which should be approached with an open mind.

Rarer infections of skin

Borrelia

Long known as a skin disease, erythema migrans, in Europe and associated with tick bites in 1910, it was not until 1970 that it was recorded in the United States. In 1975 an outbreak of 'juvenile rheumatoid arthritis' in Connecticut resulted in the description of Lyme arthritis and later an association of the arthritis with erythema migrans resulted in the acceptance of Lyme disease as a multisystem disorder. In 1982 a new spirochaete was discovered in ticks and was subsequently recognized as a new *Borrelia* species and as the cause of Lyme disease. There appears to be a real increase in the prevalence of Lyme disease but an increased interest has lead to a rapidly lengthening list of publications. The reader is referred to reviews of *Borrelia burgdorferi*.[183,184]

Prototheca

Infections with *Prototheca wickerhamii* or *P. zopfii*, achlorophyllous algae, remain very rare. The condition was well reviewed by Sudman[185] and a number of further cases were published in the mid-1970s. Further cases of infection continue to be described,[186,187] with the observation that these occur chiefly among the immosuppressed patients but that the alga itself may contribute to the immunosuppression. Skin infection also occurs in animals,[188] although infections of the udder or viscera are more common. Infection with prototheca and chlorella are described as 'water borne' but it is not apparent whether acquisition is direct from water or from wind-borne organisms of aquatic origin.[189]

Pneumocystis

A case of cutaneous pneumocystosis in an AIDS patient has been described.[190]

References

1 Noble WC. Hospital epidemiology of *Acinetobacter* species. In: Towner KJ, Bergogne-Berezin E, Fewson CR, eds. The Biology of *Acinetobacter* (FEMS Acinetobacter Symposium). New York: Plenum Press; 1991.

2 Somerville DA. The normal flora of the skin in different age groups. Br J. Dermatol 1969; 81: 248–58.

3 Gaughan M, White PM, Noble WC. Skin as a source of *Acinetobacter/Moraxella* species. J Clin Pathol 1979; 32: 1193.

4 Al Khoja MS, Darrel JH. The skin as the source of *Acinetobacter* and *Moraxella* species occurring in blood cultures. J Clin Pathol 1979; 32: 497–99.

5 Kloos WE, Musselwhite MS. Distribution and persistence of *Staphylococcus* and *Micrococcus* species and other aerobic bacteria on human skin. Appl Microbiol 1975; 30: 381–95.

6 Retailliau HF, Hightower AW, Dixon RE, Allen JR. *Acinetobacter calcoaceticus*: a nosocomial pathogen with an unusual seasonal pattern. J Infect Dis 1978; 139: 371–75.

7 Glew RH, Moellering RC, Kunz LJ. Infection with *Acinetobacter calcoaceticus* (*Herellea vaginicola*): clinical and laboratory studies. Medicine 1977; 56: 79–97.

8 Sneider JR, Gunther SF. A hand infection from *A. calcoaceticus* (*M. polymorpha*). Clin Orthopaed Rel Res 1979; 140: 184–88.

9 Bouvet PJM, Grimont PAD. Identification and biotyping of clinical isolates of *Acinetobacter*. Ann Inst Pasteur Microbiol 1987; 138: 569–78.

10 Tjernberg I, Ursing J. Clinical strains of Acinetobacter classified by DNA–DNA hybridization. APMIS 1989; 97: 595–605.

11 Musa EK, Desai N, Casewell MW. The survival of *Acinetobacter calcoaceticus* inoculated on fingertips and on formica. J Hosp Infect 1990; 15: 219–27.

12 Leyden JJ, Stewart R, Kligman AM. Experimental inoculation of *Pseudomonas aeruginosa* and *Pseudomonas cepacia* on human skin. J Soc Cosmet Chem 1980; 31: 19–28.

13 Hope YM, Clayton YM, Hay RJ, Noble WC, Elder Smith JG. Foot infection in coal miners: a reassessment. Br J Dermatol 1985; 112: 405–13.

14 Silverman AR, Nieland ML. Hot tub dermatitis: a familial outbreak of *Pseudomonas* folliculitis. J Am Acad Dermatol 1983; 8: 153–56.

15 Hogan K, Bennet R, Savoury B, Ratnam S, March S, Butler RW. Outbreak of whirlpool-associated folliculitis due to *Pseudomonas aeruginosa* serotype 0:7 – Newfoundland. Can Dis Wkly Rep 1984; 19: 73–75.

16 Jiminez-Reyes J, Palomo Arellano A, Castanada Sanz S, Castro Torres A, Barat A. Foliculitis por pseudomonas. Actas Derm Sif 1984; 75: 9–10.

17 Chandrasekar PH, Rolston KVI, Kannangara W, LeFrock JK, Binnick SA.

Hot tub-associated dermatitis due to *Pseudomonas aeruginosa*. Arch Dermatol 1984; 120: 1337–40.

18 Schleck WF III, Simonsen N, Sumarah R, Martin RS. Nosocomial outbreak of *Pseudomonas aeruginosa* folliculitis associated with a physiotherapy pool. Can Med Ass J 1986; 134: 909–13.

19 Jacobson JA. Pool-associated *Pseudomonas aeruginosa* dermatitis and other bathing-associated infections. Infect Control 1985; 6: 398–401.

20 Highsmith AK, Le PN, Khabbaz RF, Munn VP. Characteristics of *Pseudomonas aeruginosa* isolated from whirlpools and bathers. Infect Control 1985; 6: 407–12.

21 Noble WC, White PM. Pseudomonas and man. Trans St John's Hosp Dermatol Soc 1969; 55: 202–28.

22 Chapel TA, Adcock M. Pseudomonas chromonychia. Cutis 1981; 27: 601–02.

23 Dorff GJ, Geimer NF, Rosenthal DR, Rytel MW. Pseudomonas septicemia. Illustrated evolution of its skin lesion. Arch Int Med 1971; 128: 591–95.

24 Roberts R, Tarpay M, Marks MI, Nitschke R. Erysipelas-like lesions and hyperesthesia as manifestations of *Pseudomonas aeruginosa* sepsis. J Am Med Ass 1982; 248: 2156–57.

25 Sangeorzan JA, Bradley SF, Kauffman CA. Cutaneous manifestations of *Pseudomonas* infection in the acquired immunodeficiency syndrome. Arch Dermatol 1990; 126: 832–33.

26 Taplin D, Bassett DCJ, Mertz PM. Foot lesions associated with *Pseudomonas cepacia*. Lancet 1971; i: 568–71.

27 Mandell IN, Feiner HD, Price NM, Simberkoff M. *Pseudomonas cepacia* endocarditis and ecthyma gangrenosum. Arch Dermatol 1977; 113: 199–202.

28 Peel MM, Davis JM, Armstrong WLH, Wilson JR, Holmes B. *Pseudomonas paucimobilis* from a leg ulcer on a Japanese seaman. J Clin Microbiol 1979; 9: 561–64.

29 Neubert U, Braun Falco O. Mazeration der Zehenzwischen-raume und Gram negativer Fussinfekt. Hautarzt 1976; 27: 538–43.

30 Hay RJ, Clayton YM, Howell SA, Noble WC. Management of combined bacterial and fungal foot infection in coal miners. Mycoses 1988; 31: 316–19.

31 Ehrenkranz NJ, Afonso BC, Eckert DG, Moskowitz LB. *Proteeae* species bactiuria accompanying *Proteeae* species groin skin carriage in geriatric patients. J Clin Microbiol 1989; 27: 1988–91.

32 Rasmussen JE. *Haemophilus influenzae* cellulitis. Case presentation and review of the literature. Brit J Dermatol 1973; 88: 547–50.

33 Shaw RA, Plouffe JF. *Haemophilus influenzae* cellulitis in an adult. Arch Int Med 1979; 139: 368–69.

34 Sokal RJ, Bowden RA. An erysipelas-like scalp cellulitis due to *Haemophilus influenzae* type B. J Pediatr 1980; 96: 60–61.

35 Spencer RC, Barnham M. *Haemophilus influenzae* cellulitis. Brit Med J 1975; ii: 615.

36 Francis DP, Holmes MA, Brandon G. *Pasteurella multocida*: infections after domestic animal bites and scratches. J Am Med Ass 1975; 233: 42–45.

37 Elling F, Pedersen KB, Hogh P, Foged NT. Characterization of the dermal lesions induced by a purified protein from toxigenic *Pasteurella multocida*. APMIS 1988; 96: 50–55.

38 Fulghum DD, Linton WR Jr, Taplin D. Fatal *Aeromonas hydrophila* infection of the skin. Southern Med J 1978; 71: 739–41.

39 Young DF, Barr RJ. *Aeromonas hydrophila* infection of the skin. Arch Dermatol 1981; 117: 244.

40 Ryan WJ. Marine vibrios associated with superficial septic lesions. J Clin Pathol 1976; 29: 1014–15.

41 Lambert WC, Pathan AK, Imaeda T, Kaminski ZC, Reichman LB. Culture of *Vibrio extorquans* from severe chronic skin ulcers in a Puerto Rican woman. J Am Acad Dermatol 1983; 9: 262–68.

42 Wickboldt LG, Sanders CV. *Vibrio vulnificus* infection: case report and update since 1970. J Am Acad Dermatol 1983; 9: 243–51.

43 Woo ML, Patrick WGD, Simon MTP, French GL. Necrotising fasciitis caused by *Vibrio vulnificus*. J Clin Pathol 1984; 37: 1301–04.

44 West PA. The human pathogenic vibrios – a public health update with environmental perspectives. Epidemiol Infect 1989; 103: 1–34.

45 Burnett JW. *Vibrio vulnificus* infection. Cutis 1988; 42: 392–93.

46 Auerbach PS. Natural microbiologic hazards of the aquatic environment. Clin Dermatol 1987; 5: 52–61.

47 Helms CM, Johnson W, Donaldson MF, Corry RJ. Pretibial rash in *Legionella pneumophila* pneumonia. J Am Med Ass 1981; 245: 1758–59.

48 Ampel NM, Ruben FL, Norden CW. Cutaneous abscess caused by *Legionella micdadei* in an immunosuppressed patient. Ann Int Med 1985; 102: 630–32.

49 Gee-Lew BM, Nicholas EA, Hirose FM, Yoshimori RN, Keller MA. Unusual skin manifestation of brucellosis. Arch Dermatol 1983; 119: 56–58.

50 Ariza J, Servitje O, Pallares R, Viladrich PF, Rufi G, Peyri J, Gudiol F. Characteristic cutaneous lesions in patients with brucellosis. Arch Dermatol 1989; 125: 380–83.

51 Kurtz JB. Leg abscess caused by *Salmonella heidelburg*. Lancet 1976; i: 200–01.

52 Stoll DM. Cutaneous shigellosis. Arch Dermatol 1986; 122: 22.

53 Rigatos GA, Kappos-Rigatou I. Cutaneous manifestation of brucellosis. Br J Clin Pract 1977; 31: 167.

54 Berger TG, Guill MA, Goette DK. Cutaneous lesions in brucellosis. Arch Dermatol 1981; 40–42.

55 Niemi KM, Hannuksela M, Salo OP. Skin lesions in human yersiniosis. Br J Dermatol 1976; 94: 155–60.

56 Bolivar R, Abramovits W. Cutaneous infection caused by *Flavobacterium meningosepticum*. J Infect Dis 1989; 159: 150–51.

57 Redfield DC, Overturf GD, Ewing N, Powars D. Bacteria, arthritis and skin lesions due to *Kingella kingae*. Arch Dis Child 1980; 55: 411–14.

58 Zumwalt RD, Franz TJ. *Eikenella corrodens*: an unusual cause of an indolent skin infection. Arch Dermatol 1983; 119: 624–25.

59 Datar S, Shafran SD. Cellulitis of the foot due to *Eikenella corrodens*. Arch Dermatol 1989; 125: 849–50.

60 Brenner DE, Lookingbill DP. *Serratia marcescens* cellulitis. Arch Dermatol 1977; 113: 1599–600.

61 Leyden JJ, Marples RR, Mills OH, Kligman AM. Gram-negative folliculitis – a complication of antibiotic therapy in acne vulgaris. Br J Dermatol 1973; 88: 533–38.

62 Feibleman CE, Rasmussen JE. Gram-negative acne. Cutis 1980; 25: 194–99.

63 Blankenship ML. Gram negative folliculitis: follow-up observations in 20 patients. Arch Dermatol 1984; 120: 1301–03.

64 Scott MJ Jr, Scott MJ Sr. Primary cutaneous *Neisseria gonorrhoea* infection. Arch Dermatol 1982; 118: 351–52.

65 Fraser HS, Liburd AL, Figueroa JP, Nicholson GA, James OBO'L, Whitbourne F, Alleyne GAO. Gonococcaemia with arthritis, dermatitis and myocarditis. Postgrad Med J 1974; 50: 759–64.

66 Toews WH, Bass JW. Skin manifestations of meningococcal infection: an immediate indicator of prognosis. Am J Dis Child 1974; 127: 173–76.

67 Adams BC, Marrie TJ. Hand carriage of aerobic Gram-negative rods by health care personnel. J Hyg Camb 1982; 89: 23–31.

68 Adams BC, Marrie TJ. Hand carriage of aerobic Gram-negative rods may not be transient. J Hyg Camb 1982; 89: 33–45.

69 Ligtvoet EEJ, Mouton RP. Hands and nebulizers as a route of transmission for Gram-negative bacilli in an intensive care unit. Antonie van Leeuwenhoek 1982; 48: 204–05.

70 French GL, Casewell MW, Roncoroni AJ, Knight S, Phillips I. A hospital outbreak of antibiotic-resistant *Acinetobacter anitratus*: epidemiology and control. J Hosp Infect 1980; 1: 125–31.

71 Buxton AE, Anderson RL, Werdegar D, Atlas E. Nosocomial respiratory tract infection and colonization with *Acinetobacter calcoaceticus*. Am J Med 1978; 65: 507–13.

72 Allen KD, Green HT. Hospital outbreak of multiresistant *Acinetobacter anitratus*: an airborne mode of spread? J Hosp Infect 1987; 9: 110–19.

73 Casewell M, Phillips I. Hands as route of transmission for *Klebsiella* species. Br Med J 1977; 2: 1315–17.

74 Haverkorn ML, Michel MF. Nosocomial Klebsiellas. J Hyg Camb 1989; 82: 177–205.

75 Parry MF, Hutchinson JH, Brown NA, Wu C-H, Estreller L. Gram-negative sepsis in neonates: a nursery outbreak due to hand carriage of *Citrobacter diversus*. Pediatrics 1980; 65: 1105–09.

76 Casewell MW, Desai N. Survival of multiply-resistant *Klebsiella aerogenes* and other Gram-negative bacilli on fingertips. J Hosp Infect 1983; 4: 350–60.

77 Cooke EM, Edmondson AS, Starkey W. The ability of strains of *Klebsiella aerogenes* to survive on the hands. J Med Microbiol 1981; 14: 443–50.

78 Noble WC, Hope YM, Midgley G, Moore MK, Patel S, Virani Z, Lison E. Toewebs as a source of Gram negative bacilli. J Hosp Infect 1986; 8: 248–56.

79 Howell SA, Clayton YM, Phan QG, Noble WC. Tinea pedis: the relationship between symptoms, organisms and host characteristics. Microb Ecol Hlth Dis 1988; 1: 131–35.

80 Aly R, Maibach HI. Aerobic microbial flora of intertriginous skin. Appl. Environ Microbiol 1977; 33: 97–100.

81 Suter L, Rabbat RM, Nolting S. Gramnegativer Fussinfekt. Mykosen 1979; 22: 109–14.

82 Chow S, Westfried M, Lynfield Y. Immersion foot: an occupational disease. Cutis 1980; 25: 662.

83 Rietschel RL, Allen AM. Immersion foot: a method for studying the effects of protracted water exposure on human skin. Milit Med 1976; 141: 778–80.

84 McBride ME, Duncan WC, Knox JM. Physiological and environmental control of Gram negative bacteria on skin. Br J Dermatol 1975; 93: 191–99.

85 de Assis TL, Formiga LCD, Filgueira AL, de Mattos GA. Aspectos

microbiologicos dos espacos interdigitais dos pes. Ann Bras Dermatol 1984; 59: 3–8; 61–66.

86 Stackebrandt E, Woese CR. A phylogenetic dissection of the family Micrococcaceae. Curr Microbiol 1979; 2: 317–22.

87 Kloos WE, Tornabene TG, Schleifer KH. Isolation and characterization of micrococci from human skin, including two new species *Micrococcus lylae* and *Micrococcus kristinae*. Int J System Bacteriol 1974; 24: 79–101.

88 Glass M. Sarcina species on the skin of the human forearm. Trans St John's Hosp Derm Soc 1973; 59: 56–60.

89 Namavar F. Classification, epidemiology and virulence of coagulase-negative *Micrococcaceae*. [Thesis]. University of Amsterdam; 1979.

90 Noble WC. Skin carriage of the Micrococcaceae. J Clin Pathol 1969; 22: 249–53.

91 Somerville DA, Lancaster-Smith M. The aerobic cutaneous flora of diabetic subjects. Brit J Dermatol 1973; 89: 395–400.

92 Kloos WE, Zimmerman RJ, Smith RF. Preliminary studies on the characterization and distribution of *Staphylococcus* and *Micrococcus* species on animal skin. Appl Environ Microbiol 1976; 31: 53–59.

93 Nordstrom KM, McGinley KJ, Cappiello L, Zeckman JM, Leyden JJ. Pitted keratolysis; the role of *Micrococcus sedentarius*. Arch Dermatol 1987; 123: 1320–25.

94 Chomarat M, Rochette A. Signification de l'isolement de *Stomatococcus mucilaginosus*. La Press Med. 1988; 17: 537–38.

95 Shapiro S, Boaz J, Kleiman M, Kalsbeck J, Mealey J. Origin of organisms infecting ventricular shunts. Neurosurgery 1988; 22: 868–72.

96 Magee JT, Burnett IA, Hindmarch JM, Spencer RC. *Micrococcus* and *Stomatococcus* spp from human infections. J Hosp Infect 1990; 16: 67–73.

97 Spencer RC. Infections in continuous ambulatory peritoneal dialysis. J Hosp Infect 1984; 5: 233–40.

98 Wharton M, Rice JR, McCallum R, Gallis HA. Septic arthritis due to *Micrococcus luteus*. J Rheumatol 1986; 13: 659–60.

99 Carr DL, Kloos WE. Temporal study of the staphylococci and micrococci of normal infant skin. Appl Environ Microbiol 1977; 34: 673–80.

100 Klotz PG. Atypical acid fast bacilli in urine. Canad Med Ass J 1970; 103: 283–84.

101 Grange JM. Mycobacterial disease in the world: yesterday, today and tomorrow. In: Ratledge C, Stanford J, Grange JM, eds. The biology of the mycobacteria, vol 3. London: Academic Press; 1989: 3–36.

102 Kennedy DH. Extrapulmonary tuberculosis. In: Ratledge C, Stanford J, Grange JM, eds. The biology of the mycobacteria, vol. 3. London: Academic Press; 1989: 245–84.

103 Draper P, Kandler O, Darbe A. Peptidoglycan and arabinogalactan of *Mycobacterium leprae*. J Gen Microbiol 1987; 133: 1187–94.

104 Lumpkin LR, Cox GF, Wolf JE. Leprosy in five armadillo handlers. J Am Acad Dermatol 1983; 9: 899–903.

105 Truman RW, Kumaresan JA, McDonough CM, Job CK, Hastings RC. Seasonal and spatial trends in the detectability of leprosy in wild armadillos. Epidemiol Infect 1991. [In press].

106 Hastings C, Gillis TP, Krahenbuhl JL, Franzblau SG. Leprosy. Clin Microbiol Rev 1988; 1: 330–48.

107 Ganapati R, Revankar CR. Clinical aspects of leprosy. In: Ratledge C, Stanford J, Grange JM, eds. The biology of the mycobacteria, vol 3. London: Academic Press; 1989: 327–58.

108 Naafs B. Reactions in leprosy. In: Ratledge C, Stanford J, Grange JM, eds. The biology of the mycobacteria, vol 3. London: Academic Press; 1989: 359–404.

109 Waters MFR. The chemotherapy of leprosy. In: Ratledge C, Stanford J, Grange JM, eds. The biology of the mycobacteria, vol 3. London: Academic Press; 1989: 405–74.

110 Bales JD. Adult scrofula. Saudi Med J 1986; 7: 176–81.

111 Sehgal VN, Srivastava G, Khurana VK, Sharma VK, Bhalla P, Beohar PC. An appraisal of epidemiologic, clinical, bacteriologic, histopathologic and immunologic parameters in cutaneous tuberculosis. Int J Dermatol 1987; 26: 521–26.

112 Stead WW, Bates JH. Evidence of a 'silent' bacillemia in primary tuberculosis. Ann Int Med 1971; 74: 559–61.

113 Horwitz O. Lupus vulgaris cutis in Denmark 1895–1954. Acta Tubercle Scand 1960; Suppl 49.

114 Schmidt CL, Pomeranz JR. Lupus vulgaris: recovery of living tubercle bacilli 35 years after onset. Cutis 1976; 18: 221–23.

115 Warin AP, Wilson Jones E. Cutaneous tuberculosis of the nose with unusual clinical and histological features leading to a delay in diagnosis. Clin Exp Dermatol 1977; 2: 235–42.

116 Dihra P, Grattan CEM, Ryatt KS. Lupus vulgaris with numerous tubercal bacilli. Clin Exp Dermatol 1988; 13: 31–33.

117 Hart V, Weedon D. Lupus vulgaris and *Mycobacterium bovis*: a case report. Austral J Dermatol 1977; 18: 86–87.

118 Wilkins EGL, Griffiths RJ, Roberts C. Bovine tuberculosis of the skin. J Infect 1986; 12: 280–81.

119 Hruza GJ, Snow SN. Cutaneous *Mycobacterium bovis* infection of 40 years duration. Arch Dermatol 1990; 126: 123–24.

120 Marmalzat WL. Laennec and the 'prosectors wart'. Arch Dermatol 1980; 86: 74–76.

121 London ID. Primary cutaneous inoculation tuberculosis. Arch Dermatol 1972; 106: 264.

122 Goette DK, Jacobson KW, Doty RD. Primary inoculation tuberculosis of the skin. Arch Dermatol 1978; 114: 567–69.

123 Hoyt EM. Primary inoculation tuberculosis: report of a case. J Am Med Ass 1981; 245: 1556–57.

124 Wong KO, Lee KP, Chin SF. Tuberculosis of the skin in Hong Kong: a review of 100 cases. Br J Dermatol 1968; 80: 424–29.

125 Pandhi RK, Bedi TR, Kanwar AJ, Bhutani LK. Cutaneous tuberculosis – a clinical and investigative study. Indian J Dermatol 1977; 22: 99–100.

126 Cohn JR, Harris MS. Cutaneous autoinoculation by *Mycobacterium tuberculosis*. Arch Dermatol 1982; 118: 363–65.

127 van der Werf TS, van der Graf WTA, Groothuis DG, Knell AJ. *Mycobacterium ulcerans* infection in Ashanti region Ghana. Trans R Soc Trop Med Hyg 1989; 83: 410–13.

128 Dawson JF, Allen GE. Ulcer due to *Mycobacterium ulcerans* in Northern Ireland. Clin Exp Dermatol 1985; 10: 572–76.

129 Noble WC, Hay RJ, Stanford J. Mycobacterial infection of the skin. In: Ratledge C, Stanford J, Grange JM, eds. Biology of the mycobacteria, vol 3. London: Academic Press; 1989: 477–510.

130 Pimsler M, Sponsler TA, Meyers WM. Immunosuppressive properties of the soluble toxin from *Mycobacterium ulcerans*. J Infect Dis 1988; 157: 577–80.

131 Hayman J, McQueen A. The pathology of *Mycobacterium ulcerans* infection. Pathology 1985; 17: 594–600.

132 Collins CH, Grange JM, Noble WC, Yates MD. *Mycobacterium marinum* infections in man. J Hyg Camb 1985; 94: 135–49.

133 Daillaux M, Morlot M, Sirbat C. Study of factors affecting presence of atypical mycobacteria in water of a swimming pool. Rev Epidemiol Sante Publique 1980; 28: 299–306.

134 Junger H, Witzani R. 'Swimming pool granuloma' – an infection of skin with *Mycobacterium marinum*. Z Hautkr 1981; 56: 16–18.

135 Johnson JM, Izumi AK. Cutaneous *Mycobacterium marinum* infection ('swimming pool granuloma') Clin Dermatol 1987; 5: 68–75.

136 Gray SF, Stanwell Smith R, Reynolds NJ, Williams EW. Fish tank granuloma. Br Med J 1990; 300: 1069–70.

137 Arai H, Nakajima H, Nagai R. *Mycobacterium marinum* infection of the skin in Japan. J Dermatol 1984; 11: 37–42.

138 Gombert ME, Goldstein EJC, Corrado ML, Stein AJ, Butt KMH. Disseminated *Mycobacterium marinum* infection after renal transplantation. Ann Int Med 1981; 94: 486–87.

139 King AJ, Fairley JA, Rasmussen JE. Disseminated cutaneous *Mycobacterium marinum* infection. Arch Dermatol 1983; 119: 268–70.

140 Chow SP, Ip FK, Lau JHK, et al. *Mycobacterium marinum* infection of the hand and wrist: results of conservative treatment in twenty four cases. J Bone Joint Surg 1987; 69A: 1161–68.

141 Aronson JP. Spontaneous tuberculosis in salt water fish. J Infect Dis 1926; 39: 315–20.

142 Gremillion DH, Mursch SB, Levner CJ. Injection site abscesses caused by *Mycobacterium chelonei*. Infect Control 1983; 4: 25–28.

143 Kelly SE. Multiple injection abscesses in a diabetic caused by *Mycobacterium chelonei*. Clin Exp Dermatol 1987; 12: 48–49.

144 Grange JM, Noble WC, Yates MD, Collins CH. Inoculation mycobacteriosis. Clin Exp Dermatol 1988; 13: 211–20.

145 Cooper JF, Lichtenstein MJ, Graham BS, Schafner W. *Mycobacterium chelonae*: a cause of nodular skin lesions with a proclivity for renal transplant patients. Am J Med 1989; 86: 173–77.

146 Drabnick JJ, Duffy PE, Samlaska CP, Scherbenske JM. Disseminated *Mycobacterium chelonei* sub sp. *chelonei* infection with cutaneous and osseous manifestations. Arch Dermatol 1990; 126: 1064–67.

147 Young LS, Inderlied CB, Berlin OG, Gottlieb MS. Mycobacterial infections in AIDS patients with an emphasis on the *Mycobacterium avium* complex. Rev Infect Dis 1986; 8: 1024–33.

148 Barbaro DJ, Orcutt VL. Coldiron BM. *Mycobacterium avium–Mycobacterium intracellulare* infection limited to the skin and lymph nodes in patients with AIDS. Rev Infect Dis 1989; 11: 625–28.

149 Lugo-Janer G, Cruz A, Sanchez JL. Disseminated cutaneous infection caused by *Mycobacterium avium* complex. Arch Dermatol 1990; 126: 1108–10.

150 Neeley SP, Denning DW. Cutaneous *Mycobacterium thermoresistible* infection in a heart transplant recipient. Rev Infect Dis 1989; 11: 608–11.

151 Armbruster C, Junker W, Vetter N, Jaksch G. Disseminated bacille Calmette–Guerin infection in an AIDS patient 30 years after BCG vaccination. J Infect Dis 1990; 162: 1216.

152 Drewett SE, Payne DJH, Tuke W, Verrdon PE. Skin distribution of *Clostridium welchii*: use of iodophor as a sporicidal agent. Lancet 1972; 1: 1172–73.

153 Hulme JR. Localised *Clostridium welchii* wound infection (Welch abscess) following a skin abrasion. J Clin Pathol 1975; 29: 273–74.

154 Bibel DJ, Lovell DJ, Smiljanic RJ. Survival of *Bacillus licheniformis* on human skin. Appl Environ Microbiol 1978; 35: 1128–36.

155 Henrickson KJ, Shenep JL, Flynn PM, Pui C-H. Primary cutaneous *Bacillus cereus* infection in neutropenic children. Lancet 1989; i: 601–03.

156 Akesson A, Hedstrom SA, Ripa T. *Bacillus cereus*: a significant pathogen in post-operative and post-traumatic wounds on orthopaedic wards. Scand J Infect Dis 1991; 23: 71–77.

157 Turnbull PCB, ed. Anthrax: proceedings of an international workshop. Salisbury Medical Bulletin 1990; no. 68.

158 Kalb RE, Kaplan MH, Grossman RE. Cutaneous nocardiosis: case report and review. Am J Acad Dermatol 1985; 13: 125–33.

159 Landau Z, Feld S, Frumkin A, Resnitsky P. *Nocardia brasiliensis* skin infections. Israel J Med Sci 1986; 22: 397–99.

160 Stropnik Z. Isolation of *Nocardia asteroides* from human skin. Sabouraudia 1965; 4: 41–44.

161 Lacroix J, Delage G, Mitchell G. Erysipeloid in an infant. J Pediatr 1981; 99: 745–46.

162 Normann B, Kihlstrom E. *Erysipelothrix rhusiopathiae* septicaemia. Scand J Inf Dis 1985; 17: 123–24.

163 Cain DB, McCann VC. An unusual case of cutaneous listeriosis. J Clin Microbiol 1986; 23: 976–77.

164 Lloyd DH, Sellers KC, eds. Dermatophilus infection in animals and man. London: Academic Press; 1976.

165 Kaminski GW, Suter II. Human infection with *Dermatophilus congolensis*. Med J Austral 1976; 1: 443–47.

166 Rubel LR. Pitted keratolysis and *Dermatophilus congolensis*. Arch Dermatol 1972; 105: 584–86.

167 Woodgyer AJ, Baxter M, Rush-Munro FM, Brown J, Kaplan W. Isolation of *Dermatophilus congolensis* from two New Zealand cases of pitted keratolysis. Austral J Dermatol 1985; 26: 29–35.

168 Brook I. Microbiology of abscesses of the head and neck in children. Ann Otol Rhinol Laryngol 1987; 96: 429–33.

169 Bose B, Maykut F. Infected sebaceous cyst due to *Bacteroides* species. Can Med Ass J 1977; 116: 475.

170 Brook I. Microbiology of infected epidermal cyst. Arch Dermatol 1989; 125: 1658–61.

171 Buck A, Kalkoff KW. Zum nachweis von Fusobakterien aus Efflorenzenen der Perioral Dermatitis. Hautarzt 1971; 22: 433–36.

172 Adriaans B, Drasar BS. The isolation of fusobacteria from tropical ulcers. Epidem Infect 1987; 99: 361–71.

173 Adriaans B, Hay R, Drasar R, Robinson D. The infectious aetiology of tropical ulcer – a study of the role of anaerobic bacteria. Br J Dermatol 1987; 116: 31–37.

174 Daltrey DC, Rhodes B, Chattwood JG. Investigation into the microbial flora of healing and non-healing decubitus ulcers. J Clin Pathol 1981; 34: 701–05.

175 Akintewe TA, Akanji AO, Odunsan O. Hand and foot ulcers in Nigerian diabetics – a comparative study. Trop Geog Med 1983; 35: 353–56.

176 Gieler U, Vogt E. Development of bacterial flora on ulcera crurum. Z Hautkr 1984; 59: 435–42.

177 Anderson E, Hansson C, Swanbeck G. Leg and foot ulcers: an epidemiological study. Acta Dermatovener Stockh. 1984; 64: 227–32.

178 Eriksson G, Eklund AE, Kallings LO. The clinical significance of bacterial growth in venous leg ulcers. Scand J Infect Dis 1984; 16: 175–80.

179 McFarlane DE, Baum KF, Serjeant GR. Bacteriology of sickle cell leg ulcers. Trans R Soc Trop Med Hyg 1986; 80: 553–56.

180 Sapico FL, Ginunas VJ, Thornhill-Joynes M, et al. Quantitative microbiology of pressure sores in different stages of healing. Diagn Microbiol Inf Dis 1986; 5: 31–38.

181 Allman RM, Laprade CA, Noel LB, et al. Pressure sores among hospitalized patients. Ann Int Med 1986; 105: 337–42.

182 Gilchrist B, Reed C. The bacteriology of chronic venous ulcers treated with occlusive hydrocolloid dressings. Br J Dermatol 1989; 121: 337–44.

183 Asbrink E, Hovmark A. Lyme borreliosis: aspects of tick-borne *Borrelia burgdorferi* infection from a dermatologic viewpoint. Sem Dermatol 1990; 9: 277–91.

184 Malane MS, Grant-Kels JM, Feder HM, Luger SW. Diagnosis of Lyme disease based on dermatologic manifestations. Ann Int Med 1991; 114: 490–98.

185 Sudman MS. Protothecosis – a critical review. Am J Clin Pathol 1974; 61: 10–14.

186 Modley CE, Burnett JW. Cutaneous algal infection: protothecosis and chlorellosis. Cutis 1989; 44: 23–24.

187 Tyring SK, Lee PC, Walsh P, Garner JF, Little WP. Papular protothecosis of the chest. Arch Dermatol 1989; 125: 1245–52.

188 McCartney L, Rycroft AN, Hammil J. Cutaneous protothecosis in the dog: first confirmed case in Britain. Vet Rec 1988; 123: 494–96.

189 Nelson AM, Neafie RC, Connor DH. Cutaneous protothecosis and chlorellosis: extraordinary 'aquatic borne' algal infections. Clin Dermatol 1987; 5: 76–87.

190 Coulman CU, Greene I, Archibald RWR. Cutaneous pneumocystosis. Ann Int Med 1987; 106: 396–98.

10

Fungi and fungal infections of the skin

R. J. HAY

Normal fungal flora of the skin

As with bacteria, the fungal flora on the surface of the stratum corneum of otherwise healthy persons can be regarded as consisting of two types of populations – transient and resident commensals. The resident members are the *Pityrosporum* (*Malassezia*) or lipophilic yeasts, which are found on the skin surface of all adults and cluster around the openings of sebaceous glands. The existence of a transient fungal skin flora has not been as well documented as that of the bacteria, although temporary colonization of nails and hair by dermatophytes, and of other sites by *Candida* spp. is recognized. Transient colonization may also reflect contamination from another site where carriage rates are comparatively higher. For example, the isolation of yeasts from the perineum may well reflect their presence in the gastrointestinal tract and, in women, in the vagina.

Malassezia (Pityrosporum) yeasts

Members of the genus *Pityrosporum* are thick-walled yeast fungi that inhabit the superficial layers of the stratum corneum.[1] They comprise three main species or varieties – *Pityrosporum ovale*, *P. orbiculare* and *P. pachydermatis*.[2] The first two of these are found chiefly on human hosts and *P. pachydermatis* on a variety of other hosts. *Pityrosporum ovale* and *P. orbiculare* are associated with certain human diseases including pityriasis versicolor, where yeasts and short, stubby hyphae can be demonstrated in skin scrapings. These hyphae were originally named, without cultural confirmation, *Malassezia furfur*, but are now known to represent a parasitic phase of pityrosporum. The classification of these fungi, therefore, is the subject of an intense debate at present. It is possible to isolate lipophilic yeasts from the skin using special media. Generally they are either oval or round. However, there is some doubt as to the stability of such forms. It has been suggested that they can be converted from one morphological appearance to another. If this is correct, it would be more appropriate to designate all these organisms as a single species, *P. ovale*.[3] There are, however, a number of studies which show clearly that the shapes of the *Pityrosporum* spp. isolated from human skin, provided the cultures are adequately purified initially, are stable and, indeed, the oval forms, *P. ovale*, can be subdivided further into three types (A, B, and C).[2] Whether these are variants of a single *Pityrosporum* sp. or different species is not clear; however, the evidence for this subdivision into different types is based on physiological factors, antigenicity and analysis by restriction fragment length polymorphism as well as on morphology. To complicate matters further the most appropriate name for these fungi is *Malassezia furfur*, which was the original name used to describe a morphological form consisting of round yeasts and short, stubby hyphae associated with pityriasis versicolor (see above). There is also little doubt that this infection is caused by a pityrosporum yeast, usually identical to the round, *orbiculare* form.[4] Even though the original description was not based on cultured organisms, the designation used first should take precedence, making *Malassezia* the preferred name. However, given the unsolved question as to the status of the different stable varieties/species of human pityrosporum, and as it is now recognized that oval forms identical to *P. ovale* may also cause pityriasis versicolor, the terms *Pityrosporum ovale* and *orbiculare* will be used in this text, even though these fungi may ultimately turn out to be genetically identical. Fortunately the third species, *P. pachydermatis*, is a commensal and pathogen on non-human animal species, and as it has a number of distinguishing features, in particular its lack of lipophilicity, its position as a distinct species is not in question.

Pityrosporum yeasts are found on human skin from an early age.[5] While earlier studies suggested that they were uncommon in children, they have now been demonstrated in significant numbers in infants, where they have been associated with scalp scaling, cradle-cap dermatitis, and infantile seborrhoeic dermatitis.[6] The peak presence of these fungi is in the late teens and early adult life; their prevalence declines in the elderly.[2,4] They can be demonstrated in the highest numbers on areas rich in sebaceous glands such as the scalp, chest and upper back. The organisms are usually clustered around the pilosebaceous apparatus, although most are found close to the skin surface rather than deep in the glands themselves. Morphologically they are generally found as yeast forms, even though many have the capacity for mycelial transformation in vivo and in vitro.

The relationship between the pityrosporum yeasts and sebum is based on observations that their favoured sites of colonization are around the ostia of sebaceous glands as well as on their ability to cause lipolysis and the effect of certain fatty acids such as palmitic and oleic acids as growth stimulators;[7] cholesterol and cholesterol esters may also induce filamentous changes in these yeasts in vitro. The concentration of skin-surface fatty acids rises after puberty and this may explain the prevalence of these organisms in teenagers and adults rather than in younger age groups. Pityrosporum yeasts have been shown to produce a lipase, which may split these fats. In addition, in areas where they have invaded the stratum corneum, for instance in pityriasis versicolor, they have been found to induce the production of a substance, known as azaleic acid, that affects the ability of melanocytes to form pigment.[8]

There is little evidence that other fungi are permanent commensals on the skin surface of man, although some may be temporarily carried. For instance, *Candida* spp. may be found around the mouth, labia and in other body-fold areas such as beneath the breasts and in the axillae.[9] In most of these sites, however, these yeasts are only transients. Other fungi described as temporary colonists include *Trichosporon* spp. around the perianal area and dermatophytes beneath nails[10] and in the scalp.[11] In both nails and scalp it is suggested that the appearance of colonization without evidence of tissue invasion is merely a prelude to infection, although in the case of the scalp, long-term colonization has been demonstrated over 6 months without invasion of the hair shaft.

Immunity to infection

Resistance to superficial fungal infections can be divided into two main types, natural or acquired. Mechanisms of natural resistance do not require prior exposure to the same organism.[12] They include the effect of fatty acids in sebum on proliferation of the fungi, as well as other inhibitory substances (such as unsaturated transferrin) and the turnover rate of the epidermis. Microorganisms have a precarious hold in this site and any increase in the rate of epidermal growth is likely to lead to increased shedding of the fungi into the environment. In addition to these non-specific mechanisms, phagocytic cells can also engulf fungi, particularly where they invade around hair follicles. Natural killer cells similarly play a role in defence.

Serum has been known to exert some inhibitory activity against certain fungi. In the case of dermatophytes there is inhibition of penetration beyond the stratum corneum and, with candida, clumping of organisms will occur.[13] The identity of such inhibitory factors is not known, although it is likely that at least one of these is the iron carrier molecule, transferrin,[14] which is present in serum and in sweat. The relationship between the amount of transferrin and fungi causing superficial infections is a complicated one. There is evidence that with some organisms, unsaturated transferrin's inhibitory activity is mediated via direct binding of the molecule to the fungal cell. Kinetic studies indicate that the inhibitory activity is also not due to competition for iron but rather that unsaturated transferrin *per se* is an inhibitory molecule.[15] Its mode of action appears to be independent of iron-binding capacity.

A further important mode of defence is provided by the presence of fatty acids from sebaceous glands, which inhibit dermatophyte growth in vitro.[16] This activity appears to reside in saturated fatty acids containing chain lengths of 7, 9, 11 and 13 carbon residues. It has been suggested that their presence on the skin in postpubertal children may account for the spontaneous resolution of tinea capitis after this age and the rarity of new infections in adults.[17] A further potential factor is the capacity of commensal pityrosporum yeasts for lipolysis, which may increase the pool of fatty acids available for inhibitory activity. Pityrosporum yeasts themselves may grow readily in the presence of the same fatty acid residues that inhibit dermatophytes.[18]

In experimentally infected guinea-pigs, increased turnover of epidermal cells develops after candida infection, possibly through a cellular immune mechanism, although the increased turnover commences before the usual time taken for activation of immunological memory.[19] A similar phenomenon has been observed with the dermatophytes where, in man, there is evidence of increased incorporation of thymidine into nuclei of cells under the leading edge of the infection.[20] Some evidence that this process may not be entirely mediated through immunological memory has been provided by experiments using immunodeficient mice. Skin grafted on to nu nu (T-cell deficient) mice and then subsequently infected with dermatophyte fungi shows increased turnover of epidermis even in the absence of effective T lymphocyte-mediated defence.[21]

In experimental dermatophytosis, inflammatory cells including neutrophils appear within 4 h of the initiation of infection.[22] This suggests that endogenous mechanisms may attract leucocytes,[23] and the role of inflammatory mediators such as the eicosanoids in this respect needs to be investigated. It has also been found that dermatophytes are chemotactic and that they can trigger the alternative pathway of complement activation. This has been demonstrated for *Trichophyton rubrum*, *T. mentagrophytes*[23] and fungi causing endothrix scalp infections such as *T. violaceum*. The production of cytokines such as interleukin 1 by keratinocytes in the mobilization of neutrophil defences has not been investigated. It has been shown that neutrophils and to a lesser extent monocytes can kill dermatophyte conidia.[24] This activity depends on both intra- and extracellular mechanisms, and the generation of respiratory burst activity is an important stage in this process.[25] Dermatophytes produce catalase, which may act as a defence against the myeloperoxidase system of killing. Similar findings have been recorded with candida, where the organisms can be killed by either intra- or extracellular mechanisms.[26]

There is now a little evidence that natural killer cells may have an effect on destruction of certain yeasts such as cryptococci but there are no data on the efficacy of such a mechanism for mycelial fungi such as the dermatophytes.

Acquired resistance to superficial mycoses

With the dermatophytes and *Candida* spp. there is little evidence to support an active role for antibody in defence apart from, possibly, opsonization. There is, for instance, no correlation between the development of an antibody response and recovery in dermatophytosis. Indeed, patients with widespread but chronic infections such as tinea imbricata may have high antibody titres.[27] The presence of elevated levels of IgE in particular is associated with chronic infections.[28] Transfer to irradiated mice of specific serum containing a high titre of antibody does not convey immunity on the recipients.[29] It is still premature to rule out completely a role for antibody, as dermatophytes show some evidence of cytological damage when grown in the presence of specific antibody in vitro. In candidosis rather similar observations hold true. Patients with chronic mucocutaneous candidosis, a persistent form of superficial candidosis, often have high antibody titres to candida but remain infected.[30, 31] Likewise, in experimental infections it has not been possible to correlate clearance of infection with antibody formation. In systemic candidosis it has been noted that the presence of antibodies to a 47-kDa antigen correlates with recovery; patients with chronic mucocutaneous candidosis or those with AIDS who do not develop systemic candidosis usually have high titres of antibody, whereas those dying with systemic candidosis usually do not.[32] While it can be argued that the presence or absence of a particular immunodominant antibody may simply reflect the state of the immune system, it is possible that it may be protective.

There is evidence to suggest that immunity to superficial mycoses largely depends on the development of T lymphocyte-mediated immune responses. With candidosis, patients with defective T-lymphocyte function, such as those with AIDS, appear to be particularly susceptible to mucosal or cutaneous candidosis but not systemic infections.[9] Congenitally T cell-deficient mice (nu nu) do not show reproducible, increased susceptibility to systemic infection by candida. In fact, some investigators have found heightened resistance, suggesting that T-lymphocyte activity alone does not account for resistance to systemic invasion.[33] By contrast, in patients with chronic mucocutaneous candidosis the most consistent abnormalities have been those of T-lymphocyte function, even though some of these are now thought to be secondary to immunoregulation induced by the infection as they can be reversed with successful therapy.[34] Patients with defective neutrophil or macrophage function are susceptible to systemic candidosis. The activity of neutrophils and macrophages in phagocytosis and killing of candida in vitro has been demonstrated.[26] In addition, some cytokines, such as interferon-γ, appear to interact with these cells to enhance killing of the organism.[35] It seems that there is therefore substantial interplay between different immune mechanisms in defence against candidosis.

There is also evidence that the development of cellular immunity via sensitized T lymphocytes is a key factor in immunological defence in dermatophytosis. Lymphocytes bearing the T-helper phenotypic marker are responsible for transferring immunity to infection from sensitized donors to naive recipient mice.[29, 36] In man, the appearance of inflammation in ringworm correlates with the development of delayed-type skin reactivity to trichophytin.[37-39] Chronic infections are associated with poor T lymphocyte-mediated responses to specific fungal antigens, suggesting that depression of responses is the cause of the poor clinical outcome.[37, 40] Other in vitro measures of resistance, such as leucocyte migration inhibition and leucocyte adherence, may also indicate that T lymphocyte-mediated pathways are involved. Langerhans cells can act as antigen-presenting cells for dermatophyte antigens.[41]

In pityriasis versicolor, defective T-lymphocyte function has also been described, although it has been shown that small numbers of specifically reactive T cells may be responsible.[42, 43] It is interesting that, although there is a well-established association between pityriasis versicolor and disease such as Cushing's syndrome where there is defective T lymphocyte-mediated immunity,[44] pityriasis versicolor is not well established as a complication of AIDS. Conversely, seborrhoeic dermatitis – an eczema-like process affecting the skin of the scalp (dandruff), face and trunk (see below) – is a common complication of infection with human immune deficiency virus.[45] The reason for recognizing a connection between this condition and the presence of pityrosporum yeasts is that antifungal therapy is an effective treatment and the removal and re-emergence of yeasts correspond with the improvement and deterioration of the skin complaint, respectively.[46] The immunological background of seborrhoeic dermatitis is not well established, although there is some evidence that patients with this condition have higher antibody titres (IgG and IgM) against antigens of pityrosporum isolates;[47] conversely, there is no evidence of contact sensitization to the same antigens.[48] Whatever the mechanism of involvement of *Pityrosporum* spp. in this condition, it does not appear to depend on delayed-type hypersensitivity to the organisms.

There is still a problem in explaining why it is well-nigh impossible to rid the body surface of these fungi in a significant proportion of patients. Chronic infections with dermatophyte fungi are very common in clinical practice, to the extent where most infections affecting the palms and soles, caused by *Trichophyton rubrum*, fail to clear naturally. Similarly, persistent superficial candidosis and chronic pityriasis versicolor are equally common. The reasons for failure of immunity in persistent dermatophyte, or other fungal, infections and their relationship with chronicity are still not well understood. There is an association between the presence of atopy and chronic dermatophytosis, with a high proportion of those with persistent disease having atopy (usually asthma or hay fever) as well as immediate-type hypersensitivity and raised levels of Ig E.[37,49] It has been suggested that modulation of T-lymphocyte activity either locally or systemically may be responsible via a number of mechanisms including activation of histamine-responsive suppressor cells. It has also been found that dermatophyte antigens, including one which shares common epitopes with phosphorylcholine, affect expression of T-lymphocyte responses. Patients with persistent infection have detectable serum levels of this antigen.[50] Blockade of T lymphocyte-mediated responses has also been described by other investigators,[51] and it is known that dermatophyte antigens inhibit lymphocyte transformation at low concentrations.[52] These are possible factors in the regulation of immunity in dermatophytosis. However, whether these mechanisms operate in vivo has yet to be established. With chronic mucocutaneous candidosis there is also evidence to suggest that immuno-modulation may also be involved, as successful therapy may be accompanied by reversal of the immune defects that were associated with infection. It is not clear whether this is due to a circulating antigenic product of candida such as mannan,[53] which is known to affect immunoresponsiveness, or some other factor such as blocking antibody or immune complexes.

Patients with chronic infections, including dermatophytosis, are usually otherwise healthy. However, altered or chronic infections have also been noted in a number of patient groups such as those with chronic mucocutaneous candidosis and AIDS,[54] and those on corticosteroid therapy or with endogenous Cushing's syndrome. In addition to these there is the raised incidence of atopy in those with chronic dermatophytosis, suggesting that host factors may well determine the clinical course.[55] However, this is clearly not the only process involved and it has been found that where there is ample opportunity for spread of infection, for instance amongst coal miners, the incidence of atopy is no different to that seen in uninfected coworkers.[47] A further point of interest is the dominance of *T. rubrum* as a cause of chronic disease. There is some evidence to suggest that dry-type infections caused by this organism *per se* are associated with poorer lymphocyte transformation responses than to other dermatophytes.[40] Similar associations are not seen with chronic candidosis, although in the mucocutaneous type there is evidence in some cases of genetically determined susceptibility, either inherited as an autosomal dominant[56] or recessive character.[57]

Dermatophyte infections

The dermatophyte or ringworm fungi are hyphal organisms that are adapted to cause disease of the skin. Originating from keratinophilic fungi found in nature, the dermatophytes affecting man are derived from three genera, *Trichophyton*, *Microsporum* or *Epidermophyton*. They can be divided into those infections that are spread from man to man (anthropophilic), animal to man (zoophilic) or soil to man (geophilic).[58] These different routes of spread are largely responsible for determining the epidemiological features of dermatophytosis. While it is difficult to be precise about the frequency of isolation of different species on a worldwide basis, the most commonly recorded organism overall is *T. rubrum* followed by *T. violaceum*, *T. interdigitale/mentagrophytes*, *M. canis* and *M. audouinii*. However, this pattern differs in different countries. For instance the order of frequency most often seen in the United Kingdom is shown in Table 10.1. However, with specific infections such as tinea capitis the patterns of infections in different countries are strikingly different (Table 10.2).

Dermatophyte infections can occur in any patient, irrespective of age or sex.[59] Generally scalp infections are not seen in adults, except rarely in women, and tinea pedis is uncommon under the age of 10 years. Certain patterns of infection are also less common in women. These include tinea cruris (infection affecting the groins) but such a pattern will occur in females from time to time, particularly in the tropics. These data are shown in Table 10.3. There is some evidence of intrafamilial spread of tinea pedis,[60] although it does not occur in all cases and therefore other susceptibility factors, such as atopy, may regulate the occurrence of infection (see above). It has been suggested that susceptibility to one infection at least, tinea imbricata (caused by *T. concentricum*), may be conferred by an autosomal recessive trait. This is based on population genetic surveys carried out in the Gogol valley of Papua New Guinea,[61] although other surveys have failed to find a similar genetic link in a different area of the same country, Goodenough Island.[62] The genetic interpretation of such large-scale surveys, which compare real and expected ratios of infected to non-

Table 10.1. *Dermatophytes in the United Kingdom, in order of frequency of isolation*

Trichophyton rubrum
T. interdigitale
Epidermophyton floccosum
Microsporum canis
T. verrucosum
T. mentagrophytes (animal source)

T. erinacei, T. soudanense, T. violaceum, T. equinum, M. gypseum, all infrequent and sporadic isolates

Table 10.2. *Main causal agents for tinea capitis in different geographic areas*

Europe	North America	Africa	India
M. canis	*T. tonsurans*	*T. violaceum*	*T. violaceum*
	M. canis	*T. soudanense*	
	M. audouinii	*M. audouinii*	
		M. canis	
		T. yaoundei	

infected individuals within families, is difficult, particularly if the gene frequency of the putative susceptibility trait is high in the population studied. In the last of these studies an autosomal dominant trait with incomplete expression would have explained the ratios obtained. Some support for the concept of genetic susceptibility is derived from studies of inbred mice where certain strains (Balb/c) are highly susceptible to infection with the mouse pathogen *T. quinckeanum*, whereas others are resistant (C57/Bl).[36] This may explain the difficulty of establishing experimental infections in mice.

As described previously, infections due to dermatophytes are acquired from one of three main sources, animal, soil or man. Animal or zoophilic infections are usually sporadic and restricted to the areas where the host animal is found. For instance, dermatophyte infection caused by *M. persicolor*, a parasite of the European bank-vole, are mainly seen in Europe, whereas *M. simii* infections, where the natural host is the monkey, occur in India and the Far East. A further example of this is the infection caused by *T. erinacei*, which is a natural pathogen of the hedgehog; human infections are mainly seen in Europe, its original habitat, and New Zealand, where it was imported in the nineteenth century. In the case of *M. canis*, the cat and dog ringworm, fungus infections may spread widely in the community and appear to be transmissible more

Table 10.3. *Percentage distribution by age of different lesions of patients with dermatophytosis*

	Distribution in different age (years) groups (%)								
	0–4	5–9	10–14	15–19	20–24	25–29	30–34	36–39	40+
Tinea capitis[a]									
Males (160)	22.5	65.5	12			0			4
Females (136)	32.0	61.0	4			2			9
Tinea corporis[a]									
Males (154)	14	44	23	4	2	4	3	0.5	4
Females (319)	11	33	19	8	6	4	4	3.0	9
Tinea corporis[b]									
Males (1965)		48.5		16.2		13.6		9.2	12.5
Females (1020)		54.9		20.1		11.4		5.2	8.4
Tinea cruris[b]									
Males (417)		0.25		20.1		35.7		25.2	18.7
Females (13)		(7)		(7)		(31)		(15)	(18)

Based on data from: [a] Caprilli F et al. Mykosen 1979; 22: 413–420 (Rome); and [b] McAleer R. Aust J Dermatol 1980; 21: 25–46 (West Australia).
Acknowledgements to: Noble WC. Microbial skin disease: its epidemiology. London: Edward Arnold; 1983.

extensively than can be accounted for if transmission occurs directly from an infected animal. It has been found that arthrospores of *M. canis* originating from an infected cat can be isolated from furniture and carpets in the environment of an infected animal,[63] and this may provide a source of infection to humans. With anthropophilic dermatophytes the infections are spread more widely in the community and in some cases there is evidence to support the existence of a localized epidemic of infection where there are appropriate conditions for transmission. These are best seen in swimming baths, where there are opportunities for spread on floors from tinea pedis,[64] alternative sources are school changing-areas[65] and industrial shower rooms. In industry, spread of dermatophyte infection has led to the existence of a heavy rate of infection in coal miners in Europe.[66,67] In some mines the infection rate is at least 35 per cent or more. This trend, originally studied in the early 1950s, has not altered over the intervening years despite the availability of more effective therapies and the institution of measures such as the use of dedicated shower-room footwear and the removal of wooden tread boards from bath areas. The main difference between the earlier and later studies has been a shift from *T. interdigitale* (*mentagrophytes*) to *T. rubrum* as the main cause of infection.[67] Other industries with similar problems include those where protective clothing is worn regularly, such as the nuclear fuel industry. The situation is complicated by the fact that bacterial foot infection is also common in this group and may also be associated with interdigital disease.[68]

Tinea capitis in childhood is another example of spread in the community. In many countries this is a sporadic infection caused predominantly by organisms of human origin. However, in some places notably Africa,[69] certain urban areas in the United States,[70] as well as other parts of the world,[71] epidemics of this infection have been described affecting large numbers of children. Transmission can occur easily after only a short contact with an infected child. In cases in Africa and the United States the absence of gross symptoms until the later stages of disease,[39] or of obvious signs of infection, means that spread can occur easily without those involved being aware of the problem. However, it is also apparent that carriage of scalp pathogens can occur in children with seemingly normal scalps, particularly schoolchildren from classes where there are already infected cases (Table 10.4).[72] It is not known whether these pose a threat of infection to their classmates, but follow-up of such children indicates that some develop clinical infections whereas others remain carriers or become culture negative (non-carriers).

Anthropophilic infections may also be geographically restricted. One possible reason for this is best illustrated by tinea capitis, which is generally

Table 10.4. *Scalp carriage of dermatophytes by healthy schoolchildren, London*

	Carriage rates (%)	
	In classes where there are clinically infected cases	In classes where there are no clinically infected cases
Microsporum audouinii	12.1	0.8
M. rivalieri	21.1	0.8
M. canis	12.7	0.5
M. ferrugineum	31.0	1.0
Trichophyton sulphureum	17.8	1.4
T. soudanense	8.6	0.4
T. gourvillii	6.5	0.4

Based on data from Midgley and Clayton.[72]

confined to children. As children constitute a static population with less opportunity for travel and hence spread, it is likely that infections confined to this age range are less likely to be disseminated to other areas. In Africa, for instance, there are still areas that remain endemic for specific organisms, such as *T. yaoundei*, which is restricted to the Cameroons.[69] Geographic and social isolation may also account for the existence of endemic foci of other dermatophytes. *Trichophyton concentricum* is only found in isolated foci in the West Pacific, Malaysia and Central and South America.[62] Patients affected generally live in small, isolated communities, often in rain-forest areas. Presumably spread between different communities is less likely although the reason why this infection should have such a widespread geographic distribution is not clear. Favus, the infection caused by *T. schoenleinii*, may also be found in endemic pockets of disease in isolated communities such as those in the Appalachian mountains of the United States.[71]

Infections from soil are much rarer, although small outbreaks of infection, for instance associated with greenhouse workers, have been described.[73] Only one fungus, *M. gypseum*, is involved in these cases. Infections due to this organism are also seen more often in certain parts of the tropics such as the West Pacific.[74]

Pathogenesis

The initial infection probably follows contact with a desquamated scale or hair. It is known that dermatophyte arthrospores remain viable for up to 18 months in shed skin material and therefore contact with an infected host may not be necessary.[63] This is seen with cattle ringworm, where transmission from shed hairs and skin scales lodged in farm buildings seems most likely. The process of skin invasion is initiated by adherence of the arthrospore to the stratum corneum.[75] This appears to be necessary for the germination of the spore. The process in vitro takes a minimum of 2 h. Factors that affect the process of germination include the ambient carbon-dioxide tension and the humidity. Invasion of the stratum corneum is effected by the production of enzymes such as keratinases. *Trichophyton mentagrophytes*, for instance, produces at least two different keratinases.[76]

Although the clinical appearances of dermatophytosis may be altered in the immunosuppressed patient, there is little support for the view that these infections are more common in this group. This is exemplified in the case of AIDS in homosexuals, where studies show that although the prevalence of dermatophyte infections may be high, it is no higher than in an age-matched population also consisting of gay men.[54] However, atypical clinical forms are seen, including a form of nail infection of rapid onset involving the whole of the nail plate.[77]

Most dermatophyte infections are confined to the stratum corneum or specialized keratin structures such as hair or nail.[78] In the skin the infection seldom passes the granular layer unless there is invasion via a hair follicle, in which case fungal fragments may be found surrounded by phagocytes or within giant cells in the dermis in the vicinity of a destroyed follicle. In many infections the main feature is a lymphohistiocytic infiltrate around the upper dermal blood vessels, the fungus in the upper layers of the epidermis only being visible with special stains such as periodic acid–Schiff. In more inflammatory lesions, in the early phase, there is a dense neutrophil accumulation around hair follicles. Some histiocytes are found and fungal fragments can be seen in the upper dermis. In the later stages a more organized pattern of inflammation with fully developed granulomas forms, and there is a greater representation by plasma cells within the infiltrate.

Clinical features

The archetypical lesion of a dermatophyte infection is the ringworm or tinea circinata. This is a round, scaly lesion occurring in isolation or in clusters, usually on the trunk. The rim of each lesion is more inflamed than the centre and there is generally more scaling. Typically this form occurs in infections of the body, tinea corporis. Generally, a similar convention is adopted for describing all dermatophyte infection by using the Latin term 'tinea' followed by the appropriate part of the body involved, also in Latin. The different forms are tinea pedis, tinea corporis, tinea cruris, tinea capitis and tinea facei. Although the term tinea unguium is still used for nail infections, many prefer the designation onychomycosis. Tinea incognito describes an atypical dermatophyte infection often located on the face and associated with the inappropriate use of topical corticosteroids as therapy. In this case the typical features of the lesion are lost, although there are still many fungal hyphae to be found in skin scrapings.

Tinea pedis is generally caused by anthropophilic fungi such as *T. rubrum* and *T. interdigitale* (*mentagrophytes*). The earliest lesion develops as scaling between the toes, usually affecting the lateral third and fourth interdigital spaces. The cracking may spread to the undersurface of the toes. With *T. interdigitale*, in particular, there may be blister formation. With time, in *T. rubrum* infections, the organisms may also invade the soles to cause a dry, scaly rash often with a prominent rim around the margins of the foot – 'dry' or 'moccasin' type dermatophytosis. This form is the type associated with infections that persist despite treatment.

In chronic cases, involvement of the toe webs may alter in clinical appearance, with cracking of the skin, soreness rather than itching, and on occasions a greenish discoloration. This occurs when there is secondary infection by Gram-negative bacteria such as *Pseudomonas* spp. The condition has been described as dermatophytosis complex.[79] The relationship between dermatophytes and bacteria in this site is complex and often treatment of one will be followed by its replacement by the other, and vice versa.

Tinea cruris also presents with dry scaling around the groin extending on to the upper surface of the thigh. The infection is generally bilateral. There is often a raised margin and the infection may extend around the natal cleft to the perineum. This infection is mainly seen in male adults. Foot infection may coexist.

Tinea corporis may either be caused by zoophilic fungi or anthropophilic organisms, more rarely by geophilic fungi. Generally, when the fungi are zoophilic the lesion is inflammatory and more closely resembles classical tinea circinata. With anthropophilic fungi such as *T. rubrum* the margins of the lesion are ill defined and there is little erythema or scaling. The area involved may also be very extensive.

Tinea capitis usually presents in childhood with patches of hair loss and scaling in the scalp. Again, inflammation varies, although the zoophilic fungi usually produce more inflammation, with crusting and oozing. At its most extreme this type of inflammatory lesion affecting a hair-bearing area is called a kerion and, although there may be extensive formation of pustules, it represents an extreme inflammatory response to the dermatophyte rather than secondary bacterial infection.[80] The pattern of hair loss is determined, in part, by the fact that dermatophytes either form chains of arthrospores within the shaft of the hair or on its external surface. In one type of scalp invasion where the organisms form arthrospores within the shafts, known as an endothrix infection, the hair fractures at scalp level leaving a swollen stub of infected hair visible at the surface. Endothrix infections are generally anthropophilic in origin. In ectothrix infections the organisms form chains of spores outside the hair and weakened hairs break a few millimetres above the skin. Infected hairs in this type of tinea capitis can be seen to be greyish in colour and swollen. Ectothrix infections may be caused by either anthropophilic or zoophilic fungi, although in Europe and the United States the main cause is a zoophilic fungus, *Microsporum canis*. Finally, in infections caused by *T. schoenleinii*, the organisms invade the hair shaft but hyphae disintegrate leaving air spaces within the hair. Hairs may not break but an accumulation of epithelial debris and inflammatory cells forms around the hair shaft. This is known as a scutulum. Individual scutula may amalgamate to form a dense cap over the scalp. Most forms of scalp ringworm infections will slowly heal and permanent hair loss is unlikely. Scarring alopecia (hair loss) occasionally follows a severe kerion or favus.

Onychomycosis is an infection of the nail plate.[81] Dermatophytes usually invade from the distal and lateral margin to produce a thickened and discoloured nail. Onychomycosis is more common on the toe-nails than the fingers and frequently the whole nail plate is involved. Rarely, with *T. mentagrophytes*, the superior aspect of the nail is invaded, a process known as superficial white onychomycosis. Here the fungus forms into small colonies on the upper nail surface and these are found in small pits scalloped out of the superficial nail plate.

More unusual clinical patterns of dermatophytosis are also seen. A dry type of infection, usually caused by *T. rubrum*, affecting the palms may occur. Typically this involves only one palm but both soles and the principal clinical abnormality is scaling over the affected area. Patients with hereditary hyperkeratosis of the palms or soles are particularly susceptible to this pattern of dermatophytosis.[82] Tinea of the face is difficult to recognize as the infection usually spreads across both sides and it is often difficult to discern the rim of the lesion. In addition, many patients record that it flares up in sunlight.[83]

Tinea imbricata is a specific infection, caused by *T. concentricum*, seen in the West Pacific and parts of central and South America.[62] It is usually confined to remote areas of rain forest. The skin is rapidly covered with extensive scales, which form into concentric rings or solid sheets. The infection may be initiated in early childhood and persist throughout life without spontaneous remission.

Majocchi's granuloma describes the late stage of a hair-shaft invasion, where occasionally a persistent granuloma, often without visible or viable fungi, remains within the skin.

'Id' reactions are inflammatory reactions, occurring on the skin, that do not harbour infective fungi but are temporally related to a dermatophyte infection.[84] The commonest form is a type of acute vesicular eczema that develops after the appearance of inflammatory tinea pedis and is generally worse on the affected side. A disseminated papular rash may occur in concert with the development of inflammatory ringworm on the body. Histologically this appears to be a form of leucocytoclastic vasculitis. Other 'id' reactions include erythema nodosum and multiforme.

The hallmark of these reactions is the appearance of a secondary rash coincidentally with a worsening of inflammatory dermatophytosis, often after the initiation of therapy. Generally such patients have very strong delayed-type skin-test reactions to dermatophyte antigens. The immunological basis of the dermatophyte 'id' reaction is unknown.

Laboratory diagnosis

Diagnosis of dermatophyte infections is based on the demonstration of hyphal elements in skin or nail fragments taken by scraping the lesion. These can be found in material by light microscopy using 10–20 per cent potassium hydroxide as a clearant. The skin is cultured on Sabouraud's agar, which also contains antibiotics and cycloheximide. The gross and microscopic appearances of dermatophytes are usually sufficient for diagnosis, although other confirmatory tests such as the ability to penetrate hairs or the development of pigment on rice-grain medium are helpful in some cases.[58]

Treatment

Detailed consideration of therapy is beyond the scope of this chapter; however, this subject is covered in a number of articles and chapters elsewhere.[85,86] Generally the approach to treatment is fairly straightforward. Where the lesion is accessible, topically applied therapy is used; but in extensive nail or scalp infections, oral drugs are usually necessary. The main topically active drugs used include topical forms of azole antifungal drugs (such as clotrimazole, miconazole, econazole), tolnaftate or the mixture of benzoic and salicylic acids (Whitfield's ointment). The main oral drugs used are griseofulvin, itraconazole, ketoconazole or terbinafine.

Immunization has not been used as a preventative measure in human

Table 10.5. *Factors associated with candida infection*

Age – infancy, old age
Pregnancy
Epithelial abnormalities, e.g. ulceration, hyperkeratosis
Endocrine disease – diabetes mellitus
Antibiotic therapy
Immunosuppression (drugs, congenital, cancer):
Defective numbers or function of neutrophils
Defective numbers or function of T lymphocytes
Miscellaneous – zinc deficiency, iron deficiency

dermatophytosis, although it is now the subject of an extensive field study for the prevention of ringworm in cattle.

Hendersonula and *Scytalidium* infections

Hendersonula toruloidea (*Natrassia mangifera*), a plant pathogen found in the tropics and subtropics, causes an infection of the skin that mimics the dry-type infection caused by *T. rubrum*. *Hendersonula toruloidea* is a black mould fungus, which has been isolated from nail and palmar/plantar infections in man.[87] A white fungus, antigenically closely related to *Hendersonula*, called *Scytalidium hyalinum* has also been isolated from similar lesions. Both fungi are inhibited by cycloheximide, which is commonly incorporated into mycological media, and this may explain why their existence has only been established in recent years. These infections are mainly seen in immigrants from tropical areas to temperate countries, although there has recently been some evidence that infection in the tropics may be more common than previously believed. One survey in the Caribbean, for instance, showed that over 30 per cent of healthy individuals carried the organisms on their feet,[88] and a study of nail infection in Nigeria has confirmed that these organisms are common causes of onychomycosis in West Africa.[89]

The clinical pattern of infection involves scaling of soles and palms, and cracking between the toe webs; nail dystrophy is common. Infections closely resemble the dry-type infections caused by *Trichophyton rubrum* affecting the palms or soles.[90] The clinical appearances of *H. toruloidea* and *S. hyalinum* infections are indistinguishable. Lesions are often asymptomatic and only discovered on routine inspection. The nail changes start at the lateral and distal edges, and there may be extensive undermining of the nail without corresponding thickening of the plate. Paronychia, infection of the nail fold, often accompanies these changes. Occasionally there may be increased pigmentation in the nail plate, a change which is most prominent in caucasians.[91] Involvement of other parts of the skin is not found, although hair may be invaded in vitro. Rarely, cases of deep infection affecting the subcutaneous tissue, such as mycetoma, have been described.

The fungi are visible by direct microscopy of skin or nails where the hyphae are notably sinuous, changes that are best appreciated by examining material under phase contrast. The organisms grow on cycloheximide-free media.

Unfortunately neither *Hendersonula* nor *Scytalidium* infections respond to any of the topical or systemically active, antifungal drugs.

Candidal infections

Infections caused by yeasts of the genus *Candida* are common in clinical practice and they may involve the mucous membranes and/or skin, or spread internally to produce systemic infection.[9] The chief pathogen is *C. albicans*, although other species such as *C. tropicalis*, *C. parapsilosis*, *C. krusei* and *C. glabrata* may also cause human infections.

Candida spp. are normal commensals in the mouth, gastrointestinal tract and vaginal mucosa. The extent of their commensal status has varied between different studies, both with different patients investigated and the methods of sampling used. However, between 20 and 25 per cent of the adult population carry candida in their mouths, and 12–22 per cent of healthy women have vaginal carriage of these organisms. Generally, when these fungi cause disease, it is because of some change in the host. Some of these changes are listed in Table 10.5. Infants, for instance, are particularly susceptible to superficial candidosis and this probably reflects immaturity of the immune response. Vaginal candidosis is common in pregnancy and its development may follow hormonally related changes in the mucosa. Factors that alter the epithelial integrity, such as mucosal disease, also predispose to infection.[92] Antibiotic therapy, by altering the balance between competing microorganisms, may also affect the ability of candida to cause disease. Therapy or disease that alters the immune response of the host, particularly if this involves neutrophil capacity or T-lymphocyte function, will also favour the development of candidosis. AIDS is now commonly associated with candidosis of the mouth.[93] Endocrine disease may also affect this process. In particular, diabetes mellitus is associated with increased susceptibility to vaginal infection.[94]

The first phase of invasion by candida involves the adherence of the yeast to epithelial surface.[95] This is a time-dependent process, similar to that described for dermatophytes; however, it is better understood. Adherence of *C. albicans* varies with local pH, temperature and the presence of drugs. It can also be inhibited by certain sugars, such as mannose, suggesting that the interaction between surface receptors may involve a mannan receptor site.[96] *Candida albicans* also has a complement (C3d) receptor on its surface.[97] The host receptor site has not been identified but blood-group substances expressed on epithelial cells are a possible candidate.[98] Adherence is a prerequisite for the germination of yeasts to produce germ tubes and hyphal elements, which can penetrate tissue. In the case of *C. albicans*, other factors are also important. Amongst these, the production of proteinase is an important virulence factor that may determine the success of fungal invasion.[99] Mutant strains that do not produce proteinase are significantly less virulent.

Attempts to identify specific strains of *C. albicans* associated with infections have not been very successful, primarily because of the unsatisfactory nature of typing systems. There are two main approaches used to identify strain types: one involves the use of differential inhibition of different strains using a variety of compounds;[100] the second is by genetic 'fingerprinting', for instance by using restriction fragment length polymorphisms.[101] One further problem that may be relevant here is that under defined but varying conditions it is possible for a single strain of a *Candida* spp. to display different phenotypic characters such as morphology. This 'phenotypic switching' makes the analysis of data on strain typing difficult.[102] Even so, it has proved possible to trace particular strains in certain circumstances in order to link carriage and the development of disease.[103]

Pathological features

Candida spp. are not common invaders of the skin surface and most of our knowledge of the histopathological changes originates from the study of oral mucosal lesions or chronic mucocutaneous candidosis (see below). In the early stages the main changes are the infiltration of the epithelium by neutrophils with some hyper- and parakeratosis. There is an upper dermal infiltrate of lymphocytes and plasma cells.[104] In some chronic infections of the oral mucosa there is atrophy of the epithelium with dysplastic changes in the basal layers. There is a risk of the development of severe dysplastic changes and this raises the possibility that persistent oral candidosis, either on its own, or, more likely, in combination with some other factor such as smoking, may lead to the development of oral cancer.

Clinical features

Candidosis is a condition that can be divided into two distinct patterns of infection, superficial or deep. Whereas the skin is occasionally involved in the process of systemic candidosis, it will not be discussed here. Superficial candidosis principally affects the sites of carriage of the organism, such as the mouth or the vagina. Sometimes it involves the skin or the nails.

Oral candidosis can present as an acute condition in which there are white plaques and mucosal erythema affecting the buccal mucosa and the palate.[105] In some cases the white plaques are not obvious and the mucosa merely has a glazed, atrophic appearance. The corners of the mouth may be cracked – angular cheilitis. Some patients develop chronic infections where the tongue is also involved. In some this may take the form of a lozenge-shaped area of infection on the dorsal surface of the tongue – median rhomboid glossitis. In denture wearers a form of oral inflammation called denture sore mouth or denture stomatitis has been connected with candidal infection. However, in this condition it appears that the presence of other microorganisms is equally important in determining the development of symptoms, which do not appear to be due to candida alone.[106]

Vaginal candidosis presents in a similar way, with white plaques on the vaginal mucosa accompanied by itching or soreness.[107] Once again the skin is only indirectly involved when there is spread to the vulval surface and the perineum. This event presents with a prominent red rash on the upper surface of the thighs. The presence of satellite pustules and papules outside the leading edge of this rash is characteristic. Chronic or recurrent vaginal candidosis can be an important therapeutic problem.[108,109]

Infections of the skin surface caused by *Candida* spp. are less common and usually confined to the body-fold areas, except in infants, where rarely a generalized cutaneous form of candidosis arises shortly after birth. The more common variety, candida intertrigo, is seen in the body-fold areas such as the groins or under the breasts. As with secondary perineal infection occurring with vaginal candidosis, the rash is itchy and red with satellite pustules. In the groins or elsewhere, candida may also secondarily infect other skin lesions such as flexural psoriasis. The same can happen in babies with napkin (diaper) dermatitis where secondary infection with candida originating from the gastrointestinal tract is not uncommon. That attempts could be made to assess the significance of the presence of *C. albicans* in such lesions by taking quantitative cultures has been suggested but is not really practicable.[110] Generally, if present, candida should be cleared, if necessary by using topical antifungals, before the primary skin condition is treated.

Candida albicans can also cause a form of interdigital infection, either on the feet or hands. On the hands it gives rise to a white and macerated area of skin, which becomes eroded. This is mainly seen in patients who are in frequent contact with water. On the foot, interdigital candidosis may be quite common in tropical environments, where it may replace dermatophyte infections as the principal cause of foot disease. Another form of skin infection is the development of a candidal paronychium, which is an infection where the organisms proliferate in the pocket between the nail plate and the nail fold. Whereas yeasts may dominate the microflora of this area, Gram-positive and Gram-negative bacteria may also be found in large numbers here.[111,112] Generally, pure staphylococcal paronychia are mainly seen where there is pre-existing skin disease such as eczema or psoriasis. However with candidal paronychia it is not uncommon for yeasts to be replaced by Gram-negative bacteria after antifungal therapy. The key to recovery here is healing of the pocket that is colonized by microorganisms.

Infections of the skin surface due to candida occur rarely but are a well-recognized complication of the syndrome of chronic mucocutaneous candidosis. This condition is characterized by chronic oral candidosis and infection of the nails as well, and in severe cases, infection spreads on to the surface of the trunk or limbs.[113] The rash looks like a dermatophyte infection and has a slightly raised edge. In some cases there is marked hyperkeratosis, which has been inaccurately named candida granuloma. The histological feature of this pattern of infection is hyperkeratosis and epithelial hyperplasia. Patients with chronic mucocutaneous candidosis have a number of underlying abnormalities, as follows:

(1) inherited variants:
   (a) autosomal recessive,
   (b) autosomal dominant;
(2) associated with polyendocrinopathy – two basic patterns include hypoparathyroidism/hypoadrenalism and hypothyroidism, both are inherited as autosomal recessive traits;
(3) associated with thymoma;
(4) idiopathic.

The autosomal dominant and recessive forms have no obvious distinguishing features except that in the former the infection may be very severe. Patients may present with endocrinopathy after the onset of candidosis. The genetic basis for this abnormality is still unknown. Patients with chronic mucocutaneous candidosis may develop other skin infections, such as dermatophytosis or papillomavirus infections. Other complications of long-term infection include candidal oesophagitis and stricture formation. Squamous carcinomas of the mouth have been recorded in some patients with chronic mucocutaneous candidosis, particularly if they are also smokers.

Patients with AIDS develop a particularly recalcitrant form of oral candidosis with hypertrophic oral candidosis or perianal ulceration.[114] This infection may coexist with other diseases such as herpes simplex virus infections. Oesophageal involvement is also a problem in this group.[115] Infections of the skin surface itself are less common.

Laboratory diagnosis

The methods used in the diagnosis of superficial candidal infections are similar to those employed in dermatophytosis. Direct microscopy of skin scales or swabs should reveal the presence of yeasts and hyphae. The organisms grow readily on a variety of media including Sabouraud's agar. Different species can be identified by sugar assimilation patterns or simple tests such as their ability to produce germ tubes in serum. The interpretation of cultures must be undertaken with care as infection has to be distinguished from colonization. The presence of pathological signs of infection is of critical importance in assessing culture results.

Therapy

Therapy with topical antifungals is useful for acute forms of superficial candidosis. Either a polyene (amphotericin B or nystatin) or imidazole (clotrimazole, miconazole, econazole) topical formulation is usually effective. The main indication for using oral therapy is for the management of chronic infection. In this case ketoconazole, itraconazole or fluconazole are all effective methods of treatment. Detailed consideration of therapy can be found elsewhere.[116]

Malassezia infections

The pityrosporum yeasts have been described earlier. They are skin surface commensals but have also been associated with a variety of human diseases, of which the three main forms are pityriasis versicolor, pityrosporum folliculitis and seborrhoeic dermatitis and dandruff.[1] In addition these organisms rarely cause systemic infections, usually in neonates given intravenous lipid infusions.

Pityriasis versicolor

The pathogenesis of pityriasis versicolor is still ill understood. The disease occurs in young adults and older individuals but is less common in childhood. This is thought to reflect the frequency of colonization of the skin surface. Likewise the anatomical distribution of the disease reflects the distribution of organisms on the skin surface (Table 10.6). In most instances the development of the disease is accompanied by a change in the yeast flora in which many hyphal forms occur on the skin surface together with round yeasts.[44] This is

Table 10.6. *Quantitative culture of* Pityrosporum orbiculare *from lesional skin of patients with pityriasis versicolor and normal controls*

	P. orbiculare (per cm²)
Pityriasis versicolor	
Lesion on back	3522
Normal skin, same site	1644
Controls	
Upper back	327
Chest	333
Lower leg	13

Based on Faergemann.[1]

not always the case and in some forms of pityriasis versicolor oval yeasts without hyphae dominate. The appearance of hyphal forms without clinical disease has been documented in patients after renal transplantation, a finding ascribed to long-term immunosuppression; other immunosuppressed patients appear to be very susceptible to this infection. The main exception is AIDS, where infected patients do not show a higher frequency of pityriasis versicolor. However, pityriasis versicolor is a common disease in the tropics and elsewhere in otherwise healthy patients and there is no evidence of immunosuppression in these groups. Experimental pityriasis versicolor is difficult to induce in humans with any consistency and the presence of susceptibility factors, as yet not understood, seems likely.[117]

Both forms of pityrosporum yeast can be cultured from normal skin as well as skin from patients with disease such as pityriasis versicolor and dandruff. Roberts, for instance, reported finding *P. ovale* on the scalp of 97 per cent of normal subjects and *P. orbiculare* in 74 per cent of subjects. By contrast, *P. orbiculare* was more common on the chest in almost all individuals and *P. ovale* in between 80 and 90 per cent.[4] Other workers have found similar counts, although the numbers of *P. ovale* cultured from the trunk have been variable.[1] There is evidence that very high counts of pityrosporum yeasts can be isolated from the affected skin. For instance, using a modification of the Kligman wash/scrub technique, Faergemann found that the numbers of organisms in lesional skin exceeded those in normal skin by a factor of 10 (Table 10.6).[5] However, the development of this condition does not appear to depend solely on the numbers of organisms present.

Pityriasis versicolor is seen in all parts of the world, although it is most common in the humid tropics. Here the incidence may be as high as 50 per cent of the population.[74] In temperate climates far fewer people appear to be infected.[1] The reasons for this are unknown, although the disease most commonly comes to light in Europe in patients who have taken holidays in the sun and it has also been associated with exposure to ultraviolet light on sun beds. In addition, pityriasis versicolor would appear to be more common in patients with seborrhoeic dermatitis,[118] suggesting that some endogenous factors may play a part in the appearance of this condition.

The rash consists of multiple hypo- or hyperpigmented macules distributed across the upper trunk and back. The lesions are asymptomatic and scaly. Patients usually notice this infection because of its unsightly appearance.

Pityrosporum yeasts and seborrhoeic dermatitis

Lipophilic yeasts of the genus *Pityrosporum* are part of the normal skin flora and therefore any evidence that they are either directly or indirectly implicated in the pathogenesis of skin disease is often difficult to assess.[119] Pityrosporum yeasts are found in large quantities in the scales of seborrhoeic dermatitis both on the scalp, where it probably is identical to the common scaling condition, dandruff, and on skin lesions elsewhere.[1,46] This has largely been attributed in the past to hyperproliferation of the epidermis, the assumption being that the organisms were merely colonizing this particular site. However, it has become apparent that most patients with seborrhoeic dermatitis or scaling of the scalp (dandruff) respond to treatment with azole antifungal agents and that this coincides with the disappearance of the yeasts; if they relapse after therapy the organisms reappear.[120,46] The circumstantial evidence, therefore, that the two events are causally related, is strong. In animals it is possible to induce skin scaling that bears some resemblance to seborrhoeic dermatitis after the application of pityrosporum.[121] Patients with seborrhoeic dermatitis have significantly raised levels of antibody to these organisms,[47] but do not appear to develop contact sensitization to antigenic extracts. One further intriguing piece of evidence is that seborrhoeic dermatitis is one of the earliest and most consistent abnormalities seen in patients with AIDS.[48,122] All these observations reinforce the view that adult-type seborrhoeic dermatitis is directly related to pityrosporum yeasts. The relationship between infant seborrhoeic dermatitis and these organisms is less well established, although early on in life colonization with *P. ovale* has been recorded.[6] The mechanisms by which they induce the skin changes are not known and the possibilities of direct lipase activity[7] or antibody-mediated epidermal damage[47] have both been considered. It is also apparent that a small percentage of patients with typical seborrhoeic dermatitis do not respond to azole antifungals and the exact mode of pathogenesis in these cases is not clear. However, it is possible that a number of different stimuli can trigger this common condition, of which the most common is pityrosporum. A further observation is that certain patients with eczema affecting the head and neck may also respond to topically applied azole antifungals and also show immediate-type hypersensitivity to extracts of pityrosporum.[123] Patients have usually had childhood atopic disease or are atopic on family history and the condition is most often seen in young women.

Pityrosporum folliculitis

The third condition associated with pityrosporum yeasts is a form of folliculitis on the back and upper trunk. Pityrosporum folliculitis is a clinically distinct condition, most often seen in teenagers or young adult males.[124,125] Lesions are itchy papules and pustules, which are often diffusely scattered on the shoulders and back. The itching and distribution distinguishes them from acne vulgaris. Patients often report the development of lesions after a holiday in the sun. The condition responds well to oral ketoconazole or ketoconazole shampoo. Biopsies taken from typical cases show clusters of yeasts within follicles surrounded by inflammatory cells, which are distinguishable from the colonization of follicular openings that can be seen in normal individuals. The exact pathogenesis of this condition is once again unknown but treatment with appropriate antifungals is highly effective.

Diagnosis and treatment of pityrosporum infections

The diagnosis of pityriasis versicolor is achieved by microscopy of scales removed from lesions, which show the characteristic combination of small yeasts and short, stubby hyphae. Culture is not necessary. The diagnosis of both seborrhoeic dermatitis and pityrosporum folliculitis is mainly dependent on clinical features.

Therapy with a variety of topically applied antifungal drugs, such as azole antifungals or selenium sulphide solution, works well in pityriasis versicolor, although relapse is common. Oral antifungals such as ketoconazole or itraconazole may also be used. Topical azole antifungals also work well in seborrhoeic dermatitis.

Other fungi causing superficial infections

It is recognized that other fungi may also cause a variety of other skin infections. Generally these are rare, such as tinea nigra, alternariosis or white piedra. However, fungi may also attack nails, particularly where these have been altered by other disease processes including peripheral vascular disease. The mechanisms by which these organisms, which include *Aspergillus* spp., *Pyrenochaeta* spp. and *Acremonium* spp., subsist in nail are not known as none appears to be able to destroy keratin. *Scopulariopsis brevicaulis* will also invade healthy nails and occasionally the skin of the interdigital spaces. Again, the mode of pathogenesis is unknown. In practical terms it means that the isolation of fungi from nails has to be considered carefully before it is possible to exclude a pathogenic role. Generally, repeated isolations are made in order to establish that the organism is a consistent finding – and therefore more likely to be contributing to nail damage.

References

1 Faergemann J. Lipophilic yeasts in skin disease. Semin Dermatol 1985; 4: 173–84.
2 Midgley G. The diversity of *Pityrosporum* (*Malassezia*) yeasts *in vivo* and *in vitro*. Mycopathologia 1989; 106: 143–53.
3 Salkin IF, Gordon MA. Polymorphism of *Malassezia furfur*. Can J Microbiol 1977; 23: 471–73.
4 Roberts SOB. *Pityrosporum orbiculare*: incidence and distribution in clinically normal skin. Br J Dermatol 1969; 81: 264–69.
5 Faergemann J, Fredriksson T. Age incidence of *Pityrosporum orbiculare* on human skin. Acta Derm Venereol Stockh 1980; 60: 531–33.
6 Broberg A, Faergemann J. Infantile seborrhoeic dermatitis and *Pityrosporum ovale*. Br J Dermatol 1989; 120: 359–62.
7 Wilde PF, Stewart PS. A study of the fatty acid metabolism of the yeast *Pityrosporum ovale*. Biochem J 1968; 108: 225–31.
8 Nazzaro-Porro M, Passi S. Identification of tyrosinase inhibitors in cultures of *Pityrosporum*. J Invest Dermatol 1978; 71: 389–402.
9 Odds FC. Candida and candidosis. London: Bailliere Tindall; 1988.
10 Baran R, Badillet G. Primary onycholysis of the big toenails: review of 113 cases. Br J Dermatol 1982; 106: 529–31.
11 Ive FA. The carrier state of tinea capitis in Nigeria. Br J Dermatol 1966; 78: 219–21.
12 Sohnle PG. Dermatophytosis. In: Cox RA, ed. Immunology of fungal diseases. Boca Raton, FA: CRC Press; 1989: 1–27.
13 Louria DB, Smith JK, Brayton RG et al. Anticandida factors in serum and their inhibitors: 1 Clinical and laboratory observations. J Infect Dis 1972; 125: 102–14.
14 King RD, Khan HA, Foye JC, et al. Transferrin, iron and dermatophytes: 1. serum dermatophyte inhibitory component definitely identified as unsaturated transferrin. J Lab Clin Med 1975; 86: 204–12.
15 Artis WM, Patrisky E, Rastinejard F, Duncan RL. Fungistatic mechanism of human transferrin for *Rhizopus oryzae* and *Trichophyton mentagrophytes*: alternative to simple iron depletion. Infect Immun 1983: 41; 1269–76.
16 Abraham A, Mohapatra LN, Kandhari KC et al. The effects of some hair oils and unsaturated fatty acids on experimentally induced dermatophytosis. Dermatologica 1975; 151: 144–49.

17 Rothman S, Smiljanic A, Shapiro AL, Weitkamp AW. The spontaneous cure of tinea capitis in puberty. J Invest Dermatol 1947; 8: 81–98.

18 Marples RR, Downing DT, Kligman AM. Influence of *Pityrosporum* species on the generation of free fatty acids in human surface lipid. J Invest Dermatol 1972; 58: 155–62.

19 Sohnle PG, Frank MM, Kirkpatrick CH. Mechanisms involved in elimination of organisms from experimental cutaneous *Candida albicans* infections in guinea pigs. J Immunol 1976; 117: 523–29.

20 Berk SH, Penneys NS, Weinstein G. Epidermal activity in annular dermatophytosis. Arch Dermatol 1976; 112: 485–88.

21 Green F, Lee KW, Balish E. Chronic *T. mentagrophytes* dermatophytosis of guinea pig skin grafts on nude mice. J Invest Dermatol 1982; 79: 125–31.

22 Hay RJ, Calderon RA, MacKenzie CD (1988) Experimental dermatophytosis in mice; correlation between light and electron microscopic changes in primary, secondary and chronic infections. Br J Exp Pathol; 69: 703–16.

23 Davies RR, Zaini F. Drugs affecting *Trichophyton rubrum* induced neutrophil chemotaxis *in vitro*. Clin Exp Dermatol 1988; 13: 228–31.

24 Calderon RA, Hay RJ. Fungicidal activity of human neutrophils and monocytes on dermatophyte fungi, *Trichophyton quinckeanum* and *Trichophyton rubrum*. Immunology 1986; 61: 289–95.

25 Calderon RA, Shennan G. Susceptibility of *Trichophyton quinckeanum* and *Trichophyton rubrum* to products of oxidative metabolism. Immunology 1986; 61: 283–88.

26 Lehrer RI. The fungicidal mechanisms of human monocytes: 1. Evidence for myeloperoxidase linked and myeloperoxidase independent candidacidal mechanisms. J Clin Invest 1975; 55: 338–46.

27 Hay RJ, Reid S, Talwat E, et al. Immune responses of patients with tinea imbricata. Br J Dermatol 1983; 108: 581–89.

28 Kaaman T, von Stedingk LV, von Stedingk M, et al. ELISA-determined serological reactivity against purified trichophytin in dermatophytosis. Acta Derm Venereal Stockh 1981; 61: 313–17.

29 Calderon RA, Hay RJ. Cell-mediated immunity in experimental murine dermatophytosis: II Adoptive transfer of immunity to dermatophyte infection by lymphoid cells from donors with acute or chronic infections. Immunology 1984; 53: 405–10.

30 Kirkpatrick CH, Rich RB, Bennett JE. Chronic mucocutaneous candidiasis; model building in cellular immunology. Ann Intern Med 1971; 74: 955–78.

31 Dwyer JM. Chronic mucocutaneous candidiasis. Ann Rev Med 1981; 32: 491–97.

32 Mathews R, Burnie J, Smith D, et al. Candida in AIDS: evidence of protective antibody. Lancet 1988; ii: 263–66.

33 Lee KW, Balish E. Systemic candidiasis in germ free, flora defined and conventional nude and thymus-bearing mice. J Reticuloendothelial Soc 1981; 29: 71–77.

34 Drouhet E, Dupont B. Laboratory and clinical assessment of ketoconazole in deep seated mycoses. Am J Med 1983; 74 (1B): 30–47.

35 Djeu JY, Blanchard DK, Halkias D, Friedman H. Growth inhibition of Candida albicans by human polymorphonuclear neutrophils: activation of interferon gamma and tumour necrosis factor. J Immunol 1986; 137: 2980–84.

36 Calderon RA, Hay RJ. Cell mediated immunity in experimental murine

dermatophytosis: 1. Temporal aspects of T suppressor activity caused by *Trichophyton quinckeanum*. Immunology 1984: 53: 457–64.

37 Jones HE, Reinhardt JH, Rinaldi MG. Acquired immunity to dermatophytosis. Arch Dermatol 1974; 109: 840–48.

38 Jones HE, Reinhardt JH, Rinaldi MG. Model dermatophytosis in naturally infected subjects. Arch Dermatol 1974; 110: 369–74.

39 Rasmussen JE, Ahmed AR. Trichophytin reactions in children with tinea capitis. Arch Dermatol 1978; 371–72.

40 Hay RJ, Shennan G. Chronic dermatophyte infections: II. Antibody and cell-mediated immune responses. Br J Dermatol 1982; 106: 191–95.

41 Braathen LR, Kaaman T. Human epidermal Langerhans cells induce cellular immune responses to trichophytin in dermatophytosis. Br J Dermatol 1983; 109: 295–99.

42 Sohnle PG, Collins-Lech C. Cell mediated immunity to *Pityrosporum orbiculare* in pityriasis versicolor. J. Clin Invest 1978; 62: 45–50.

43 Sohnle PG, Collins-Lech C. Analysis of the lymphocyte transformation response to *Pityrosporum orbiculare* in patients with tinea versicolor. Clin Exp Immunol 1982; 49: 559–66.

44 Roberts SOB. Pityriasis versicolor; a clinical and mycological investigation. Br J Dermatol 1969; 81: 315–26.

45 Soeprono FF, Schinella RA, Cockerell CJ, et al. Seborrheic-like dermatitis of acquired immunodeficiency syndrome. J Am Acad Dermatol 1986; 14: 242–48.

46 Shuster S. Aetiology of dandruff and the mode of action of therapeutic agents. Br J Dermatol 1984; 111: 235–42.

47 Midgley G, Hay RJ. Serological responses to *Pityrosporum* (*Malassezia*) in seborrhoeic dermatitis demonstrated by ELISA and Western blotting. Bull Soc Franc Med Mycol, 1988; 17: 267–78.

48 Nicholls D, Midgley GM, Hay RJ. Patch testing against *Pityrosporum* antigens. Clin Exp Dermatol, 1990; 15: 75.

49 Hay RJ, Campbell CK, Wingfield R, Clayton YM. A comparative study of dermatophytosis in coal miners and dermatological outpatients. Br J Indust Med 1983; 40: 353–55.

50 Mayou SC, Calderon RA, Goodfellow A, Hay RJ. Deep (subcutaneous) dermatophyte infection presenting with unilateral lymphoedema. Clin Exp Dermatol 1987; 12: 385–88.

51 Allen DE, Snyderman R, Meadows L, et al. Generalized *Microsporum audouinii* infection and depressed cellular immunity associated with a missing plasma factor required for lymphocyte blastogenesis. Am J Med 1977; 63: 991–1000.

52 MacGregor J, Hamilton AJ, Hay RJ. Inhibition of human lymphocyte blastogenesis by a factor derived from *Trichophyton rubrum*. Br J Dermatol 1990; 123: 826.

53 Durandy A, Fischer A, Le Deist F, et al. Mannan specific and mannan induced T-cell suppressive activity in patients with chronic mucocutaneous candidosis. J Clin Immunol 1987; 7: 400–10.

54 Torssander J, Karlsson A, Morfeldt-Mason L, et al. Dermatophytosis and HIV infection – study in homosexual men. Acta Derm Venereol Stockh 1988; 68: 53–59.

55 Jones HE, Reinhardt JH, Rinaldi MG. A clinical, mycological and immunological survey of dermatophytosis. Arch Dermatol 1973; 108; 61–68.

56 Sams WM, Jorizzo JL, Snyderman R, et al. Chronic mucocutaneous candidiasis; immunological studies of three generations of a single family. Am J Med 1979; 67: 948–59.

57 Wells RS, Higgs JM, MacDonald D, et al. Familial chronic mucocutaneous candidiasis. J Med Genet 1972; 9: 642–43.

58 Rebell G, Taplin D. Dermatophytes: their recognition and identification. 2nd ed. Miami: University of Miami Press; 1970.

59 Blank F, Mann SJ. *Trichophyton rubrum* infection according to age, anatomical distribution and sex. Br J Dermatol 1975; 92: 171–74.

60 Rothman S, Knox G, Windhorst D. Tinea pedis a source of infection in the family. Arch Dermatol 1957; 75: 270–71.

61 Serjeantson S, Lawrence G. Autosomal recessive inheritance of susceptibility to tinea imbricata. Lancet 1977; i: 13–15.

62 Hay RJ. Tinea imbricata. In: Current topics in medical mycology, vol 2. New York: Springer-Verlag; 1987: 55–72.

63 de Vroey C. Epidemiology of ringworm (dermatophytosis) Semin Dermatol 1985; 4: 185–200.

64 Gentles JC, Evans EGV. Foot infection in swimming baths. Br Med J 1973; 3: 260–62.

65 English MP, Gibson MD. Studies in the epidemiology of tinea pedis: I and II. Tinea pedis in school children. Br Med J 1959; i: 1442–45; 1446–48.

66 Gentles JC, Holmes JG. Foot ringworm in coal miners. Br J Indust Med 1957; 14: 22–29.

67 Hope YM, Clayton YM, Hay RJ, et al. Foot infection in coal miners; a reassessment. Br J Dermatol 1985; 112: 405–13.

68 Howell SA, Clayton YM, Phan OG, Noble WC. Tinea pedis: the relationship between symptoms and host characteristics. Microb Ecol Hlth Dis 1988; 1: 131–38.

69 Verhagen AR. Distribution of dermatophytes causing tinea capitis in Africa. Trop Geogr Med 1973; 26: 101–20.

70 Branson DM, Desai DR, Barsky S, Foley SM. An epidemic of infection with *Trichophyton tonsurans* revealed in a 20 year old survey of fungal infections in Chicago. J Am Acad Dermatol 1983; 8: 322–30.

71 Rippon JW. Epidemiology and emerging patterns of dermatophyte species. In: Current topics in medical mycology, vol 1. New York: Springer-Verlag; 1985: 208–34.

72 Midgely G, Clayton YM. Distribution of dermatophytes and Candida spores in the environment. Br J Dermatol 1972; 86 (Suppl 8): 69–77.

73 Philpot CM. Geographic distribution of the dermatophytes – a review. J Hyg Camb 1978; 80: 301–13.

74 Marples MJ. Microbiological studies in Western Samoa: II. The isolation of yeast-like organisms from the mouth with a note of some dermatophytes isolated from tinea. Trans R Soc Trop Med Hyg 1960; 54: 166–70.

75 Zurita J, Hay RJ. The adherence of dermatophyte microconidia and arthroconidia to human keratinocytes *in vitro*. J Invest Dermatol 1987; 89: 529–34.

76 Yu RJ, Harmon SR, Grappel SF, Blank F. Two cell-bound keratinases of *Trichophyton mentagrophytes*. J Invest Dermatol 1971; 56: 27–32.

77 Weismann K, Knudsen EA, Pedersen C. White nails in AIDS/ARC due to *Trichophyton rubrum* infection. Clin Exp. Dermatol 1988; 13: 24–27.

78 Graham JH, Barrosos-Tobila C. Dermatophytosis. In: Banker RD, ed. The pathologic anatomy of the mycoses. Berlin: Springer; 1971: 211–35.

79 Leyden JJ, Kligman AM. Interdigital athletes foot: the interaction of dermatophytes and residual bacteria. Arch Dermatol 1978: 1466–72.

80 Birt AR, Wilt JC. Mycology, bacteriology and histopathology of suppurative ringworm. Arch Dermatol 1957; 69: 441–48.

81 Zaias N. Onychomycosis. Arch Dermatol 1972; 105: 262–74.

82 Elmros T, Liden S. Hereditary palmoplantar keratoderma; incidence of dermatophyte infections and the results of topical treatment with retinoic acid. Acta Derm Venereal Stockh 1983; 63: 254–57.

83 Ive A, Marks R. Tinea incognito. Br Med J 1968; iii: 216–21.

84 Kaaman T, Torssander J. Dermatophytid – a misdiagnosed entity. Acta Derm Venereol Stockh 1983; 63: 404–08.

85 Roberts SOB. Treatment of superficial and subcutaneous mycoses. In: Speller DCE, ed. Antifungal chemotherapy. Chichester: John Wiley, 1980: 255–83.

86 Hay RJ. Antifungal agents. Semin Dermatol 1990; 9: 309–317.

87 Moore MK. Morphological and physiological studies of isolates of *Hendersonula toruloidea* Nattrass cultured from human skin and nail samples. J Med Vet Mycol 1988; 26: 25–39.

88 Allison VY, Hay RJ and Campbell CK. *Hendersonula toruloidea* and *Scytalidium hyalinum* infections in Tobago. Br J Dermatol 1984; 111: 371–72.

89 Gugnani HC, Nzelibe FK, Osunkwo IC. Onychomycosis due to *Hendersonula toruloidea* in Nigeria. J Med Vet Mycol 1986; 24: 239–41.

90 Hay RJ, Moore MK. Clinical features of superficial fungal infections caused by *Hendersonula toruloidea* and *Scytalidium hyalinum*. Br J Dermatol 1984; 100: 677–83.

91 Jones SK. White JE, Jacobs PH, et al. *Hendersonula toruloidea* infection of the nails in Caucasians. Clin Exp Dermatol 1985; 10: 444–47.

92 Simon M, Hornstein OP. Prevalence rate of *Candida* in the oral cavity of patients with lichen planus. Arch Dermatol Res 1980; 267: 317–18.

93 Torssander J, Morfeldt-Manson L, Biberfeld G, et al. Oral *Candida albicans* in HIV infection. Scand J Infect 1987; 189; 291–95.

94 Knight L, Fletcher J. Growth of *Candida albicans* in saliva: stimulation by glucose associated with antibiotics, corticosteroids and diabetes mellitus. J Infect Dis 1971; 123: 371–77.

95 Douglas, LJ. Adhesion to surfaces. In: Rose AH, Harrison JS, eds. The yeasts, vol 2. London: Academic Press; 1987: 239–80.

96 MacCourtie J, Douglas LJ. Relationship between cell surface composition, adherence and virulence of *Candida albicans*. Infect Immun 1984; 45: 6–12.

97 Calderone RA, Lineham L, Wadsworth E, et al. Identification of C3d receptors on *Candida albicans*. Infect Immun 1988; 56: 252–58.

98 Blackwell CC, Thom SM, Weir DM, et al. Host–parasite interactions underlying non-secretion of blood group antigens and susceptibility to infection by *Candida albicans*. In: Lark DL, ed. Protein carbohydrate interactions in biological systems. London: Academic Press; 1986: 231–33.

99 MacDonald F, Odds FC. Virulence for mice of a proteinase secreting strain of *Candida albicans* and a proteinase-deficient mutant. J Gen Microbiol 1983; 129: 431–38.

100 Warnock DW, Speller DCE, Milne JD, et al. Epidemiological investigation of

patients with vulvovaginal candidosis: application of a resistogram method for strain differentiation of *Candida albicans*. Br J Vener Dis 1979; 55: 357–61.

101 Magee BB, D'Souza TM, Magee PT. Strain and species identification by restriction fragment length polymorphisms in the ribosomal DNA repeat of *Candida* species. J Bacteriol 1987; 169: 1639–43.

102 Soll DR. The regulation of cellular differentiation in the dimorphic yeast, *Candida albicans*. BioEssays 1986; 5: 5–10.

103 Burnie JP, Odds FC, Lee W, et al. Outbreak of systemic *Candida albicans* in an intensive care unit caused by cross infection. Br Med J 1985; 290: 746–48.

104 Chandler FW, Watts JC. Pathologic diagnosis of fungal infections. Chicago: ASCP Press; 1987: 97–112.

105 Samaranayake LP, MacFarlane TW, eds. Oral candidosis. London: Wright; 1990.

106 Budtz-Jorgensen E. The significance of *Candida albicans* in denture stomatitis. Scand J Dent Res 1974; 82: 151–90.

107 Kaufman RH, ed. Vulvovaginal candidiasis: a symposium. J Reproduct Med 1986; 31: 639–72.

108 Sobel JD. Recurrent vulvovaginal candidiasis. N Engl J Med 1986; 315: 1455–58.

109 Sobel JD. Vulvovaginal candidiasis – what we do and do not know. Ann Intern Med 1984; 101: 390–92.

110 Rebora A, Leyden JJ. Napkin (diaper) dermatitis and gastrointestinal carriage of *Candida albicans*. Br J Dermatol 1981; 105: 551–55.

111 Frain-Bell W. Chronic paronychia: short review of 590 cases. Trans St John's Hosp Derm Soc 1957; 38: 29–30.

112 Stone OJ, Mullins JF. Chronic paronychia: microbiology and histopathology. Arch Dermatol 1962; 86: 324–27.

113 Wells RS. Chronic mucocutaneous candidiasis: a clinical classification. Proc R Soc Med 1973; 66: 801–02.

114 Klein RS, Harris CA, Small CB, et al. Oral candidiasis in high risk patients as the initial manifestation of the acquired immunodeficiency syndrome. N Engl J Med 1984; 311: 354–57.

115 Travitian A, Raufman JP, Rosenthal Le. Oral candidiasis as a marker for esophageal candidiasis in the acquired immunodeficiency syndrome. Ann Intern Med 1986; 104: 54–55.

116 Hay RJ, Kalter DC. Superficial *Candida* infection. In: Jacobs PH, Nall L, eds. Antifungal drug therapy. New York: Marcel Dekker; 1990: 37–42.

117 Burke RC. Tinea versicolor: susceptibility factors and experimental infections in human beings. J Invest Dermatol 1961; 36: 398–402.

118 Faergemann J, Fredriksson T. Tinea versicolor with regard to seborrheic dermatitis. Arch Dermatol 1979; 115: 966–68.

119 Bergbrant I-M, Faergemann J. The role of *Pityrosporum ovale* in seborrhoeic dermatitis. Semin Dermatol 1990; 9: 262–68.

120 Gosse RM, Vanderwyk RW. The relationship of a nystatin resistant strain of *Pityrosporum ovale* to dandruff. J Soc Cosmet Chem. 1969; 20: 603–09.

121 Faergemann J, Fredriksson T. Experimental infections in rabbits and humans with *Pityrosporum orbiculare* and *P. ovale*. J Invest Dermatol 1981; 77: 314–18.

122 Mathes BM, Douglas MC. Seborrheic dermatitis in patients with acquired immunodeficiency syndrome. J Am Acad Dermatol 1985; 13: 947–51.

123 Hjorth N, Clemmensen OJ. Treatment of dermatitis of the head and neck with ketoconazole in patients with type 1 hypersensitivity for *Pityrosporum orbiculare*. Semin Dermatol 1983; 2: 26–29.

124 Potter BS, Burgoon CF, Johnson WC. Pityrosporum folliculitis. Arch Dermatol 1970; 102: 388–91.

125 Back O, Faergemann J, Hornquist R. Pityrosporum folliculitis: a common disease of the young and middle aged. J Am Acad Dermatol 1985; 12: 56–61.

11

Bacterial and fungal skin disease in animals

D. H. LLOYD

Introduction

The range of bacterial and fungal skin disease in animals is very wide and involves many pathogens that also have significant systemic effects. Comprehensive consideration of all of these infections is beyond the scope of this review and attention will be concentrated on infections of terrestrial mammals and on diseases of the general body surface. Infections of specialized skin regions, such as the ear, vulva, prepuce and skin glands, will be considered more briefly and no attempt will be made to cover mastitis. Similarly, diseases in which the skin signs form a minor part will only be mentioned briefly. Zoonotic infection is not considered here.

The skin is an efficient defensive organ and the great majority of animals have a healthy looking skin and coat. Despite this, careful examination will usually reveal the presence of minor lesions and virulent pathogens can often be demonstrated on the skin in absence of any signs of disease. These will seldom lead to clinically significant infection but are an indication of the constant battle that goes on between skin immunity and external challenges, particularly those associated with microorganisms. In animals, as in man, clinical skin infection generally results only after the equilibrium between the skin, its normal flora and fauna, and the external environment has been disturbed (see other chapters in this book) or, less commonly, following access of pathogens to the skin via the systemic route.[1-3] Thus very few microorganisms can be considered to be truly primary skin pathogens. Nevertheless, in most cases of animal skin infection, the principal pathogens can be distinguished from those that are secondary invaders, although the secondary organisms may still play an important part in exacerbating the pathological process. In addition, a need for symbiotic association is apparent between organisms that are not individually pathogenic before certain diseases, such as ovine foot-rot,[4,5] can occur. In this review, primary and secondary agents will be differentiated where possible but the main emphasis will be placed on those organisms that play a principal role in the pathogenesis of skin disease.

The skin microflora in animals is dominated by Gram-positive bacteria and, in healthy individuals, Gram-negative organisms are generally found as transients or short-term colonizers of moist or contaminated skin.[2] They seldom cause infection in the absence of prior invasion by Gram-positive species.

The normal skin flora of animals is less fully investigated than in humans. The skin flora of healthy cats and dogs has been described as comprising, respectively, 7 and 22 per cent coagulase-positive staphylococci, 11 and 7 per cent coagulase-negative staphylococci, 27 and 17 per cent *Micrococcus* spp., 20 and 21 per cent alpha-haemolytic streptococci, 23 and 26 per cent acineto-bacters, 9 and 2 per cent other Gram-negative bacilli and the remainder Gram-positive rods.[6] More details are available of the composition of the staphylococcal flora (Table 11.1); these data may suffer from changes in our understanding of staphylococcal taxonomy but are generally acceptable.

Skin diseases associated with bacteria

The Gram-positive cocci
Pathogenic staphylococci

These are probably the most common cause of skin infection in domestic animals and include the coagulase-positive species, *Staphylococcus aureus*, and *S. intermedius* (formerly *S. aureus* biotypes E and F[11]), and the coagulase-variable species *S. hyicus*.[12,13] A variety of other staphylococcal species has also been isolated from skin infections in animals but, in most instances, their status as pathogens is unclear.[14]

In dogs, staphylococcal pyoderma is one of the most common problems seen in veterinary practice. *Staphylococcus intermedius* is carried at oral, nasal or anal sites by most normal dogs[10,15,16] and is the principal bacterial pathogen in over 90 per cent of cases of pyoderma. *Staphylococcus aureus* accounts for most of the remainder but *S. hyicus* and coagulase-negative species generally considered to be non-pathogenic are also isolated occasionally in pure culture from lesions.[17,18]

Canine staphylococcal skin infection varies from mild, localized, superficial disease to severe, generalized, life-threatening conditions.[19] Impetigo, which is characterized by subcorneal pustules affecting the interfollicular epidermis of the relatively hairless abdominal and axillary skin, is seen in immature dogs

Table 11.1. *Staphylococcal flora of the skin or hair coat of domestic animals*

	Cattle[a]	Goats[a]	Sheep[a]	Pigs[a]	Pigs[b]	Cats[c]	Dogs[d]
S. chromogenes	22	1	0	17	5	0	0
S. cohnii	6	6	0	2	1	0	< 1
S. epidermidis	29	1	0	0	4	17	8
S. gallinarum	0	8	0	0	0	0	0
S. haemolyticus	9	0	0	4	2	3	3
S. hyicus	5	2	0	6	14	1	< 1
S. intermedius	0	0	0	0	0	14	33
S. lentus	9	15	27	27	4	0	0
S. saprophyticus	2	5	5	0	3	1	1
S. sciuri	3	42	60	22	36	2	6
S. simulans	7	0	0	4	1	44	5
S. warneri	7	0	0	2	2	2	13
S. xylosus	10	15	10	9	23	11	19
Unspeciated or other	1	5	0	5	5[e]	5[f]	11[g]
Number speciated	189	100	62	120	111	827	464

Based on: [a] ref. 7; [b] ref. 8; [c] ref. 9; [d] ref. 10.

[e] Others comprise one isolate each *S. arlettae*, *S. auricularis*, *S. capitis* and *S. equorum* and three of *S. hominis*.

[f] Others comprise 41 isolates of *S. aureus* and 8 of *S. capitis*.

[g] Others comprise 24 isolates of *S. aureus*, 22 of *S. hominis* and 9 of *S. capitis*.

and at puberty, and often resolves spontaneously. Folliculitis and furunculosis affecting the chin ('canine acne') also occurs in young dogs and may resolve at puberty. Superficial folliculitis is seen in dogs of all ages and can extend to involve the deeper parts of the follicle and, after follicular rupture, the dermis and hypodermis as a furunculosis and cellulitis. This may be localized or generalized. Localized pyoderma affecting the feet, muzzle, perianal region and ears occurs quite commonly and may be conditioned by poor local conformation, notably where this leads to friction, poor ventilation and excessive moisture. Secondary infection with other organisms, including Gram-negative genera such as *Proteus*, *Pseudomonas* and coliforms, may occur,[12] especially in severely affected skin. Pathogenic staphylococci are also sometimes associated with nodular and fistulating, deep granulomatous infections in which granular masses of bacteria are found in pockets of pus, so-called botriomycosis.[12] A similar syndrome can also be associated with infections by other bacteria such as *Actinomyces* and *Actinobacillus* spp. Breed predispositions to severe pyoderma, particularly in German Shepherd dogs, have been described.[20] Surface populations of coagulase-positive staphylococci are also larger than normal in other canine skin diseases including seborrhoea and atopy.[21, 22]

A wide variety of underlying causes is known to predispose to pyoderma in dogs but the pathogenesis is poorly understood.[18, 22] Little is known of the virulence of pathogenic staphylococci affecting dogs and epidemic strains are not recognized, although enterotoxins A and C, and protease production, are known to differ between isolates of *S. intermedius*.[23–25] Skin splitting activity has not been demonstrated in canine isolates of *S. intermedius* and *S. aureus*, and dog skin is not susceptible to the epidermolytic toxin of *S. aureus*,[26] although Love and Davies[27] have described a condition in greyhounds that resembled human staphylococcal scalded-skin syndrome both clinically and histologically.

In cats, bacterial skin disease is uncommon, although abscesses involving Gram-negative bacteria often occur after bite wounds. *Staphylococcus aureus* is commonly isolated from skin lesions, although *S. intermedius* and *S. hyicus* are also sometimes present.[28, 29] Devriese and colleagues[29] found that most *S. aureus* isolates were human ecovars and concluded that coagulase-positive staphylococci were not endogenous to cats.

In ruminants, pigs and horses, *S. aureus* is the principal pathogenic staphylococcus but isolation of *S. intermedius* and *S. hyicus* is now being reported with increasing frequency.[11, 30–34] In pigs, *S. hyicus* causes exudative epidermitis (see below); Devriese and Derycke[35] suggest that this organism is a member of the normal skin flora of cattle and have shown that it induces a necrotizing, exfoliative epidermitis when inoculated on to scarified bovine skin. Ishihara[36] has reported an exfoliative skin disease caused by *S. aureus* in a colony of laboratory guinea-pigs. The disease could be reproduced in guinea-pigs by subcutaneous inoculation of one of the isolates. Phage typing showed that the causative organisms were not of phage group 2, which is responsible for scalded-skin syndrome in man. *Staphylococcus aureus* also causes an exudative dermatitis in young rabbits and abscesses in adults.[37]

Staphylococcal impetigo commonly occurs in cattle, sheep and goats, affecting the udder and sometimes extending to the teats and adjacent areas of the ventral abdomen, medial thighs, perineum and ventral surface of the tail.[13] Stress and poor husbandry are predisposing factors. Folliculitis and furunculosis are also common in sheep and goats but relatively uncommon in cattle and pigs.[13, 38] Lesions tend to occur on the face, ears, perineum, tail, ventral abdomen, medial thighs and limbs. In 3- to 4-week-old lambs, a transient pustular skin disease affecting the lips and perineum occurs.[39] A more severe syndrome is seen in sheep of any age, affecting the head, and this may spread through a flock.[40]

In horses, folliculitis and furunculosis are quite common, particularly over the area covered by the saddle and girths; the dorsal surface of the tail and the distal, caudal parts of the limbs (pasterns and fetlocks) are also affected. Lesions can be quite severe and painful, with dermal nodules, oedema, urticaria, crusting, draining tracts, ulceration and scarring.[13, 41] The prevalence is higher during the spring and summer, and lesions tend to occur in areas that are occluded, remain moist or are subject to trauma. Streptococci can sometimes also be isolated from the lesions.

In pigs, staphylococcal folliculitis is seen in piglets less than 8 weeks old as a generalized, mild, transient pustular dermatitis. Facial dermatitis secondary to damage caused by immature teeth is also seen in young pigs. A characteristic disease syndrome, porcine exudative epidermitis ('greasy pig disease') is caused by *S. hyicus*. It occurs particularly in piglets under 8 weeks old and leads to the formation of reddish, macular lesions, which then become exudative as epidermal necrosis, vesicle formation and exfoliation induced by the exfoliative toxin that it produces occur.[42-44] In severe infections, vesicles also appear in the mouth, on the lips and around the coronets; systemic infection occurs and the pigs die in 3–8 days. *Staphylococcus hyicus* is a member of the normal flora in pigs, which may carry both virulent and non-virulent variants. Studies in gnotobiotic piglets show that the onset of disease is related to the population levels that individual strains can achieve on the skin; disease induced by virulent strains can be prevented by prior inoculation of an avirulent strain.[45, 46] Dual infection of pigs with *S. hyicus* and *Dermatophilus congolensis* has been reported.[47]

Streptococci

Streptococci, particularly alpha-haemolytic species, can commonly be isolated from normal skin in domestic animals[1, 6, 48, 49] and are an important cause of mastitis, particularly in cattle. Skin populations are known to be raised in hot and humid conditions in cattle and it has been suggested that this may influence the epidemiological features of bovine mastitis.[2, 48]

Streptococci are seldom implicated as the causative agents in bacterial skin disease in animals. In pigs, contagious pyoderma of unweaned piglets has been associated with infection by beta-haemolytic, chiefly Lancefield group C, strains. Pustules develop on the head, trunk and tail after a period of pyrexia and depression. In sows the udder and teats may be affected.[13, 50] In horses, *Str. equi* is the cause of strangles, a severe purulent infection of the upper respiratory tract and draining lymph nodes, which may form abscesses. Hypersensitivity to *Str. equi* may lead to purpura haemorrhagica, urticaria and dermatitis in infected animals.[13] In guinea-pigs, Group C streptococci are a principal cause of streptococcosis, a submandibular lymphadenitis in which rupture of the affected lymph nodes may lead to a localized dermatitis at the point of drainage.[51] *Peptostreptococcus tetradius* has been reported as the cause of abscesses in a puppy.[52]

In camels, streptococci, particularly Lancefield Group B strains, are the most commonly reported isolates from contagious skin necrosis, a disease characterized by skin necrosis, abscessation, sinus formation and enlargement of local lymph glands. However, a variety of other bacterial species has also been recovered and the role of streptococci in this disease is not clear.[53]

Gram-positive rods and filamentous bacteria
Erysipelothrix

In pigs, infection with *E. rhusiopathiae* is associated with the development of an urticarial reaction resulting in the formation of characteristic raised, red, rectangular or rhomboid macules, which may become necrotic and slough or resolve spontaneously. In acute infections, red or purple discoloration of the skin may also be observed.[54]

Bacillus spp.

These are found on the skin of animals and populations have been found to increase substantially under conditions of high temperature and humidity in cattle.[2,6] However, only *Bacillus anthracis* is associated with skin disease. In ruminants, the disease is usually peracute and results in sudden death with the extravasation of tarry blood from body orifices. In horses, oedematous swellings of the throat, neck and shoulders are often seen. In pigs and dogs, localized infection is more common. Pharyngeal involvement leads to oedema of the head and neck. When infection occurs via the skin, localized oedematous lesions occur but the disease usually becomes generalized.[54]

Clostridium spp.

Clostridial infection of animal skin is most commonly associated with malignant oedema, which principally affects the subcutaneous and adjacent intermuscular connective tissue with production of much gelatinous exudate 12–48 h after wound infection with *Cl. septicum*, *Cl. novyi*, *Cl. perfringens* and *Cl. sordellii*.[12,13,54–56] The condition is seen in ruminants, pigs and horses. Clinically, soft, rapidly expanding swellings are observed, which pit on pressure and subsequently become hot and painful; gas production may be seen. There is toxaemia and a high fever, and death usually occurs within 2 days. Extensive necrosis and sloughing of affected skin may occur. A particular syndrome ('big head') is seen in rams infected with *Cl. novyi* in which subcutaneous oedema first affects the head and spreads to the neck. Infection of wounds during fighting is believed to be responsible.

Clostridium chauvoei is the cause of 'blackleg' in the same range of hosts.[57] In cattle and pigs, the route of infection is believed to be oral, with dissemination of the organism into the liver and muscle via the circulation. In sheep, wound infection after tail docking, shearing or lambing often occurs. Disease does not manifest itself until the infected tissue is damaged. Rapid myonecrosis associated with the necrotizing and spreading effects of the alpha toxin and hyaluronidase produced by the organism cause the affected tissue to become dark brown or black. Initially, lesions are crepitant, swollen and painful but subsequently sensation is lost. Death normally occurs within 2 days.

In dogs, clostridia are occasionally associated with anaerobic cellulitis, either in pure culture or mixed infections. Lesions are painful and progress rapidly, with gas production and crepitation; systemic toxaemia follows. Such infections are normally associated with predisposing factors such as severe trauma, the presence of foreign bodies, neoplasia, immunodeficiency and bite wounds.[12, 58] In cats, *Cl. villosum* has been reported in subcutaneous abscesses associated with fight wounds.[59]

The genera Corynebacterium *and* Rhodococcus

The only member of the genus *Corynebacterium* now recognized as a significant cause of skin disease is *C. pseudotuberculosis*. 'C. pyogenes' and 'C. equi' have been reclassified and are considered under *Actinomyces pyogenes* and *Rhodococcus equi*, respectively.

Corynebacterium pseudotuberculosis is the cause of caseous lymphadenitis in sheep and goats. The infection enters via a wound or abrasion from infected fomites or directly by contact with other affected animals. The initial wound infection is mild and usually unnoticed but the organism becomes established in the regional lymph nodes, which enlarge and form abscesses filled with a green, odourless pus that ultimately becomes thick and caseous. Lymphadenitis and abscess formation may also occur at deeper sites, including the lungs, mediastinal and mesenteric lymph nodes. Affected animals become weak and emaciated.[60]

In horses and uncommonly in cattle, *C. pseudotuberculosis* causes ulcerative lymphangitis, a disease that clinically resembles equine farcy (*Pseudomonas mallei* infection). Other organisms, including *Rhodococcus equi*, *Actinomyces pyogenes*, *Pasteurella haemolytica*, *Pseudomonas aeruginosa*, *Fusobacterium necrophorum* and *Actinobacillus equuli*, are also occasionally isolated in pure or mixed culture from lesions in this disease.[13,41] Hard or fluctuating, nodular lesions form on the limbs, particularly around the fetlocks, and break down to form ulcers that discharge thick, green pus. These lesions heal over a period of about 2 weeks but others continue to appear. Associated lymph vessels tend to become corded. The disease may continue for months to years but some cases resolve spontaneously within weeks. The occurrence of the disease is associated with poor hygiene and husbandry. Transmission may involve insects.[13]

Large subcutaneous abscesses in the inguinal, pectoral and ventral abdominal regions may also be caused in horses ('bastard strangles') and more rarely in ruminants.[13,41,61] Lesions sometimes become generalized and the condition may be fatal. Transmission by flies or ticks may be involved. *Corynebacterium pseudotuberculosis* is also a rare cause of folliculitis and furunculosis in the horse.[13]

In rams, posthitis associated with *C. renale* infection of the prepuce is believed to be due to irritation caused by ammonia released by the urease produced by this bacterium.[54]

R. equi causes pneumonia in foals. Lymphadenitis is common and abscessation of the affected lymph nodes sometimes occurs.[54] The organism has also been isolated from lesions of suppurative lymphadenitis in pigs,[62] and from a granulomatous lymphadenitis[63] and a fistulating abscess in the cat.[64]

The actinomycete genera

Dermatophilus, Nocardia and *Actinomyces* are the causes of a variety of skin diseases in domestic animals. *Dermatophilus* tends to cause superficial lesions that are normally confined to the epidermis but the other two genera are associated with deep, pyogranulomatous infections. Nodular, pyogranulomatous disease has been reported also in two goats from which *Actinomadura madurae* was isolated. In a third goat an organism resembling *Actinomadura pelletierii* was observed in histological sections.[65]

Dermatophilus

Dermatophilus congolensis is the only species within the genus *Dermatophilus*. It has a complex life-cycle[66] in which the infective stage, a motile coccus, swims in films of water on the skin surface and is chemotactically attracted towards carbon dioxide diffusing through the skin. This is believed to lead it to points where the stratum corneum is thin or damaged and thus more susceptible to invasion. Here it germinates and produces a branching filament, which invades the living epidermis. The host reaction leads to the formation of a new epidermis and a scab, composed of neutrophils and a new stratum corneum. Repeated cycles of hyphal invasion and scab formation at an infected site lead to the formation of laminated scabs that can be 3 cm or more in thickness. Scab formation lifts the organism away from its nutrient source, stimulating maturation of the filaments, which become transversely and longitudinally septate. Within each septum a coccus is formed and remains dormant until the scab is wet, stimulating motility and its escape from the scab.

Dermatophilus congolensis causes skin disease in all the domestic animals but is relatively uncommon in pigs.[67] Infection is promoted by wet conditions and by factors that damage the stratum corneum, including thorny vegetation and ectoparasites. Concurrent infection with other pathogens, particularly viruses, has been reported. In temperate regions the disease is common in sheep and horses, whereas in the tropics it is a major problem in cattle but also occurs in other ruminants and equidae. The lesions most commonly are distributed dorsally, at tick predilection sites, or at the extremities and on the head. In healthy animals, lesions tend to be localized and transient; recovery is promoted if animals are sheltered from rainfall. However, depressed immunity, caused by intercurrent disease, malnutrition, the immunosuppressive effects of the bites of the tick, *Amblyomma variegatum*[68] and other stress factors, can lead to generalized skin infection and death.

Oral lesions have been described in cattle, buffaloes and cats, and subcutaneous infection has been reported in cattle (reviewed by Lloyd[67]). It is likely that the infection goes undiagnosed in some of these deep infections.

Actinomyces spp.

Actinomycosis, caused by *Actinomyces* spp., occurs in a wide variety of animal species. Actinomyces are normal inhabitants of the oropharynx and gut, and invade via the dental alveoli, oral lesions or skin wounds contaminated by saliva or faeces.[12,54] In cattle, *A. bovis* infection typically presents as a rarefying osteomyelitis of the jaw. Fistulous tracts may develop and allow pus to discharge via the skin. In pigs, actinomycosis caused by *A. suis* affects the udders of suckling sows and is thought to be inoculated through wounds caused by the sharp teeth of the piglets. Actinomycosis in other ruminants and the horse is uncommon but presents as in cattle.[13]

In dogs and cats, actinomycosis may occur in a variety of clinical forms including granulomas, subcutaneous abscesses and osteomyelitis.[12,69] *Actinomyces viscosus*, an inhabitant of the oropharynx, is often involved. The infection is particularly common after wounds in hunting dogs. Pus from lesions of actinomycosis typically has a yellow-green colour and contains yellowish granules up to 4 mm in diameter, the so-called sulphur granules, formed by colonies of the causative organism. Pyogranulomatous inflammation with the production of granular accumulations of bacteria ('botriomycosis') is also seen in skin infections with other bacteria including pathogenic staphylococci and *Actinobacillus* spp.

Actinomyces pyogenes is found on the normal mucous membranes of ruminants and pigs and also in the udder, tonsils and retropharyngeal lymph nodes of healthy heifers. It is commonly associated with pyogenic processes in ruminants and pigs. Infection usually follows stress or trauma caused by a wide variety of factors including other bacterial infections. It is an important cause of mastitis in dairy cattle. The organism can be inoculated and transmitted by flies.[54]

Nocardia spp.

Nocardiosis affecting the skin occurs in cattle, goats, horses, dogs and cats. Most nocardial species are soil saprophytes and, in large animals, infection occurs via contaminated wounds. In cattle, the disease is caused by *Nocardia farcinica* and is a particular problem in the Sudan.[70,71] However, an identical syndrome has been described in West Africa caused by *Mycobacterium farcinogenes* and *M. senegalense*,[72] and it is possible that these species have been wrongly identified as *N. farcinica*.[73] The disease is characterized by the formation of slowly growing, hard, painless, subcutaneous nodules and by thickening and enlargement of associated lymph vessels and nodes. Lesions are commonly found on the head and neck, medially on the limbs, and in sites of tick attachment such as the perineum and groin. Nodules may liquefy and ulcerate, discharging an odourless, cheesy and sometimes granular material that hardens and may be found adhering to the skin around old wounds. Healing is followed by continuing development of underlying lesions. Secondary infection with other bacteria may occur. The course may be prolonged with little effect on general health or may generalize rapidly, leading to cachexia and death.

The disease is uncommon in other species of domestic animals and may involve nocardial species including *N. asteroides*, *N. caviae* and *N. brasiliensis*. In dogs and cats, nodules, sinuses, abscesses and cellulitis may occur.[12] *Nocardia asteroides* uncommonly causes dermatitis in the horse,[74] and mycetoma in the goat has been reported.[54]

The genus *Mycobacterium*

Tuberculosis caused by *M. tuberculosis* and *M. bovis* is uncommon in domestic animals in countries where effective eradication programmes have been instituted, such as the United Kingdom and United States. In animals, the infection is most often recognized in cattle but transmission of infection from man is an important feature, particularly in urban areas.[75, 76] Skin lesions are quite rare in cases of tuberculosis in animals and are seen as nodules, plaques, abscesses and ulcers in animals that normally also show signs of systemic disease. The lesions are typically tuberculoid granulomas with caseation, necrosis and mineralization. Numbers of organisms present in the lesions may be small and difficult to find. Infection with the *M. avium–intracellulare* complex is recognized, particularly in countries where disease due to *M. tuberculosis* and *M. bovis* is rare. It is principally a bird pathogen but all domestic animals are susceptible and the infection is seen particularly in pigs.[77] Infection also occurs quite commonly in cattle, which it sensitizes to the intradermal tuberculin test but in which it causes minimal lesions in the lymph nodes. Mammary gland infection with prolonged shedding of the organism but no visible lesions has been reported.[78] Skin lesions are rare.

Feline leprosy is a granulomatous, nodular skin disease. Nodules may ulcerate and chronic abscesses or fistulae may form but the lesions remain localized. Nasal and buccal lesions may occur and peripheral lymph nodes may be affected. The disease is caused by acid-fast bacteria that have not been isolated in vitro.[12] Inoculation of cats with fresh tissue from cases causes typical localized skin and lymph node lesions containing acid-fast bacilli,[79] and in rats this procedure may result in generalized granulomatous infection. However, the causative organism is probably not *M. lepraemurium*, the cause of murine leprosy, which can be isolated in tissue culture.[80] The disease tends to occur on the head in cats less than 3 years old; transmission of the causative organism by arthropod vectors has been proposed.[79]

Animals are also affected by a variety of non-tuberculous mycobacteria. In cattle, 'skin tuberculosis' is seen throughout the world. Papular or nodular lesions, often associated with corded lymphatics, are seen and may ulcerate discharging thick, greyish-yellow pus. The lesions tend to occur on the distal parts of the limbs and spread dorsally. Affected animals remain otherwise healthy but may develop positive reactions to the intradermal tuberculin test. The causative organisms are usually not identified but *M. kansasii* has been isolated in some cases.[81] In Africa, 'M. farcinogenes' is a cause of bovine farcy, described earlier (see *N. farcinica*).

In dogs and cats, infections by *M. fortuitum*, *M. chelonei*, *M. phlei*, *M. xenopi*, *M. thermoresistible* and *M. smegmatis* have been reported. They cause chronic, localized, subcutaneous abscesses and fistulae after injury or injection; these may resolve spontaneously after a period of months.[12] Lesions tend to occur on the head but may also affect the trunk. Systemic signs of illness are uncommon.

Gram-negative bacteria
Actinobacillus spp.

Actinobacillus lignierisii is the cause of slowly developing, thick-walled abscesses affecting particularly the head and neck of ruminants but which can affect any part of the body. In cattle it causes a syndrome known as 'wooden tongue'. The organism is a commensal of the buccal cavity and infection develops after penetration via a wound. The abscesses contain a viscous pus with soft yellow granules ('sulphur granules') formed by colonies of the organism and discharge eventually through the skin, forming chronic ulcers. The disease bears clinical similarities to actinomycosis, which generally affects bony structures. In dogs, infections by *A. lignierisii* or closely related organisms have been reported.[82, 83]

In the horse, *A. equuli* normally causes systemic disease in foals but has been reported as a cause of botriomycosis in adults.[13] *Actinobacillus lignierisii* has been isolated from lesions of the tongue.

In pigs, *A. lignierisii* is uncommonly a cause of abscesses affecting the udder in sows. Infection with *A. equuli* and *A. suis* is associated with the appearance of multiple haemorrhages in the skin, particularly over the ears and abdomen, and with necrosis of the tail and skin over the joints.[84]

Pseudomonas spp.

Pseudomonas mallei is an obligate parasite of equidae. It is the cause of glanders, a highly fatal disease of equines and of carnivores that consume infected meat.[54] The organism penetrates the nasopharyngeal or intestinal mucosa and spreads via the regional lymphatics. Nodular lesions are found, particularly in the lungs and upper respiratory tract; these rupture and a purulent nasal discharge is a common feature of the disease. The skin form ('farcy') involves cording of the lymphatics and the formation of nodules that ulcerate to discharge a honey-like infectious exudate. The disease is restricted to Eastern Europe, North Africa and Asia.

A similar disease is caused by *Ps. pseudomallei*, which is widely distributed in soil and water in endemic areas. The disease occurs in South-East Asia but has also been reported in Australia, France and the Caribbean. It was a particular problem in military dogs during the Vietnam war.[85] Natural infection occurs primarily in rodents but is transmissible to a wide variety of animals. Infection occurs by inhalation or through wounds, including insect bites. The lesions are small, caseous nodules, which may coalesce or break down to form abscesses sometimes affecting the skin. Most infections are subclinical but the disease is always severe in rabbits and guinea-pigs.[54]

Pseudomonas aeruginosa is often associated with suppurative infections in domestic animals. In dogs, it is one of the most common bacteria isolated from cases of otitis externa[86] and is also found as a secondary invader in cases of deep pyoderma. In sheep, it appears to be the principal causative organism in 'fleece rot'. This is a disease occurring in the fleeces of sheep subjected to prolonged wetting; occurrence of lesions is related to the population density of the organism. *Pseudomonas maltophila* can also be isolated from lesions of fleece rot but its role in the pathogenesis of the disease is not clear. Fleece rot predisposes sheep to myiasis caused by *Lucilia cuprina*, which is attracted to odours produced in the lesions. Other bacterial species appear to potentiate the attractiveness of the lesions to the flies, particularly *Proteus mirabilis*. The central role of *Ps. aeruginosa* in these two conditions is indicated by the fact that both fleece rot and myiasis can be prevented with vaccines prepared from this bacterium (reviewed by Burrell[87]).

Borrelia spp.

Borreliosis is a cause of skin lesions in both pig and dogs. In the pig, *Borrelia suilla* infection occurs particularly in young pigs in association with poor hygiene and trauma to the skin but the pathogenesis of the condition is not well understood. The lesions are characterized by the development of granulomas and ulcers, which are most common on the head but may affect any part of the body. Secondary infection of the lesions with other bacteria including *Fusobacterium necrophorum*, *Actinomyces pyogenes*, streptococci and coliforms is believed to be a contributory factor. These organisms are also the cause of infectious foot-rot of pigs.[88, 89]

In dogs, *Borrelia burgdorferi* is the cause of Lyme disease. The causative organism is known to be transmitted by ixodid ticks but other bloodsucking arthropods are probably involved; clinical signs develop shortly after exposure to tick bites. Signs of shifting lameness and localized dermatitis commonly occur and may be accompanied by fever and lymphadenopathy.[12, 54, 90]

Fusobacterium and *Bacteroides*

Bacteria belonging to these two genera are commonly associated with foot-rot in ruminants. *Fusobacterium necrophorum* is a gut commensal in many mammalian species and can survive for over 10 months on contaminated pasture.[91] Infections are more common under conditions of poor hygiene and where penetration of the bacteria is promoted by wounds, maceration or primary infection by other microorganisms.[54] In cattle, *F. necrophorum* infection is associated with a number of different clinical syndromes of digital and interdigital dermatitis.[92] However, experimental inoculation of pure cultures does not induce infection and concurrent infection with other bacteria appears to be necessary to induce clinical disease. In severe bovine foot-rot, infection with *Actinomyces pyogenes* and *Bacteroides nodosus* is often found. *Fusobacterium necrophorum* is also a cause of cheilitis and stomatitis in rabbits, and of subcutaneous infection of the facial skin in pigs ('bullnose'), which often follows the fitting of a ring in the nose.[54]

Bacteroides nodosus is an obligate parasite of the hooves of cattle, sheep and goats.[54] In sheep, it is the cause of foot-rot but depends on prior colonization of the stratum corneum by *F. necrophorum*. Subsequently, *F. necrophorum* promotes tissue destruction in the lesions, an effect which is in turn promoted by the presence of *Actinomyces pyogenes*.[5] *Bacteroides nodosus* produces a powerful extracellular protease, which digests the hoof horn. Benign and virulent strains of *B. nodosus* can be differentiated by their protease isoenzyme patterns and preliminary studies indicate that vaccination with an appropriate protease antigen will protect sheep against foot-rot. Vaccines prepared from *B. nodosus* pili have also been used to control foot-rot but have been limited in their effectiveness by variation in the piliary antigens between different strains.[93]

In cats and dogs, *Bacteroides* and *Fusobacterium* spp. are found in abscesses, bite wounds and cellulitis, often in association with other aerobic and anaerobic bacteria.[12, 58]

Other Gram-negative species

A variety of other Gram-negative species is involved in skin wounds. Amongst the enterobacteriaceae, *Proteus* spp. and *Escherichia coli* are found as secondary invaders in deep folliculitis, furunculosis and cellulitis, and in otitis in dogs. *Klebsiella pneumoniae* and *Serratia marcescens* are found in cases of anaerobic cellulitis.[12] *Pasteurella multocida* is found in cat bite wounds.

Skin lesions are also seen as part of systemic disease syndromes. In pigs, *Salmonella choleraesuis* septicaemia can lead to blue discoloration of the ears and abdomen associated with capillary dilation and congestion. Vascular thrombosis may lead to necrosis of patches of skin, particularly at the extremities.[94] Enterotoxaemia associated with haemolytic *E. coli* causes subcutaneous oedema of the head and neck in addition to a progressive paralysis.[95] *Yersinia pestis* infection causes multiple subcutaneous abscesses affecting the limbs, head and neck in cats; lymphadenopathy, fever and malaise also occur and there is a high mortality.[96]

Brucellosis caused by *Brucella canis* in dogs has been associated with chronic exudative lesions affecting the limbs and scrotum.[12]

Mycoplasmas

Skin lesions associated with the mycoplasmas are very rarely diagnosed in animals although several species, most commonly *Mycoplasma bovis*, can cause bovine mastitis. Keane[97] reported chronic abscesses in two cats from which organisms resembling mycoplasmas could be cultured but failed to grow on subculture. The cases responded to tetracycline therapy. Experimental inoculation of material aspirated from lesions in one cat into another caused abscess formation but no organisms could be cultured from them. Mycoplasmas have been isolated from cases of cellulitis and an abscess in the goat.[98]

Rickettsias

Two rickettsial diseases are associated with skin diseases in animals. In dogs, Rocky Mountain spotted fever, caused by *Rickettsia rickettsii*, is a disease characterized by malaise and fever. Skin signs may include erythema, oedema particularly affecting the extremities, and petechial haemorrhages. Necrosis and ulceration of mucous membranes and of the pinnae of the ears and the ventral trunk skin may occur. Histological examination reveals a necrotizing vasculitis.[12, 99]

In cats, signs of cutaneous hyperaesthesia and alopecia areata were reported by Gretillati[100] in acute and chronic infections with *Haemobartonella felis* in France, but these findings have not been substantiated.

Skin disease associated with fungi

Fungal skin diseases of animals can be conveniently classified according to the depth of infection within the skin and the origin of the infection. Superficial mycoses are those that infect only the keratinized tissues, including the stratum corneum, the coat and the claws. The so-called subcutaneous mycoses affect the deeper layers of the skin and subcutaneous tissue and may also affect other tissues including the lymphatics. They normally enter the skin via wounds. Systemic mycoses are diseases in which primary infection usually occurs by inhalation and disseminates from the lung to the internal organs; skin infection is secondary; however, the diseases may not be noticed until skin lesions appear. The division between the subcutaneous and systemic mycoses is sometimes arbitrary.

Table 11.2. *Dermatophytes infecting domestic animals*

Dermatophyte species	Animal species						
	Horse	Cow	Sheep	Goat	Pig	Dog	Cat
M. audouinii[a]						+	+
M. canis	+	+	+	+	+	★	★
M. cookei	+	+				+	+
M. distortum						+	+
M. equinum	+						
M. gallinae						+	+
M. gypseum	+	+	+	+	+	+	+
M. nanum		+			★	+	
M. persicolor						+	
M. vanbreuseghemii						+	+
T. ajelloi[b]	+	+	+			+	
T. equinum	★	+				+	
T. erinacei						+	+
T. megninii						+	+
T. mentagrophytes	+	+	+	+	+	+	+
T. quinckeanum	+	+	+			+	+
T. rubrum	+	+	+		+	+	+
T. schoenleinii	+		+	+		+	+
T. simii						+	
T. terrestre	+	+				+	+
T. tonsurans	+				+		
T. verrucosum	+	★	★	★	+	+	+
T. violaceum		+				+	+
E. floccosum[c]				+			

[a] *M.*, *Microsporum*; [b] *T.*, *Trichophyton*; [c] *E.*, *Epidermophyton*.
★, Commonest infections in each species.
Based on references 12, 13.

Dermatophytes

A wide variety of dermatophytes is known to affect domestic animals (Table 11.2),[12,13,101] but only a few of these are commonly involved. Dual dermatophyte infections have been recorded in some animal species. The zoophilic dermatophytes, e.g. *Trichophyton verrucosum*, *T. equinum*, *Microsporum canis*, *M. distortum*, are parasites of the skin of animals and do not normally live in the soil whereas the anthropophilic species (see Chapter 10), which are parasites of human skin, are better adapted to survival in soil. Geophilic species, such as *M. nanum* and *M. gypseum*, live in the soil; infections with these organisms are related to exposure to the external environment.[102] Infections of dogs with *M. gypseum* derived from soil are influenced by the presence of hair in the soil promoting the infectivity of the fungus.[103] The occurrence of the disease is often related to environmental factors and management but the effects of these differ between the different types and species of dermatophyte.[102] Survival of the dermatophyte arthrospores is greatly reduced in dry conditions and at high environmental temperatures.[104]

In both large and small domestic animals, dermatophytosis tends to be more severe in the young but is self-limiting, with recovery generally occurring within 4–16 weeks of onset. In cattle and horses, the disease has been successfully controlled using live vaccines containing *T. verrucosum* mycelium.[105,106] Contamination of animal accommodation and the presence of healthy carriers[107–109] frequently leads to repeated infection as young stock is introduced to the premises. Lesions vary from thick, circular, discrete areas of scaling and crusting, sometimes with suppuration and ulceration, to more diffuse areas of hair loss with or without associated scales and crusts. Occasionally, deeper infections are seen, in which folliculitis and furunculosis, with the formation of kerions or nodular granulomas (pseudomycetomas), involve the dermis and/or subcutaneous tissue.

In the horse, dermatophytosis is relatively common and most cases involve infection with *T. equinum*. Lesions often resemble those of equine dermatophilosis, with discrete papules or thick, circumscribed crusts affecting particularly areas of skin covered by the saddle, girths or harness. Much milder infections are generally seen with *M. equinum* and *M. canis*.

In ruminants, dermatophytosis usually involves infection with *T. verrucosum*. Lesions vary in severity but often appear as thick, circular, scaling and crusting areas, which may become ulcerated, particularly affecting the head, neck and caudal trunk. In less severe infections, circular zones of hair loss and scaling are seen. The disease is uncommon in sheep but is an endemic problem on many cattle farms.

In pigs, *M. nanum* is most commonly involved. Lesions appear as circular, reddish areas with thin, loose, brown crusts. They are commonly located behind the ears but may appear on any part of the body.

In cats and dogs, the great majority of cases involve *M. canis* but infections with *M. gypseum* and *T. mentagrophytes* also occur quite commonly in the dog. *Microsporum canis* infections normally cause diffuse alopecia and scaling; lesions can sometimes be difficult to find, particularly in long-haired cats, which quite often develop chronic, inapparent infections. Infections with trichophyton and *M. gypseum* tend to be more severe and may cause confluent, extending areas of crusting and alopecia. Infection of the claws also occurs but is relatively rare. Infected claws are brittle, tend to split or crumble, and become deformed. The occurrence of granulomatous dermal lesions (pseudomycetomas) caused by both microsporum and trichophyton have been reported in cats.[110]

Pityrosporum canis (Malassezia pachydermatis)

This is a normal inhabitant of the ear canals and is commonly associated with otitis externa in dogs and cats.[111] It can also be found in large numbers at the skin surface associated with generalized or localized seborrhoeic dermatitis in dogs.[112] Scott and Miller[113] have described a clinical syndrome involving epidermal dysplasia and infection with this organism within the superficial layers of the stratum corneum of the interfollicular regions and hair follicles in West Highland White terriers. However, the role of the yeast in the pathogenesis of these conditions is not clear. Response of such conditions to treatment with systemic and topical antimicrobial agents effective against pityrosporum suggests that the yeast does play a part in exacerbating the dermatosis.[112-114]

Candida spp.

Candida is also rarely associated with skin disease in both large and small animals. Often, predisposing factors likely to reduce immunity, causing skin damage or excessive wetness are implicated. *Candida guilliermondi* has been reported as causing mastitis and nodular, granulomatous lesions in a mare,[115] and exudative dermatitis in pigs held in insanitary conditions has been associated with *Candida albicans* infection.[116]

Scott[13] has reported a generalized exfoliative dermatitis in protein-deficient goats associated with a yeast infection resembling candidiasis. In dogs and cats, lesions tend to be moist, red and ulcerated or eroded, and affect relatively hairless areas of the skin or those adjacent to mucocutaneous junctions.[12] Infections with *Candida albicans* and *C. parapsilosis* have been reported.[117,118]

Trichosporon spp.

Infection of the forelock, mane and tail with *Trichosporon beigelii* causing whitish nodules along the hair shafts ('white piedra') has been reported in the horse;[119] granulomatous lesions of the skin caused by *Trichosporon* spp. have also been reported in cats.[120]

Subcutaneous mycoses

Subcutaneous mycoses in animals are generally uncommon in domestic types. Infection is derived from the environment, often soil or decaying organic material. Where favourable environments promote proliferation of the individual fungal species or where animals have close contact with contaminated soil or water, a higher incidence of infection may be found.

True fungal mycetomas, characterized by swelling, the presence of granules formed by the fungal mycelium, and draining tracts, have been reported in horses in Africa, Australia and Europe, caused by *Curvularia geniculata* and *Pseudoallescheria boydii*.[121–123]

Phaeohyphomycosis, caused by dematiaceous fungi, causes subcutaneous nodular lesions that may develop fistulae and ulcers; in contrast to the mycetomas, granules are not formed. Infections have been reported with *Drechslera spicifera*, *Moniella suaveolens*, *Exophiala jeanselmei*, *Phialophora verrucosa*, *Stemphylium* sp. and *Cladosporium* sp. in cats and with *D. spicifera*, *Phialemonium obovatum* and *Pseudomicrodochium suttonii* in dogs;[12] and with *D. spicifera* and *Phaeoscera dematoides* in cattle, with *Peyronella glomerata* in goats, and with *D. spicifera* and *Hormodendrum* spp. in horses.[13]

Infection with *Pythium* spp. (pythiosis) occurs in areas where animals are exposed to warm temperatures and moist conditions, particularly if they have frequent access to, or prolonged contact with water. Lesions tend to occur on the limbs and ventral trunk; they manifest initially as nodules and may grow very rapidly with ulceration and fistulation. In horses the lesions are characterized by the elaboration within them of gritty, elongate masses formed by the fungal hyphae and host reaction, which resemble coral ('kunkers' or 'leeches');[13,41] these are not found in canine infections.[12] The disease is seen particularly in horses and dogs but has also been reported in cattle.[12,13,124]

Sporotrichosis is caused by infection with *Sporothrix schenckii*, a common saprophyte on decaying vegetation. Infection via a wound leads to the formation of small nodules that may affect only the skin, tend to ulcerate and may become crusted. Spread may occur to the lymphatics, leading to cording of the vessels with nodule formation and ulceration. More rarely there is dissemination to other, deeper tissues. The disease occurs in a wide variety of animals including cattle, pigs, horses, camels, dogs, cats and rodents. It is most commonly reported in equidae.[12,13,125,126]

Zygomycosis includes diseases caused by a number of species belonging to the *Zygomycota*. In horses, *Basidiobolus haptosporus* causes large, ulcerative, granulomatous lesions located on the trunk, head and neck, particularly laterally; *Conidiobolus coronatus* causes similar lesions affecting the external nares and nasal mucosa.[127] In pigs, *Rhizopus oryzae* has been reported, causing granulomas and draining tracts affecting the subcutis, stomach and lymph nodes.[128]

Alternaria spp. are commonly present in specimens from skin but can seldom be implicated in disease processes. However, Coles and coworkers[129] reported a nodular dermatitis in a horse from which *Alternaria tenuis* could be consistently isolated.

Systemic mycoses

The systemic mycoses are caused by fungi that are either primary pathogens (*Blastomyces dermatitidis*, *Coccidioides immitis* and *Histoplasma* spp.) able to invade healthy animals, or cause infection only in animals in which immunity is depressed (*Aspergillus* spp., *Cryptococcus neoformans*, *Paecilomyces* spp.).[12] The fungi are saprophytes living in soil enriched with organic matter including faeces. Infection commonly occurs by inhalation of the infective phase but primary skin infection can occur. The majority of infections by the primary pathogens are inapparent and skin involvement by either type of infection does not necessarily arise.

Blastomycosis occurs in dogs and cats and causes chronic, ulcerating, papular and nodular granulomatous lesions and draining tracts particularly affecting the head, legs, chest and scrotum, often with marked local lymph node enlargement.[12] It has been reported causing granulomatous lesions and abscesses of the udder and perineal region in a horse.[130]

Coccidioidomycosis is a problem associated with desert rodents that excrete large numbers of *Coccidioides immitis* spherules in their faeces, resulting in the abundant production of arthroconidia, which are concentrated around the rodent burrows.[131] The disease affects a wide variety of domestic animals. It causes severe systemic disease in some animals and skin lesions, which are uncommon, appear as granulomas, abscesses and fistulas. Primary infection of the skin has been reported in the dog and cat.[132] In the horse, an abscess involving the sternum has been reported in a case of disseminated coccidioidomycosis.[133]

Histoplasma farciminosum is the cause of epizootic lymphangitis, a disease of horses and mules that is endemic in countries bordering the Mediterranean, in central and southern Africa, and in parts of Asia and the Soviet Union.[54] Lesions appear initially as nodules, particularly affecting the head and neck, which rupture to discharge a greenish exudate and form chronic, granulating ulcers that gradually increase in size. The disease often spreads to the lymph vessels, which become corded with the development of nodules along them. General health is usually unaffected and some animals recover spontaneously. Histoplasmosis caused by *H. capsulatum* can affect a wide variety of animal species, causing severe systemic disease, but rarely involves the skin. Firm nodules that eventually ulcerate have been reported in small animals.[12,134]

Aspergillus spp. are opportunistic pathogens of animals with depressed immunity; they are rarely associated with skin disease. Skin lesions often involve the mucocutaneous junctions of the eyelids and nostrils in small animals.[12] Lesions vary from erythema and pruritus to granulomas, abscesses and ulcers. In large animals, aspergillus has been described as causing granulomatous lesions in a cow and a goat, and a papular dermatitis in pigs.[135-137]

Cryptococcosis is the most common systemic mycosis in cats[134] and also affects a wide variety of other animal species. Infection generally occurs by inhalation but invasion via the skin or teat canal in cattle and goats is also common.[54] The great majority of infections are subclinical and frank disease is normally associated with depressed immunity. In cats, skin lesions tend to affect the head and are seen as dermal and subcutaneous nodules, which may ulcerate.[134]

Opportunistic infection by *Paecilomyces* spp. has also been reported as causing an ulcerated nodular lesion on the paw of a cat,[138] and chronic otitis developing into internal otitis and systemic disease in a dog.[139]

References

1 Dubos RJ. Biochemical determinants of microbial diseases. Massachusetts: Harvard University Press; 1954.
2 Lloyd DH. The inhabitants of the mammalian skin surface. Proc R Soc Edinb 1980; 79B: 25–42.
3 Noble WC. Microbial skin disease: its epidemiology. London: Edward Arnold; 1983.
4 Egerton JR, Roberts DS, Parsonson IM. The aetiology and pathogenesis of ovine foot-rot. II. A histological study of the bacterial invasion. J Comp Pathol 1969; 79: 207–15.
5 Roberts DS, Egerton JR. The aetiology and pathogenesis of ovine foot-rot. III. The pathogenic association of *Fusiformis nodosus* and *F. necrophorus*. J Comp Pathol 1969; 79: 217–27.
6 Krogh HV, Kristensen S. A study of skin diseases in dogs and cats. II. Microflora of the normal skin of dogs and cats. Nordisk Vet-Med 1976; 28: 459–63.
7 Devriese LA, Schleifer KH, Adegoke GO. Identification of coagulase-negative staphylococci from farm animals. J Appl Bacteriol 1985; 58: 45–55.
8 Noble WC, Allaker RP. Staphylococci on the skin of pigs: isolates from two farms with different antibiotic policies. Vet Rec 1992; 130: 466–68.
9 Cox HU, Hoskins JD, Newman SS, Turnwald GH, Foil CS, Roy AF, Kearney MT. Distribution of staphylococcal species on clinically healthy cats. Am J Vet Res 1985; 46: 1824–28.
10 Cox HU, Hoskins JD, Newman SS, Foil CS, Turnwald GH. Temporal study of staphylococcal species on healthy dogs. Am J Vet Res 1988; 49: 747–51.
11 Hajek V. *Staphylococcus intermedius*, a new species isolated from animals. Int J System Bacteriol 1976; 26: 401–08.

12 Muller GH, Kirk RW, Scott DW. Small animal dermatology. 4th ed. Philadelphia: WB Saunders; 1989.

13 Scott DW. Large animal dermatology. Philadelphia: WB Saunders; 1988.

14 Devriese LA. Staphylococci in healthy and diseased animals. J Appl Bacteriol 1990 (Symp Suppl); 71S–80S.

15 Hajek V, Marsalek E. A study of staphylococci isolated from the upper respiratory tract of different animal species. I. Biological properties of *Staphylococcus aureus* strains of canine origin. Zentralbl Bakteriol Parasitenk Infektionskr Hyg Abt 1 Orig 1969; 212: 60–67.

16 Allaker RP, Lloyd DH, Bailey RM. Population sizes and frequency of staphylococci at mucocutaneous sites on normal dogs. Vet Rec 1992; 130: 303–04.

17 Medleau L, Long R, Brown J, Miller WH. Frequency and antimicrobial susceptibility of *Staphylococcus intermedius* species isolated from canine pyodermas. Am J Vet Res 1986; 47: 229–31.

18 Lloyd DH. Therapy for canine pyoderma. In: Kirk RW, ed. Current veterinary therapy XI. Philadelphia: WB Saunders; 1992. (In press).

19 White SD, Ihrke PJ. Pyoderma. In: Nesbitt GH, ed. Contemporary issues in small animal practice. Volume VIII: Dermatology. New York: Churchill Livingstone; 1987: 95–121.

20 Buerger RC. Staphylococci and German Shepherd Dog pyoderma. In: Kirk RW, ed. Current veterinary therapy X. Philadelphia: WB Saunders; 1989: 609–13.

21 Ihrke PJ, Schwarzman RM, McGinley K, Horwitz LN, Marples RR. Microbiology of normal and seborrhoeic canine skin. Am J Vet Res 1978; 39: 1487–89.

22 Mason IS, Lloyd DH. The role of allergy in the development of canine pyoderma. J Small Anim Pract 1986; 30: 216–18.

23 Kaji Y, Kato E. Occurrence of enterotoxigenic staphylococci in household and laboratory dogs. Jap J Vet Res 1980; 28: 86–94.

24 Shimuzu A, Kawano J, Hazue S, Fujinami T, Kumara S, Sugihara K. Pathogenicity of *Staphylococcus intermedius* for mice. Sci Rep Fac Agri, Kobe Univ 1989; 18: 213–20.

25 Allaker RP, Lamport AI, Lloyd DH, Noble WC. Production of 'virulence factors' by *Staphylococcus intermedius* isolates from cases of canine pyoderma and healthy carriers. Microb Ecol Hlth Dis 1991; 4: 169–73.

26 Elias PM, Fritsch P, Mittermayer H. Staphylococcal toxic epidermal necrolysis: species and tissue susceptibility and resistance. J Invest Dermatol 1976; 66: 80–89.

27 Love DA, Davies PA. Isolation of *Staphylococcus aureus* from a condition in Greyhounds resembling 'staphylococcal scalded skin syndrome' of man. J Small Anim Pract 1980; 21: 351–57.

28 Medleau L, Blue JL. Frequency and antimicrobial susceptibility of *Staphylococcus* spp. isolated from feline skin lesions. J Am Vet Med Assoc 1988; 193: 1080–81.

29 Devriese LA, Nzuambe D, Godard C. Identification and characterisation of staphylococci isolated from cats. Vet Microbiol 1984; 9: 279–85.

30 Philips WE, Kloos WE. Identification of coagulase-positive *Staphylococcus intermedius* and *Staphylococcus hyicus* subsp. *hyicus* isolates from veterinary clinical specimens. J Clin Microbiol 1981; 14: 671–73.

31 Takeuchi S, Kobayashi Y, Morozumi T, Niibori S. Isolation and some properties of *Staphylococcus hyicus* subsp. *hyicus* from pigs, chickens and cows. Jap J Vet Sci 1985; 47: 841–43.

32 Adegoke GO. Characteristics of staphylococci isolated from man, poultry and some other animals. J Appl Bacteriol 1986; 60: 97–102.

33 Devriese LA, Thelissen M. *Staphylococcus hyicus* in donkeys. Vet Rec 1986; 118: 76.

34 Hazarika RA, Mahanta PN, Dutta GN, Devriese LA. Cutaneous infection associated with *Staphylococcus hyicus* in cattle. Res Vet Sci 1991; 50: 374–75.

35 Devriese LA, Derycke J. *Staphylococcus hyicus* in cattle. Res Vet Sci 1979; 26: 356–58.

36 Ishihara C. An exfoliative skin disease in guinea pigs due to *Staphylococcus aureus*. Lab Anim Sci 1980; 30: 552–57.

37 Okerman L, Devriese LA, Maertens L, Okerman F, Godard C. Cutaneous staphylococcosis in rabbits. Vet Rec 1984; 114: 313–15.

38 Martin WB. Staphylococcal dermatitis in sheep. Vet Ann 1983; 23: 104–08.

39 Parker BNJ, Bonson MD, Carroll PJ. Staphylococcal dermatitis in unweaned lambs. Vet Rec 1983; 113: 570–71.

40 Scott FMM, Fraser J, Scott GR. Pyodermas. In: Martin WB, ed. Diseases of Sheep. Oxford: Blackwell Scientific; 1983: 193–97.

41 Pascoe RR. A colour atlas of equine dermatology. London: Wolf; 1990.

42 Amtsberg G. Nachweis von Exfoliation auslösenden Substanzen in Kulturen von *Staphylococcus hyicus* des Schweines und *Staphylococcus epidermidis* Biotyp 2 des Rindes. Zentralbl Veterinarmed 1979; 26: 257–72.

43 Blood DC, Jubb KV. Exudative epidermitis of pigs. Austral Vet J 1957; 33: 126–67.

44 Allaker RP, Lloyd DH, Lamport A. Studies on the virulence of *Staphylococcus hyicus*. Vet Dermatol 1990; 1: 197–99.

45 Allaker RP, Lloyd DH, Smith IM. Prevention of exudative epidermitis in gnotobiotic piglets by bacterial interference. Vet Rec 1988; 123: 597–98.

46 Lloyd DH, Allaker RP, Smith IM, Mackie A. Colonisation of gnotobiotic piglets by *Staphylococcus hyicus* and the development of exudative epidermitis. Microb Ecol Hlth Dis 1990; 3: 15–18.

47 Lomax LG, Cole JR. Porcine epidermitis and dermatitis associated with *Staphylococcus hyicus* and *Dermatophilus congolensis* infections. J Am Vet Med Assoc 1983; 183: 1091–92.

48 Cullen GA. *Streptococcus uberis*: a review. Vet Bull 1969; 39: 155–65.

49 Devriese LA, De Pelsmaecker K. The anal region as a main carrier site of *Staphylococcus intermedius* and *Streptococcus canis* in dogs. Vet Rec 1987; 121: 302–03.

50 Hare T, Fry RM, Orr AB. First impressions of the beta haemolytic *Streptococcus* infection of swine. Vet Rec 1942; 54: 267–69.

51 Collins BR. Dermatologic disorders of common small nondomestic animals. In: Nesbitt GH, ed. Contemporary issues in small animal practice. Volume VIII: Dermatology. New York: Churchill Livingstone; 1987: 235–94.

52 Price PM. Pyoderma caused by *Peptostreptococcus tetradius* in a pup. J Am Vet Med Assoc 1991; 198: 1649–50.

53 McGrane JJ, Higgins AJ. Infectious diseases of the camel. In: Higgins AJ, ed. The camel in health and disease. London: Bailliere Tindall; 1986: 92–110.

54 Timoney JF, Gillespie JH, Scott FW, Barlough JE. Hagan and Bruner's

microbiology and infectious diseases of domestic animals. 8th ed. Ithaca: Comstock; 1988.

55 Smith LDS, Safford JW, Hawkins WW. *Clostridium sordelli* infection in sheep. Cornell Vet 1962; 52: 62–68.

56 Bergeland ME. Clostridial infections. In: Leman AD, Straw B, Glock RD, Mengeling WI, Penny RHC, Scholl E, eds. Diseases of swine. Ames: Iowa State Univ Press; 1986: 557–70.

57 Morgan CO. Blackleg. In: Howard JL, ed. Current veterinary therapy: food animal practice. Philadelphia: WB Saunders; 1981: 684–87.

58 Dow SW, Jones RJ, Adney WS. Anaerobic bacterial infections and response to treatment in dogs and cats: 36 cases (1983–1985). J Am Vet Med Assoc 1986; 189: 930–34.

59 Love DN, Jones RF, Bailey M. *Clostridium villosum* sp. nov. from subcutaneous abscesses in cats. Int J System Bacteriol 1979; 29: 241–44.

60 Ayers JL. Caseous lymphadenitis in goats and sheep: a review of diagnosis, pathogenesis and immunity. J Am Vet Med Assoc 1977; 171: 1251–54.

61 Hughes JP, Biberstein EL. Chronic equine abscesses associated with *Corynebacterium pseudotuberculosis*. J Am Vet Med Assoc 1959; 135: 559.

62 Woodroofe GM. Studies on strains of *Corynebacterium equi* isolated from pigs. Austral J Exp Biol Med Sci 1950; 28: 399.

63 Jang SS, Lock A, Biberstein EL. A cat with *Corynebacterium equi* lymphadenitis clinically simulating lymphosarcoma. Cornell Vet 1975; 65: 233–39.

64 Higgins R, Paradis M. Abscess caused by *Corynebacterium equi* in a cat. Can Vet J 1980; 21: 63–64.

65 Guma SA, et al. Mycetoma in goats. Sabouraudia 1978; 16: 217.

66 Roberts DS. *Dermatophilus* infection. Vet Bull 1967; 37: 513–21.

67 Lloyd DH. Dermatophilosis: a review of the epidemiology, diagnosis and control. In: Proceedings of the CARDI/CTA Seminar–cowdriosis and dermatophilosis of livestock in the Caribbean Region. [St John, Antigua, November 1990]. St Augustine, Trinidad: Caribbean Agricultural Research and Development Institute; 1991: 99–111.

68 Martinez D. Workshop on dermatophilosis. In: von Tscharner C, Halliwell REW, eds. Advances in veterinary dermatology, vol I. London: Bailliere Tindall; 1990: 410.

69 Bestetti G, Buhlmann V, Nicolet J, Frankhauser R. Paraplegia due to *Actinomyces viscosus* infection in a cat. Acta Neuropathol Berl 1977; 37: 231–35.

70 Shigidi MTA, Mirgham T, Mura MT. Characterisation of *Nocardia farcinica* isolated from cattle with bovine farcy. Res Vet Sci 1980; 28: 207–11.

71 Lloyd DH. Bovine farcy. In: Howard JL, ed. Current veterinary therapy: food animal practice. Philadelphia: WB Saunders; 1981: 1136.

72 Chamoiseau G. Aetiology of farcy in African bovines: nomenclature of the causal organisms, *Mycobacterium farcinogenes* (Chamoiseau) and *Mycobacterium senegalense* (Chamoiseau) comb. nov. Int J Syst Bacteriol 1979; 29: 407–10.

73 El Sanousi SM, Tag El Din MH. On the aetiology of bovine farcy in the Sudan. J Gen Microbiol 1986; 132: 1673–75.

74 Biberstein EL, et al. *Nocardia asteroides* infection in horses: a review. J Am Vet Med Assoc 1985; 186: 273–77.

75 Parodi A, Fontaine M, Brion A, Tisseur H, Goret P. Mycobacteriosis in the domestic carnivora: present-day epidemiology of tuberculosis in the cat and dog. J Small Animal Pract 1965; 6: 309–26.

76 Foster ES, Seavelli TD, Greenlee PG, Gilbertson SR. Tuberculosis in a dog. J Am Vet Med Assoc 1986; 188: 1188–90.

77 Windsor RS, Durrant DS, Burn KJ, Blackburn JT, Duncan W. Avian tuberculosis in pigs: miliary lesions in bacon pigs. J Hyg Camb 1984; 92: 129–38.

78 Timoney JF. Avian tuberculosis in the cow. Vet Rec 1939; 51: 191–96; 239–43.

79 Schiefer HB, Middleton DB. Experimental transmission of feline mycobacterial skin disease (feline leprosy). Vet Path 1983; 20: 460–71.

80 Rees RJW, Tee RD. Studies on *Mycobacterium lepraemurium* in tissue culture. II. The production and properties of soluble antigens from *Myco. lepraemurium* in tissue culture. Br J Exp Pathol 1962; 43: 480–87.

81 Jarnagin JL, Himes EM, Richards WD, Luchsinger DW, Harrington R Jr. Isolation of *M. kansasii* from lymph nodes of cattle in the United States. Am J Vet Res 1983; 44: 1853–55.

82 Fletcher RB, Linton AH, Osborne AD. Actinobacillosis of the tongue of a dog. Vet Rec 1956; 68: 645–46.

83 Carb AV, Liu S. *Actinobacillus lignierisii* infection in a dog. J Am Vet Med Assoc 1969; 154: 1062–67.

84 Windsor RS. *Actinobacillus lignierisii* infection in a litter of pigs and a review of previous reports on similar infections. Vet Rec 1973; 92: 178–80.

85 Moe JB, Stedham MA, Jennings PB. Canine melioidosis. Am J Trop Med Hyg 1972; 21: 351–55.

86 Grono LR. Otitis externa. In: Kirk RW, ed. Current veterinary therapy VII. Philadelphia: WB Saunders; 1980: 461–66.

87 Burrell DH. In: von Tscharner C, Halliwell REW, eds. Advances in veterinary dermatology, vol I. London: Bailliere Tindall; 1990: 347–58.

88 Albiston HE. Spirochaetal granuloma of swine. In: Seddon HR, ed. Diseases of domestic animals in Australia. 2nd ed, Pt 5, vol 2. Canberra ACT: Commonwealth Bureau of Health; 1965.

89 Penny RHC, Osborne AD, Wright AI. Foot-rot in pigs: observations on the clinical disease. Vet Rec 1965; 77: 1101–07.

90 von Tscharner C. Cutaneous lesions of borreliosis (Lyme disease). In: von Tscharner C, Halliwell REW, eds. Advances in Veterinary Dermatology, vol I. London: Bailliere Tindall; 1990: 440.

91 Marsh H, Tunnicliff EA. Experimental studies of foot-rot in sheep. Montana Agric Exp Station Bull 1934; 285: 3–16.

92 Berg JN. 'Foot rot' complex in cattle. In: Howard JL, ed. Current veterinary therapy: food animal practice. Philadelphia: WB Saunders; 1981: 1104–06.

93 Stewart DJ, Kortt AA, Lilley GG. New approaches to foot rot vaccination and diagnosis utilizing the proteases of *Bacteroides nodosus*. In: von Tscharner C, Halliwell REW, eds. Advances in veterinary dermatology, vol I. London: Bailliere Tindall; 1990: 359–69.

94 Penny RHC, Muirhead MR. Skin. In: Leman AD, Straw B, Glock RD, Mengeling WL, Penny RHC, Scholl E, eds. Diseases of swine. 6th ed. Ames: Iowa State Univ Press; 1986: 82–101.

95 Nielsen NO. Edema disease. In: Leman AD, Straw B, Glock RD, Mengeling

WL, Penny RHC, Scholl E, eds. Diseases of swine. 6th ed. Ames: Iowa State University Press; 1986: 528–40.

96 Rollag OJ, Skeels MR, Nims LJ, Thilsted JP, Mann JM. Feline plague in New Mexico: report of five cases. J Am Vet Med Assoc 1981; 179: 1381–83.

97 Keane DP. Chronic abscesses in cats associated with an organism resembling *Mycoplasma*. Can Vet J 1983; 24: 289–91.

98 Yedloutschnig RJ, Taylor WD, Dardiri AM. Isolation of *Mycoplasma mycoides* var *capri* from goats in the United States. Proc US Anim Hlth Assoc 1971; 75: 166–75.

99 Green CE. Rocky Mountain spotted fever. J Am Vet Med Assoc 1987; 191: 666–71.

100 Gretillati S. Feline haemobartonellosis. Feline Pract 1984; 14: 22–27.

101 Ainsworth GC, Austwick PKC. Fungal diseases of animals. 2nd ed. Farnham Royal, UK: Commonwealth Agricultural Bureaux; 1973: 10–34.

102 Kaplan W, Ivens MS. Observations on seasonal variations in incidence of ringworm in dogs and cats in the USA. Sabouraudia 1961; 1: 91–102.

103 Kushida T. Studies on dermatophytosis in dogs. III. An experimental study on some factors for establishment of infection with *Microsporum gypseum* of soil origin. Jap J Vet Sci 1978; 40: 1–7.

104 Hoshimoto T, Blumenthal HJ. Survival and resistance of *Trichophyton mentagrophytes* arthrospores. Appl Environ Microbiol 1978; 35: 274–77.

105 Sarkisov AK, Petrovitch SV. Immunity of horses to spontaneous and experimental ringworm caused by *Trichophyton equinum*. Veterinarii 1976; 11: 39–40.

106 Naess B, Sandvik O. Early vaccination of calves against ringworm caused by *Trichophyton verrucosum*. Vet Rec 1981; 109: 199–200.

107 Krivanek K, Dvorak J, Hanak F. Dermatophytosis in cattle caused by *Trichophyton equinum*. Zentralb Veterinaermed 1978; 25B: 356–62.

108 Woodgyer AJ. Asymptomatic carriage of dermatophytes by cats. NZ Vet J 1977; 25: 67–69.

109 Van Cutsem J, De Keyser H, Rochette F, Van Der Flaes M. Survey of fungal isolates from alopecia and asymptomatic dogs. Vet Rec 1985; 116: 568–69.

110 Tuttle PA, Chandler FW. Deep dermatophytosis in a cat. J Am Vet Med Assoc 1983; 183: 1106–08.

111 Sanguinetti V, Tampieri MP, Morganti L. A survey of 120 isolates of *Malassezia pachydermatis*. Mycopathologica 1984; 85: 93–95.

112 Mason KV, Evans AG. Dermatitis associated with *Malassezia pachydermatis* in 11 dogs. J Am Anim Hosp Assoc 1991; 27: 13–27.

113 Scott DW, Miller WH Jr. Epidermal dysplasia and *Malassezia pachydermatis* infection in West Highland White terriers. Vet Dermatol 1989; 1: 25–36.

114 Dufait R. Two cases of canine yeast infection treated with ketoconazole. Vlaams Diergeneesk Tijdsch 1985; 54: 419–23.

115 Nicolet J, Steck W, Gerber H. *Candida guilliermondi* als wahrscheinliche Ursache einer disseminierten Hautgranulomatose beim Pferd. Schweizer Archiv fur Tierheilkunde 1965; 107: 185–96.

116 Reynolds IM, Miner PW, Smith RE. Cutaneous candidiasis of swine. J Am Vet Med Assoc 1968; 152: 182–86.

117 Dale JE. Canine dermatosis caused by *Candida parapsilosis*. Vet Med Small Anim Clinic 1972; 67: 548–49.

118 Pilcher ME, Gross TL. Cutaneous and mucocutaneous candidiasis in a dog.

Compendium on Continuing Education for the Practising Veterinarian 1985; 7: 225–30.

119 Mullowney PC, Fadok VA. Dermatologic diseases of horses. Part III. Fungal skin diseases. Compendium on Continuing Education for the Practicing Veterinarian 1984; 6: S324–S331.

120 Doster AR, Erickson ED, Chandler FW. Trichosporonosis in two cats. J Am Vet Med Assoc 1987; 190: 1184–86.

121 Schiefer B, Mehnert B. Maduromykose beim Pferd in Deutschland. Berl Münch Tierarztl Wochenschr 1965; 78: 230–34.

122 Boomker J, Coetzer JAW, Scott DB. Black grain mycetoma (maduromycosis) in horses. Onderstepoort Vet Res 1977; 44: 249–51.

123 Miller RI, Norton JH, Summers PM. Black grained mycetoma in two horses. Austral Vet J 1980; 56: 345–48.

124 Miller RI, Olcott BM, Archer M. Cutaneous pythiosis in beef cattle. J Am Vet Med Assoc 1985; 186: 984–85.

125 Attleberger MH. Subcutaneous and opportunistic mycoses; systemic mycoses; and actinomycosis, nocardiosis, and dermatophilosis. In: Kirk RW, ed. Current veterinary therapy VIII. Philadelphia: WB Saunders; 1983: 1177–80.

126 Morris P. Sporotrichosis. In: Robinson NE, ed. Current therapy in equine medicine. Philadelphia: WB Saunders; 1983: 555–56.

127 Miller RI. Equine phycomycosis. Compendium on Continuing Education for the Practicing Veterinarian 1983; 5: S472–S479.

128 Sandford SE, Josephson GKA, Waters EH. Submandibular and disseminated zygomycosis (mucormycosis) in feeder pigs. J Am Vet Med Assoc 1985; 186: 171–74.

129 Coles BM, Steven DR, Hunter RL. Equine nodular dermatitis associated with *Alternaria tenuis* infection. Vet Pathol 1978; 15: 779–80.

130 Benbrook EA, Bryant JB, Saunders LZ. A case of blastomycosis in the horse. J Am Vet Med Assoc 1948; 112: 475–78.

131 Reed RE, Converse JL. The seasonal incidence of canine coccidioidomycosis. Am J Vet Res 1966; 27: 1027–30.

132 Wolf AM. Primary cutaneous coccidioidomycosis in a dog and a cat. J Am Vet Med Assoc 1979; 174: 504–06.

133 Crane CS. Equine coccidioidomycosis: case report. Vet Med 1962; 57: 1073–74.

134 Holzworth J. Diseases of the cat. Vol 1. Philadelphia: WB Saunders; 1987.

135 Davis CL, Schafer WB. Cutaneous aspergillosis in a cow. J Am Vet Med Assoc 1962; 141: 1339–43.

136 Guha AN. *Aspergillus fumigatus* infection in goats. Indian Vet J 1959; 36: 252–54.

137 Tabuchi K, et al. Papular dermatitis in pigs. Therapeutic trials against *Aspergillus*. Bull Azabu Vet Coll 1963; 11: 67.

138 Elliot GS, Whitney MS, Reed WM, Tuite JF. Antemortem diagnosis of paecilomycosis in a cat. J Am Vet Med Assoc 1984; 184: 93–94.

139 Patterson JM, Rosendal S. A case of disseminated paecilomycosis in a cat. J Am Vet Med Assoc 1983; 19: 569.

12

Viral skin disease in man

P. MORGAN-CAPNER

Apart from bacteriophage, which can readily be demonstrated in sebaceous material expressed from glands on the face,[1] viruses cannot be considered a component of the normal flora of the skin. They are rarely, if ever, detected on the surface of the skin in the absence of clinically apparent lesions. Virus may be present in the deeper layers of the skin during the later incubation period after infection, or there may be latent infection with viruses such as papillomavirus. This is unlike the mucous membranes of the oropharynx, genitalia and gastrointestinal tract, where infective viruses may often be detected in the absence of clinical disease. For instance, herpes simplex virus (HSV) cannot be isolated from normal skin, although it may be found in the oropharynx of about 1 per cent of normal healthy adults;[2] early studies suggesting its presence in uncomplicated eczemas[3] have been contradicted.[4]

The skin is a frequent site of manifestation of virus infection. Lesions may be localized or widespread as part of a systemic infection.

Microbiology

All viruses are obligate intracellular parasites and are characterized by containing only one type of nucleic acid, either DNA or RNA, which may be double or single stranded. These provide the main criteria for the classification of viruses. The virion comprises the nucleocapsid, which may be contained within an envelope derived from the cell membrane of the cell in which it replicated. The core of the virus containing the nucleic acid and possibly other proteins, such as enzymes, is surrounded by a capsid made up of individual protein capsomeres. The capsomeres are arranged in icosahedral or helical symmetry, or their arrangement is complex. The characteristic features of those viruses associated with skin disease are given in Table 12.1 and are described in detail elsewhere.[5]

Table 12.1 *Viruses that involve the skin*

Virus family	Virus genus	Virus and disease		Nucleic acid	Symmetry	Diameter (nm)	Envelope
Herpetoviridae	Herpesvirus	Herpes simplex	Stomatitis, genital herpes, etc.	ds DNA	Icosahedral	100–200	Yes
		Varicella–zoster	Chickenpox, shingles				
		Herpes simiae (B)					
		Herpesvirus type 6	Roseola infantum				
Poxviridae	Orthopoxvirus	Variola	Smallpox	ds DNA	Complex	200–250 ×300–350	Yes
		Vaccinia					
		Cowpox					
		Monkey pox					
	Unclassified	Molluscum contagiosum					
		Tanapox					
	Parapoxvirus	Orf				150 × 300 –350	
		Pseudocowpox					
Papovaviridae	Papillomavirus	Papillomavirus	Warts	ds DNA	Icosahedral	50–55	No
Picornaviridae	Enterovirus	Coxsackievirus A, B	Hand, foot and mouth disease	ss RNA	Icosahedral	27	No
		Echovirus					
Paramyxoviridae	Morbillivirus	Measles		ss RNA	Helical	120–250	Yes
Togaviridae	Rubivirus	Rubella		ss RNA	Icosahedral	60	Yes
Parvoviridae	Parvovirus	Parvovirus B19	Erythema infectiosum, aplastic crisis	ss DNA	Icosahedral	22	No

Diagnosis

Although histological appearances, such as the presence of intranuclear inclusions in HSV lesions, may be of great help in diagnosis, the small size of viruses means that they can only be directly observed under the high magnification afforded by the electron microscope. Such direct observation still has a major role in the diagnosis of some skin lesions, such as those due to HSV, varicella–zoster virus (VZV) and orf. The high magnification of electron microscopy means this approach has a limited sensitivity, with a concentration of about 10^6 virions/mm^3 of material being required for reliable detection. Although the appearance by electron microscopy may be sufficient to ascribe any virus seen to a particular group, members within the same group, such as HSV and VZV, cannot be distinguished. Electron microscopy is a rapid technique, with results being available within an hour of receipt of specimen.

Electron microscopy is usually applied to the diagnosis of vesicular lesions; a number of approaches to collection and transport of vesicular fluid have been suggested. Although transport in a sealed capillary would be the choice of many, the problems of specimen collection remote from the investigating laboratory, of finding appropriate capillaries locally and of drying in transit mean that a more simple approach is beneficial. An intravenous needle may be used to puncture the vesicle, fluid being taken into the lumen of the needle by capillary action, and the bevelled edge of the needle being used to gently scrape the base of the vesicle. Fluid and cell debris may be transferred to a microscope slide by gently placing the bevelled edge of the needle on the slide and spreading it over an area of 0.5–1 cm in diameter. After being allowed to air-dry for a few minutes the preparation is stable and there is no need for urgent transport. Care needs to be taken, however, that an appropriate slide box is used for transport so that the surface of the slide is not rubbed. On receipt in the laboratory the material on the slide can be resuspended in a drop of distilled water before mixing with a negative stain prior to electron microscopy.

The detection of virus-specific antigen provides another approach to rapid diagnosis. A source of specific antisera is required and the advent of monoclonal antibodies has revived interest in such techniques. The eradication of smallpox means that use of immunodiffusion for detection of VZV or variola antigen is no longer of interest. This technique has now been superseded by enzyme-linked immunosorbent assay (ELISA), which is being used for detection of HSV antigen. This approach is now rivalling culture for diagnosis of genital herpes as it is rapid and reasonably specific, although it may lack some sensitivity.[6] Importantly, cell culture services are not required and retaining viability of the virus during transport is not critical. Such approaches

Table 12.2 *Approaches to diagnosis for the main virus infections*
involving the skin

Infection	Diagnosis
Herpes simplex	Electron microscopy
	Cell culture
	Antigen detection
	Polymerase chain reaction detection of genome in cerebrospinal fluid
	Serology (for primary or systemic infection)
Varicella–zoster	Electron microscopy
	Cell culture
	Serology
Cowpox/monkeypox	Electron microscopy
	Cell culture
	Culture on chorioallantoic membrane of fertile hens' eggs
Orf/pseudocowpox	Electron microscopy
Molluscum contagiosum	Electron microscopy
Papillomavirus	DNA detection
Hand, foot and mouth	Cell culture (faeces, throat swab)
Measles	Antigen detection (in immunocompromised children)
	Cell culture
	Serology
Rubella	Serology
Parvovirus B19	Serology
Human herpesvirus type 6	Serology

are likely to progressively replace cell culture isolation for the diagnosis of certain viruses such as HSV and VZV.

Certain viruses of major importance in skin disease, such as some poxviruses and the papillomaviruses, cannot be isolated in routine cell culture, with diagnosis usually being achieved by electron microscopy. Although this is a useful approach for poxviruses, it is very insensitive and time consuming for the diagnosis of papillomavirus infection, and is unable easily to differentiate the many types. The diagnosis of papillomavirus infection was revolutionized by techniques to detect viral DNA by hybridization.[7] These techniques also enabled the infecting papillomavirus type to be identified, but have largely remained a research tool, and are not generally available as yet.

Isolation remains the cornerstone of diagnosis of HSV and enterovirus infections, and is also applicable to a range of other viruses, such as VZV and certain poxviruses. The chorioallantoic membrane of fertile hens' eggs was an essential requisite for the diagnosis of smallpox, vaccinia, and disseminated poxvirus infections. With the eradication of smallpox, and vaccinia no longer being used, this diagnostic approach has been discontinued, except rarely to differentiate HSV types 1 and 2. Many cell lines can be used and infection usually becomes apparent within a few days as a cytopathic effect. Confirmation of the identity of the virus isolated can be achieved by electron microscopy, but is usually by neutralization or immunofluorescent antigen detection using specific antisera.

For a number of infections, diagnosis is best achieved by testing for the antibody response of the infected patient to show seroconversion or a rising titre, or by detecting specific IgM. Numerous techniques such as haemagglutination inhibition, complement fixation, ELISA and radioimmunoassay have been developed, and which technique is used will depend on the infection being investigated and local interest and expertise. The main approaches to diagnosis for each of the virus groups are given in Table 12.2.

Systemic virus infections

Systemic virus infection with maculopapular rashes

Many common systemic virus infections are clinically apparent, mainly as a generalized skin rash. For these virus infections, after an initial replication phase in or close to the site of infection, the oropharynx, there is a systemic viraemia with seeding of the skin. It is probable that the rash is immune mediated. Rubella virus has been isolated from areas of the skin unaffected by the rash, and measles virus is absent from the lesions themselves. Measles, rubella, parvovirus B19 and some enteroviruses produce generalized maculopapular rashes and it may not be easy to distinguish between them clinically, particularly infection with the latter three. Transmission is by the respiratory route for measles, rubella and parvovirus B19, but is faeco-oral for the enteroviruses.

Measles

Measles has an incubation period of some 10–11 days, the rash being preceded by a 2- to 3-day prodrome of fever, coryza and conjunctivitis, with the appearance of the characteristic elevated white Koplik's spots on the buccal mucosa. The rash usually starts around the head and spreads to the trunk and extremities, with resolution after a few days. Complications are not uncommon, arising in about 3–4 per cent of cases, and include bacterial pneumonia and otitis media. In the developing world, where malnutrition is common, complications, including cancrum oris, may be particularly severe and there is a significant fatality rate. Postinfectious encephalitis occurs at a rate of about 1 in 2000–5000 cases and carries a significant mortality. Subacute sclerosing panencephalitis (SSPE) occurs after an interval of some years in about one in a million cases. It reflects a persistent infection with measles virus and is uniformly fatal. Patients present with intellectual impairment and progress to motor dysfunction, coma and death. In the immunocompromised child, measles may occur without a rash but lead to encephalitis or giant-cell pneumonia, which have high fatality rates.[8]

The use of live attenuated vaccines given in the second year of life has led to a great decline in incidence of measles in those countries with a high uptake. This is exemplified by the situation in the United Kingdom. Despite the introduction of measles vaccine in the late 1960s, biannual epidemics were still occurring up to the late 1980s. The introduction of mumps, measles and rubella (MMR) vaccine in 1988,[9] together with more active promotion of the benefits of immunization, led to an increased uptake of vaccine. Thus 1990, rather than being an epidemic year, has seen the lowest number of notified cases on record. This follows the example set by the United States, where measles is now a very uncommon disease, although still presenting occasional problems of institutional outbreaks in adolescents who were not immunized or had vaccine failure.

Rubella

Rubella has a somewhat longer incubation period of 16–17 days and, particularly in children, is a very benign disease, often being asymptomatic. The pink macular rash usually starts on the face, spreads centrifugally, and lasts only 2–3 days. The most common complication, which is particularly manifest in adult women, is arthralgia of the fingers, wrists and ankles. This usually lasts only a few days, but may rarely persist for months. The major complication of rubella, however, is intrauterine infection and fetal damage if infection occurs during the first 4 months of pregnancy.[10] The main features of congenital rubella are deafness, cataract, cardiovascular abnormalities and mental retardation, but most organs and systems can be affected. Persistent infection with rubella virus can lead to immunopathological problems presenting after birth, such as pneumonitis. Live attenuated rubella vaccines have been available since the early 1970s to prevent congenital rubella. They have been used in two ways. First, to selectively immunize girls at 10–14 years of age to ensure that no woman becomes pregnant still susceptible to rubella. The second approach is to offer immunization to all children at 1–2 years of age, as well as to older girls, to try to eradicate rubella from the community. Both approaches also strive to identify and immunize susceptible adult

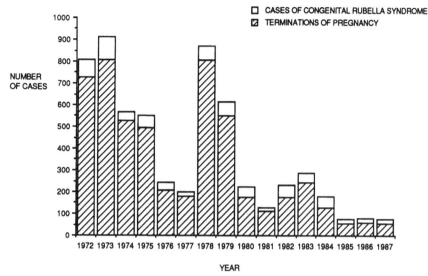

Fig. 12.1. Rubella related to pregnancy in the United Kingdom

women. As it became apparent that with the first approach there would always be a small group of women becoming pregnant whilst susceptible (Fig. 12.1), it is the second approach that is now favoured.[9]

Parvovirus B19

Erythema infectiosum had been recognized as a childhood exanthemata since the turn of the century, but the causative virus, parvovirus B19, was not identified until 1983.[11]

Infection with parvovirus B19 cannot be differentiated clinically from rubella in the adult.[12] In the child, but not in the adult, the rash, erythema infectiosum (or Fifth disease), is usually accompanied by malar erythema leading to the alternative name of 'slapped cheek syndrome'. The rash has a characteristic reticulate appearance, and often recrudesces after initially fading if the environmental temperature is changed.[11] As in rubella, arthralgia is a common complication in adults.[13] In patients with haemolytic anaemias, such as sickle cell disease and hereditary spherocytosis, the transient inhibitory effect of parvovirus B19 on the bone marrow may lead to aplastic crisis.[14] Occasional cases have been reported in which a major effect has been on platelet production, leading to thrombocytopenia and purpura.[15] Infection during pregnancy does not lead to fetal damage, although hydrops fetalis, intrauterine death and stillbirth may occur after infection in the second trimester.[16] No vaccine is available.

Erythema infectiosum is usually recognized when occurring as outbreaks related to primary schools. Indeed, the identification of parvovirus B19 as the

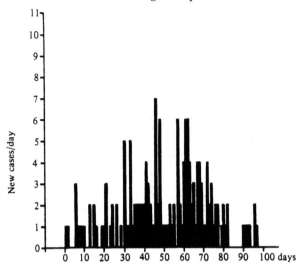

Fig. 12.2. Distribution of 162 cases of erythema infectiosum by date of onset of rash in a north London primary school of 430 pupils[11] (reproduced with the permission of the Editors of Epidemiology and Infection).

causative agent was first made when an outbreak in a primary school of a rash illness (Fig. 12.2) was investigated.[11] To demonstrate how difficult clinical diagnosis can be, this outbreak was initially thought to be scarlet fever, and general practitioners had offered a wide variety of diagnoses.[11] It is known, however, that infection is endemic throughout the year, although peaking in the spring, and 50–70 per cent of adults will have been infected at some time.

Measles, rubella and parvovirus B19 infection are usually diagnosed serologically, although cell culture isolation can be performed for the former two. Parvovirus B19 cannot be isolated in routine cell cultures. The immunocompromised patient will often not respond serologically to measles infection and diagnosis is best achieved by immunofluorescent detection of antigen in exfoliated cells of the nasopharynx obtained by aspiration.

Human herpesvirus type 6

Like erythema infectiosum, roseola infantum was accepted as a distinct childhood illness characterized by a high fever that resolves with the appearance of a pinkish macular rash. This illness occurs in children under the age of 3 years and there are no significant complications. In 1988 it was shown that the illness was a result of primary infection with human herpesvirus type 6 (HHV-6),[17] which was first reported in 1986.[18] Other significant manifestations of infection with HHV-6 have not been reported, although infection is common, with almost all people being infected early in life.

Others

Enteroviruses, such as echoviruses and coxsackieviruses B, may account for some cases of generalized rashes. Diagnosis is by isolation of virus from faeces and throat, with serology being of little value. A wide range of arboviruses may present with a maculopapular rash; of particular note are dengue, sindbis and West Nile virus.

Systemic virus infections with vesicular rashes
Smallpox and vaccinia

The greatest success of infectious disease control has been the eradication of smallpox. The last naturally occurring case was in Somalia in 1977, with two laboratory-associated cases occurring in the United Kingdom in 1978. Smallpox virus is held now in only two high-security laboratories in the United States and Soviet Union and these stocks will be destroyed by 1994.[19] This major achievement of mankind was possible because of the rarity of subclinical infection, a characteristic illness, no animal reservoirs, and an effective live attenuated vaccine, vaccinia, which left a mark visible on the arm of the vaccinee for many years. The story of the eradication of smallpox is detailed by Fenner and colleagues.[20]

Consequently there was a progressive decline in the early 1980s in the use of vaccinia, such that in most countries of the world vaccination has not taken place for some years. Vaccinia itself used to carry a significant risk of complications, such as disseminated vesicular lesions, recently described in military personnel infected with human immunodeficiency virus (HIV),[21] eczema vaccinatum and locally progressive infection (vaccinia gangrenosum). Vaccinia virus has recently attracted attention as a possible vector for immunizing epitopes for other infectious agents.[22]

Monkeypox

During the smallpox eradication campaign there was anxiety about another disseminated vesicular rash disease, monkeypox, which was described in Africa.[23] Clinically, infection with monkeypox could be extremely difficult to differentiate from smallpox, and had appreciable mortality. Infection outside Africa has not been recorded.

Fortunately, monkeypox is transmitted person-to-person less readily than smallpox, with only about 10 per cent of contacts of the index case being infected. Further transmission from such secondary cases is rare. Infection is usually in children under the age of 10 years, and vaccination offers significant protection, the mortality being about 10 per cent in the unvaccinated compared with no deaths in the vaccinated.[24] Although, as the name suggests, monkeys are affected by the virus, they do not seem to be the natural reservoir, which may be the African squirrel.

Varicella–zoster

The only disseminated virus infection of importance that presents as a vesicular rash is VZV infection. Infection is by the respiratory route. Primary infection with VZV manifests as varicella (chickenpox), with a latent infection of posterior root and cranial nerve ganglia being established. Later in life the latent virus in ganglia may reactivate and present as zoster (shingles).

Varicella is a common childhood infection with an incubation period of 14–16 days. Macules mature rapidly to papules and then vesicles and are present predominantly on the face and trunk. The vesicles appear in crops, and hence may be seen at various stages simultaneously. After 5–7 days the vesicles dry and crust; a few days later the crusts separate. Varicella is a benign illness in the immunocompetent child, but overwhelming disseminated infection can occur in the immunocompromised.[25] Fortunately VZV is sensitive to acyclovir but treatment is not always successful. Susceptible children may be offered live attenuated VZV vaccine.[26] In adults, varicella presents a higher risk of complications such as viral pneumonia, encephalitis and skin sepsis. Varicella in the first 5 months of pregnancy may occasionally cause fetal damage, about a 4 per cent risk, and varicella in the neonate also presents a major risk, although the mortality rate of 20 per cent is almost certainly an overestimate due to selective reporting.[27]

Recurrent VZV infection presents as zoster, which is usually limited to one unilateral dermatome, and has recently been reviewed by Hope-Simpson.[28] Occasionally more than one dermatome may be involved, and not uncommonly scanty disseminated vesicles may be seen. Reactivation becomes more common with age (Table 12.3), although it does occur in childhood, and is particularly common in the immunocompromised, whether due to therapy or an underlying disorder. The virus is reactivated in the sensory nerve ganglia and travels peripherally down the neurone to involve the skin of the dermatome. The dermatomes usually involved are the lower cervical, thoracic and lumbar. The trigeminal nerve, particularly the ophthalmic division, is also frequently affected (Table 12.4). If the facial nerve is involved, there may be facial palsy together with vesicles in the external auditory meatus, the Ramsay Hunt syndrome.

The skin lesions are usually accompanied by local pain, which often precedes the lesions, and indeed pain may occur without visible lesions (zoster

Table 12.3. *Age distribution of people with shingles in general practice in*
Cirencester, UK, 1947–62[28]

Age group (years)	Population	Shingles	Rate/1000/ annum
0–9	510	6	0.74
10–19	455	10	1.38
20–29	412	17	2.58
30–39	491	18	2.29
40–49	492	23	2.92
50–59	454	37	5.09
60–69	350	38	6.79
70–79	263	27	6.42
80+	107	16	9.35
Total	3534	192	3.39

Reproduced by kind permission of the Editor, PHLS Microbiology Digest.

Table 12.4. *Anatomical distribution of shingles rashes in Cirencester, UK.*[28]
Only two cranial nerves were involved, V and VII (V has three ganglia). The
total omits four cases in which area not recorded, but includes three in which
the area but not the side was recorded

Area of body	Number of pairs of ganglia	Right side		Left side		Total	
		Cases	No. per ganglion	Cases	No. per ganglion	Cases	No. per ganglion
Cranial	4	13	3.2	12	3.0	26	3.2
Cervical	8	12	1.5	14	1.7	27	1.6
Thoracic	12	51	4.3	52	4.3	103	4.3
Lumber	5	12	2.4	12	2.4	24	2.4
Sacral	5	2	2.4	5	1.0	8	0.8
Total	34	90	2.6	95	2.8	188	2.8

Reproduced by kind permission of the Editor, PHLS Microbiology Digest.

sine herpete). The most severe complication in normal individuals is persistent pain, which may last for several months, at the site of the lesions. Some benefit may be seen from early use of acyclovir, but whether this influences the post-herpetic neuralgia has been debated.[29] In the immunocompromised individual, zoster may disseminate with visceral involvement.[25] Once again acyclovir provides appropriate therapy. Zoster in pregnancy present no hazard to the fetus or neonate.

Rarely, reactivation of HSV may occur and give a clinical appearance identical to zoster. This seems particularly to occur in the sacral region.

Rapid diagnosis of varicella and zoster may be achieved by electron microscopy of vesicle fluid, although this will not distinguish VZV from HSV infection. The virus may be isolated in cell culture, although failure to isolate is not uncommon, particularly if there is delay before the specimen is inoculated into cell culture. Serology provides a reliable approach to diagnosis of VZV infection, although specific IgM is detected after both varicella and zoster.[30]

Hand, foot and mouth disease

As the name suggests, hand, foot and mouth disease is characterized by vesicular lesions on the hands, feet and mucous membranes of the mouth, although those in the mouth rapidly break down to form ulcers. Several enteroviruses have been implicated, usually strains of coxsackievirus A and B, but it is often due to coxsackievirus A16. Infection commonly occurs in epidemics in the late summer and autumn, with intrafamilial spread being common. Transmission to contacts occurs at a high rate, with up to 40 per cent of nursery-school contacts developing the disease. Although the majority will be asymptomatic,[31] 70–80 per cent of school and household contacts may be infected. Recovery is almost always uncomplicated, although myocarditis and spontaneous abortion may occur rarely. Diagnosis is by isolation of the virus in cell culture from faeces and throat swab, although for some strains of coxsackievirus A isolation in suckling mice is required. Neutralizing antibody tests have been described for coxsackievirus A16, and may be useful for diagnosis, although having limited availability.[32]

Localized virus infections

Papillomavirus infections

During the last decade increasing attention has been paid to papillomaviruses and the conditions they cause. This interest has largely been due to the advances that have been made in detection and characterization of nucleic acids, as papillomavirus cannot be isolated in any routine cell cultures, and the association with cervical carcinoma. Human papillomaviruses (HPV) contain double-stranded DNA and are classified into types on the basis of the relatedness of their nucleotide sequences. If a papillomavirus has less than 50 per cent homology on nucleotide pairing with an existing HPV type it is designated as a new type. There are now at least 60 human HPV types, sequentially numbered from 1, with some being further divided into subtypes alphabetically if distinctive endonuclease restriction patterns are seen.

Warts

The types of HPV are associated with the particular consequences of infection.[33] Infection is primarily of the squamous epithelium, and although there are many manifestations, the common wart (verruca vulgaris), plantar warts, and plane warts are the usual presentations. It has been estimated that 10 per cent of children and young adults have common warts at any one time, with the peak incidence being in 10- to 16-year-olds (Fig. 12.3).[34] The principal sites are on the hands and feet, and they are a major cause of dermatological consultation. Most common and plantar warts are due to HPV-1, -2, -4, -31, and -32. The incubation period is usually about 4–6 months, with transmission by direct contact or by fomite. The natural history is of regression, with about two-thirds resolving within 2 years. Other benign non-genital skin lesions include flat warts (HPV-3 and -12) and butchers warts (HPV-7).

Epidermodysplasia verruciformis This is a rare condition where there is an HPV-specific disorder of cell-mediated immunity resulting in disseminated warty lesions that persist for life.[35] An autosomal recessive mode of inheritance is probable. Up to 23 types of HPV infect these patients, such as HPV-5, -8, -9, and -12, and most do not give lesions in the normal person. The flat wart and pityriasis-like lesions are refractory to treatment, and in about one-third of patients malignant change occurs, probably with ultraviolet radiation as a cofactor.

Genital warts These have attracted great attention because of the association with genital cancers, and as a presenting feature of sexual abuse in children. The common type of genital wart is the condyloma acuminatum, which is due to infection with HPV-6 or -11. The incubation period is some 1–6 months and they may occur not only on the external genitalia, but also the mucosal surfaces of the vagina and urethra. They rarely become malignant and usually spontaneously resolve. Condylomata acuminata are sexually transmitted and dramatic increases in prevalence have been seen in the last 20 years. Infection may often be asymptomatic, so the possibilities of transmission are enhanced as the infected person does not seek treatment.

As for any sexually transmitted disease, the occurrence of condylomata acuminata in prepubertal children raises the likelihood of sexual abuse. HPV infection may also have been acquired from non-sexual close contact, or from the mother, probably at the time of delivery, so genital warts do not provide unequivocal evidence of sexual abuse.[36]

Condylomata acuminata may enlarge rapidly during pregnancy, and rarely

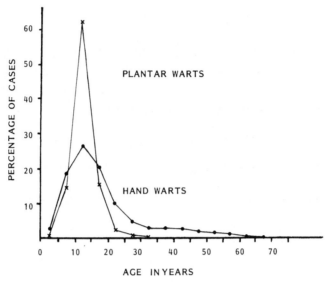

Fig. 12.3. Age distribution of plantar and hand warts (based on Barr and Coles[34]).

may present a danger of obstructing delivery.[37] The mother with genital warts may present a further risk to her child. Transmission of HPV-6 or -11 from mother to neonate may occur and later present in childhood as recurrent respiratory papillomatis.[38] Most cases are diagnosed before 5 years of age, and it may occasionally be life threatening. Although the papillomas are usually on the laryngeal mucosa, they may occasionally occur in the oropharynx or lower down the respiratory tract. There are often recurrences after surgical resection, although spontaneous regression is more usual. The risk of developing this complication in the child born to a mother with condylomata acuminata has not been quantitated, but is considered so low that prophylactic caesarian section is not recommended,[39] and indeed infection has occurred even when caesarian section has been done.[38]

Papillomaviruses and cancer

The malignant potential of papillomaviruses has been recognized for many years in species such as the rabbit and cow, but it is only in the last 10 years that they have become a prime candidate for involvement in a human cancer, namely carcinoma of the cervix. It has been established for many years that an increased risk of cervical carcinoma is associated with an early age of first sexual experience and an increased number of sexual partners, hence suggesting that a sexually transmissible agent was involved. In the early 1980s, attention focused on genital herpes, but the ability to detect HPV DNA by hybridization techniques demonstrated HPV, particularly HPV-16 and -18, in a range of cervical lesions from carcinoma *in situ* to invasive cervical carcinoma. In malignant cells, the HPV genome has been integrated into the cell genome, rather than remaining extrachromosomal. These HPV types also occur very commonly in sexually active women with no cervical lesions, so the role of detection of HPV-16 and -18 in the management of women with a clinically and cytologically normal cervix remains to be defined.[40] Other factors, such as smoking, are implicated in the development of cervical carcinoma, and coincident infection with other agents, such as herpes simplex may be important. Papillomaviruses have also been implicated in other human malignancies of the skin, such as squamous cell carcinoma in patients with epidermodysplasia verruciformis, and a similar carcinoma may occur in the immunocompromised renal transplant recipients, who have a high risk of developing warts.[41]

Herpesvirus infections

HSV is probably the most common virus infecting the skin, with almost everyone having been infected by late adulthood. HSV is divided into type 1 and 2 by a number of features including DNA fragment sizes after endonuclease restriction analysis, type-specific proteins, and size of pocks when cultured on the chorioallantoic membrane. Classically, type 1 was associated with lesions above the waist, and type 2 with genital herpes. This distinction has become increasingly blurred, however, with up to 50 per cent of genital herpes being due to type 1, although type 2 is still an infrequent cause of oral herpes infection. All aspects of HSV and the infections it causes have been recently reviewed by Mindel.[42]

Primary HSV infection

Primary infection with HSV-1 usually occurs in childhood and is often asymptomatic, although it can present as a stomatitis, occasionally severe enough to warrant admission to hospital. Such stomatitis due to primary infection can also occur in young adults, and it seems probable that asymptomatic infection is less likely if primary exposure is delayed until adulthood. After primary oral infection, the virus becomes latent in the neurones of the trigeminal ganglia, with reactivation being likely later in life. Reactivation is manifest as the ubiquitous 'cold sore', the most common clinically obvious lesion of humans due to a single virus, with 20–45 per cent of people suffering a recurrence at some time, and about 5–10 per cent having more than two attacks each year.[43] Reactivation may be precipitated by many external factors, such as stress, other febrile illness, menstruation, exposure to ultraviolet radiation and immunosuppression. The natural history is of a few hours non-specific tingling, followed by development of vesicles, scabbing, and resolution over a few days. Cold sores usually occur at the mucocutaneous junction of the lip, although reactivated herpes simplex lesions may also occur at other sites on the face, such as the cheek and chin, and rarely at intraoral sites such as on the palate. There may be recurrences distressingly often, and although there is debate about the usefulness of antivirals, such as acyclovir, for the sporadic cold sore, continuous oral therapy is often recommended to attempt suppression of recurrence.[44]

Infection with herpes simplex, even in those already latently infected, may occur at a range of other skin sites. Herpetic paronychia, or infection at other sites on the hand,[45] are a well-recognized occupational hazard of certain health care workers, such as dentists, anaesthetists and intensive care nurses. All these groups frequently have contact with oral secretions, and up to 1 per cent of adults at any one time may be asymptomatically excreting virus into the oropharynx.[2] The herpetic lesions on the hands may be multiple and it is therapeutically important that an herpetic cause is considered as surgery is then contraindicated and acyclovir is the required treatment. Full recovery may take some weeks.

HSV infection in eczema and other skin lesions

Eczematous skin is particularly prone to herpes simplex infection and this may involve large areas. Primary infection may be life threatening. Clinically distinguishing eczema herpeticum, or Kaposi's varicelliform eruption, from superimposed staphylococcal infection may be difficult and indeed the two infections may coexist.[42] Electron microscopy and culture are required to identify the causative agent to ensure appropriate therapy. Herpes simplex can also present problems of superinfection in a number of other chronic dermatological conditions, such as pemphigus and Darier's disease. One particular form of HSV infection has earned the title 'herpes gladiatorum', a facial herpes occurring in wrestlers, or scrumpox in rugby players, with transmission occurring by close facial contact during the sporting activity.[46]

Herpes encephalitis

Herpes encephalitis is almost always a result of reactivation, with the temporal and occipital lobes of the brain being usually affected. The high fatality and residual illness associated with herpes encephalitis have been significantly improved by the availability of antiviral therapy, in particular acyclovir, although to have a major impact it must be initiated soon after onset of the illness.[47] The diagnosis of herpes encephalitis may be achieved by examining a brain biopsy,[48] or in convalescence, by detection of specific antibodies in the cerebrospinal fluid (CSF).[49] The development and application of the polymerase chain reaction for genome detection in the CSF offers an exciting prospect for rapid and specific diagnosis.[50] The presence or absence of herpetic lesions on the skin is of no help in diagnosis, nor is the detection of virus in the oropharynx or CSF. Indeed it is a characteristic of herpes encephalitis that viable virus cannot be found in the CSF.[48]

Ophthalmic herpes

Infection with herpes simplex can have various manifestations in the eye, it being the most frequent cause of corneal blindness. Infection may be primary or due to reactivation, and about a quarter will have a recurrence in the year after their first attack. The range of ophthalmic infections includes keratitis, with or without conjunctival involvement, and uveitis. The damage that occurs in iridocyclitis appears associated primarily with the consequence of the immune response.

Erythema multiforme

This may be precipitated by herpes simplex infection, and indeed this is probably one of the most common initiating factors. The erythema multiforme is presumably immune mediated and occurs some 3 weeks after the infection, with both oral and genital herpes capable of being responsible.

Genital herpes

In the early 1980s, genital herpes attracted much attention, with the number of cases presenting at clinics for sexually transmitted diseases in the UK increasing fourfold to 20000 per annum between 1972 and 1984.[42] A first attack of genital herpes is usually more severe than a recurrence, and primary infection is usually more severe than a first attack in someone who has previously had primary oral herpes. The herpetic vesicles and ulcers of the external genitalia are often accompanied by a systemic febrile illness and inguinal lymphadenopathy in a first attack, and may be sufficiently severe to result in urinary retention.[51] Occasionally there may be an associated meningitis in which virus can be isolated from the CSF.[52] Recurrences are more frequent with HSV-2 than with HSV-1 infection, and may be sufficiently frequent to warrant suppressive acyclovir therapy.[53] Asymptomatic reactivation may occur in the urethra and cervix, and result in transmission. Both first attack and recurrent herpes can also occur anally, and is a particular problem for homosexual men.

An aspect of genital HSV infection that has caused particular concern is the possible association with cervical carcinoma, although the degree of this association is still a matter for debate.[42]

Neonatal HSV infection

Although rare in the United Kingdom, neonatal herpes simplex is a devastating infection with a high fatality rate and considerable complications in survivors. Infection of the neonate is occasionally nosocomial from their attendants, but is usually acquired from the mother at the time of delivery. Intrauterine infection is very rare. Generalized systemic infection occurs, as well as more localized infection of the skin, and infection can occur without externally obvious lesions. Primary infection at delivery presents a major risk compared to a reactivation.[54] Caesarian section is certainly indicated if primary infection is present and the membranes have not been ruptured for more than 4 h, but whether caesarian section is indicated for reactivation or asymptomatic virus excretion is still a matter of debate.[55] Equally, the proposal that women with a history of genital herpes should be virologically screened at weekly intervals during the late stages of pregnancy[56] has also been disputed,[57] and indeed in one series the mothers of most babies with neonatal herpes did not give a history of genital herpes.[58]

Herpesvirus simiae (B virus)

B virus is enzootic in certain species of monkey, and seems to behave in them rather like herpes simplex does in man. Intermittent reactivation and shedding occurs, particularly when monkeys are immunocompromised or stressed, as they may well be when in captivity. Although infection in man is rare, it can cause encephalitis and be fatal,[59] although acyclovir treatment appears effective. The initial clinical manifestation is often a vesicular lesion at the site of inoculation, often on the hand.[59]

Poxvirus infections
Molluscum contagiosum

Despite the eradication of smallpox and the consequent cessation of use of vaccinia, there are a number of other poxviruses that cause skin infections in man. Probably the most common is molluscum contagiosum, which has been reviewed by Postlethwaite.[60] It has an incubation period from 1 week to 6 months. The lesions vary in number from one to many hundreds, and develop from papules to flesh-coloured or pearly nodules, which often have an umbilicated centre. Systemic symptoms are rare. In adults they usually occur on the trunk, genital area and thighs, and infection may be sexually transmitted. In children, in whom infection is more common, the lesions are predominantly on the trunk and proximal extremities. The disease usually lasts 6–9 months, although individual lesions persist for only about 2 months. The lesions are circumscribed and the core may be expressed as a cheesy material. The virus has not been cultured and specific diagnosis, if needed, is by electron microscopy.

Parapox infections

Parapox infections are common in domesticated farm animals such as sheep and cattle. Infections in sheep and goats are usually referred to as orf or contagious pustular dermatitis, and the lesions in the animal's mouth may be sufficiently severe to inhibit feeding and have adverse commercial consequences.

Transmission to members of the farming community or abattoir workers is not infrequent, and is probably much underreported. The skin lesions may be single or multiple and usually occur on the hands, although other sites may be affected.[61] Infection presumably occurs by direct inoculation through damaged skin, and second or more attacks may occur. After a few days' incubation the lesion starts as an erythematous papule, which progresses through a 'target' stage, an erythematous centre and outer ring separated by a pale zone, to a modular state, then to a granulomatous stage before healing. The lesion usually takes 6–8 weeks before full resolution, and there is anecdotal evidence that topical therapy with idoxyuridine may speed healing.[62] The lesions are rarely painful and systemic illness is uncommon, but a severe flu-like illness can occur, as can erythema multiforme. Rarely the lesion may progress in size, and such massive lesions have been called 'giant orf'.[63] Occasionally amputation has been performed.[64] The virus can be isolated in cell culture only with great difficulty, and specific diagnosis is by electron microscopy.

The virus from cattle is very similar to orf, and they can only be separated by minor differences on detailed DNA analysis.[65] The infection in cattle is termed pseudocowpox, paravaccinia or milker's nodes, with human infection being similarly labelled. The infection in humans is clinically indistinguishable from that described for orf.

Cowpox

Cowpox is a very uncommon infection in humans, but its occurrence in people with no contact with cattle may be explained by the recognition of infection in domestic cats.[66] The lesion is very similar to that induced by vaccination and is usually on the hand. Systemic illness is common, and fatal dissemination has been described.[67]

Tanapox

Tanapox is a virus infection of monkeys, with human infection being recognized only in a small area of central Africa.[68] Vesicular lesions, usually numbering only one or two, may present anywhere on the body, but complications are rare.

Retrovirus infections

Human T-lymphotrophic virus type 1 (HTLV-1) was the first retrovirus shown to cause disease in humans.[69] It has primarily been associated with two diseases, adult T-cell leukaemia/lymphoma (ATLL)[70] and tropical spastic paraparesis, which is a progressive multiple sclerosis-like syndrome. ATLL may present with skin lesions[71] but more recently infection has been associated with infective dermatitis in Jamaican children;[72] the virus is endemic in part of the West Indies, the south-east United States and southern Japan. Transmission may occur by blood transfusion but naturally transmission is probably mother-to-infant or sexual.

Mycoplasmas

The possible role of mycoplasmas in skin disease was discussed at length in the previous edition of this book. Ten years later, however, the only mycoplasma of importance in skin disease is *Mycoplasma pneumoniae*. Infection may present with a range of skin lesions, such as Stevens–Johnson syndrome, erythema multiforme, maculopapular rashes, and erythema nodosum.[73] *Mycoplasma pneumoniae* has only rarely been isolated from skin lesions, and they are likely to be a consequence of the immune response. Diagnosis is serological.

Infections in the immunocompromised

The immunocompromised patient, whether a consequence of therapy or underlying problems, such as lymphoma or human immunodeficiency virus HIV infection, presents many additional problems with respect to viral skin infections. Those infections, such as HSV and VZV, in which a latent state is established are more likely to reactivate and disseminate rather than remain as a localized lesion. Varicella and measles may be life threatening. Rubella seems to present no particular risk, however, and parvovirus B19 and enteroviruses only rarely present problems. Dissemination of warts can occur, as it may of molluscum contagiosum.

Persons infected with HIV are presenting new dermatological manifestations and these have recently been reviewed.[74–76]

In conclusion the last decade has seen exciting developments in identifying aetiological agents for syndromes manifest in the skin, but there are still more for which a viral cause seems likely. An example is pityriasis rosea, an infective background being considered because of the clinical presentation and case clustering, although virological investigation has been unsuccessful to date.[77,78] It has been suggested that Kaposi's sarcoma has an infective cause distinct from HIV,[79] and such notions are there to tantalize investigators for the next decade.

References

1 Puhvel SM, Amirian DA. Bacterial flora of comedones. Br J Dermatol 1979; 101: 543–48.

2 Lindgren KM, Douglas RC Jr, Couch RB. Significance of herpes virus hominis in respiratory secretion of man. N Engl J Med 1968; 278: 517–23.

3 Husain MH, Sommerville RG. Presence of herpes simplex virus on eczematous skin. Lancet 1964; ii: 391–92.

4 Leyden JJ, Baker, DA. Localized herpes simplex infections in atopic dermatitis. Arch Dermatol 1979; 115: 311–12.

5 Fields BN, Knipe DM. Virology. 2nd edn. New York: Raven Press; 1990.

6 Clayton AL, Roberts C, Godley M, Best JM, Chantler SM. Herpes simplex virus detection by ELISA: effect of enzyme amplification, nature of lesion sampled and specimen treatment. J Med Virol 1986; 20: 89–97.

7 Southern E. Detection of specific sequences among DNA fragments separated by gel electrophoresis. J Mol Biol 1975; 98: 503–17.

8 Kernahan J, McQuillin J, Craft AW. Measles in children who have malignant disease. Br Med J 1987; 295: 15–18.

9 Badenoch J. Big bang for vaccination. Br Med J 1988; 297: 750–51.

10 Miller E, Cradock-Watson JE, Pollock TM. Consequences of confirmed maternal rubella at successive stages of pregnancy. Lancet 1982; ii: 781–84.

11 Anderson MJ, Lewis E, Kidd IM, Hall SM, Cohen BJ. An outbreak of erythema infectiosum associated with human parvovirus infection. J Hyg Camb 1984; 93: 85–93.

12 Anderson MJ, Kidd IM, Morgan-Capner P. Human parvovirus and rubella-like illness. Lancet 1985; ii: 663.

13 Reid DM, Brown T, Reid TMS, Rennie JAN, Eastmond CJ. Human parvovirus-associated arthritis: a clinical and laboratory description. Lancet 1985; i: 422–25.

14 Pattison JR, Jones SE, Hodgson J, Davis LR, Stroud CE, Murtaza L. Parvovirus infections and hypoplastic crisis in sickle-cell anaemia. Lancet 1981; i: 664–65.

15 Mortimer PP, Cohen BJ, Rossiter MA, Fairhead SM, Rahman AFMS. Human parvovirus and purpura. Lancet 1985; ii: 730–31.

16 Public Health Laboratory Service Working Party on Fifth Disease. Prospective study of human parvovirus (B19) infection in pregnancy. Br Med J 1990; 300: 1166–70.

17 Yamanishi K, Okuno T, Shiraki K et al. Identification of human herpesvirus-6 as a causal agent for exanthem subitum. Lancet 1988; i: 1065–66.

18 Salahuddin SZ, Ablaski DV, Markham PD, et al. Isolation of a new virus, HBLV in patients with lymphoproliferative disorders. Science 1986; 234: 596–601.

19 Godlee F. Smallpox virus to be destroyed. Br Med J 1991; 302: 373.

20 Fenner F, Henderson DA, Arita I, Jezek K, Ladnyi ID. Smallpox and its eradication. Geneva: World Health Organization; 1988.

21 Redfield RR, Wright DC, James WD, et al. Disseminated vaccinia in a military recruit with human immunodeficiency virus (HIV) disease. N Engl J Med 1987; 316: 673–76.

22 Hruby DE, Thomas G. Use of vaccinia virus to express biopharmaceutical products. Pharmaceut Res 1987; 4: 92–97.

23 Jezek Z, Fenner F. Human monkeypox. In: Monographs in virology, vol 17. Basel: Karger; 1988.

24 Jezak Z, Grab B, Szczeniowski M, Paluku KM, Mutombo M. Clinico-epidemiological features of monkeypox patients with an animal or human source of infection. Bull WHO 1988; 66: 459–64.

25 Morris DJ. Viral infections in children with cancer. Rev Med Microbiol 1990; 1: 49–57.

26 Kangro HO. Varicella vaccine. Rev Med Microbiol 1990; 1: 205–212.

27 Cradock-Watson, JE. Chickenpox in pregnancy. PHLS Microbiol Digest 1990; 7: 40–45.

28 Hope-Simpson RE. The biological significance of shingles. PHLS Microbiol Digest 1989; 6: 105–10.

29 Anonymous. Postherpetic neuralgia. Lancet 1990; 336: 537–38.

30 Chandler C, Meurisse EV, Wreghitt TG. Herpesvirus. In: Wreghitt TG, Morgan-Capner P, eds. ELISA in the clinical microbiology laboratory. London: Public Health Laboratory Service; 1990: 62–86.

31 World Health Organization. Coxsackievirus A16. Weekly Epidemiol Rec 1981; 56: 39–40.

32 Urquhart GED. A survey of coxsackie A16 virus antibodies in human sera. J Hyg Camb 1984; 93: 205–12.

33 McCance DJ, Gardner SD. Papovaviruses: papillomaviruses and polyomaviruses. In: Zuckerman AJ, Banatvala JE, Pattison JR, eds. Principles and practice of clinical virology. 2nd edn. Chichester: John Wiley; 1990: 531–60.

34 Barr A, Coles RB. Warts: a statistical survey. Trans St John's Hosp Dermatol Soc 1966; 52: 226–38. [and] Warts on the hands: a statistical survey. Trans St John's Hosp Dermatol Soc 1969; 55: 69–73.

35 Jablonska S, Orth G. Epidermodysplasia verruciformis. Clin Dermatol 1985; 3: 83–96.

36 Herman-Giddens ME, Gutman LT, Benson NL, et al. Association of coexisting vaginal infections and multiple abusers in female children with genital warts. Sex Transm Dis 1988; 15: 63–67.

37 Young RL, Acosta AA, Kaufman RH. The treatment of large condylomata acuminata complicating pregnancy. Obstet Gynecol 1973; 41: 65–73.

38 Steinberg BM. Laryngeal papillomas: clinical aspects and *in vitro* studies. In: Salzman NP, Howley PM, eds. The papovaviridae. 2. The papillomaviruses, New York: Plenum; 1987; 265–92.

39 Cobb MW. Human papillomavirus infection. J Am Acad Dermatol 1990; 22: 547–66.

40 Singer A, Jenkins D. Viruses and cervical cancer. Br Med J 1991; 302: 251–52.

41 Barr BBB, Benton EC, McLaren K, et al. Human papillomavirus infection and skin cancer in renal allograft recipients. Lancet 1989: i: 124–28.

42 Mindel A. Herpes simplex virus. London: Springer-Verlag; 1989.

43 Young SK, Rowe NH, Buchanan RA. A clinical study for the control of facial mucocutaneous herpes virus infections. Oral Surg 1976; 41: 498–507.

44 Meyrick Thomas RH, Dodd HJ, Yeo JM, Kirby JP. Oral acyclovir in the suppression of recurrent non-genital herpes simplex virus infection. Br J Dermatol 1985; 113: 731–35.

45 Gill MJ, Arlette J, Buchan K. Herpes simplex virus infection of the hand: a profile of 79 cases. Am J Med 1988; 84: 89–93.

46 Shute P, Jeffries DJ, Maddocks AC. Scrumpox caused by herpes simplex virus. Br Med J 1979; 2: 1692.

47 Whitley RJ, Alford CA, Hirsch MS, et al. Vidarabine versus acyclovir therapy in herpes simplex encephalitis. N Eng J Med 1986; 314: 144–49.

48 Whitley RJ, Soong S-J, Linneman C, Liu C, Pazin G, Alford CA. Herpes simplex encephalitis. JAMA 1982; 247: 317–20.

49 Klapper PE, Laing I, Longson M. Rapid non-invasive diagnosis of herpes encephalitis. Lancet 1981; ii: 607–09.

50 Aurelius E, Johansson B, Skoldenberg B, Staland A, Forsgren M. Rapid diagnosis of herpes simplex encephalitis by nested polymerase chain reaction assay of cerebrospinal fluid. Lancet 1991; 337: 189–92.

51 Nahmias AJ, Roizman B. Infection with herpes simplex virus 1 and 2. N Eng J Med 1973; 289: 781–89.

52 Corey L, Adams HG, Brown ZA, Holmes KK. Genital herpes simplex virus infections: clinical manifestations, course, and complications. Intern Med 1983; 98: 958–72.

53 Kinghorn GR, Jeavons M, Rowland M, et al. Acyclovir prophylaxis of recurrent genital herpes: a randomised placebo controlled crossover study. Genitourin Med 1985; 61: 387–90.

54 Prober CG, Sullender WM, Yasukawa LL, Au DS, Yeager AS, Arvin AM. Low risk of herpes simplex virus infections in neonates exposed to the virus at the time of vaginal delivery to mothers with recurrent genital herpes simplex virus infections. N Engl J Med 1987; 316: 240–44.

55 Lissauer T, Jeffries D. Preventing neonatal herpes infection. Br J Obstet Gynecol 1989; 9: 1015–23.

56 Committee on Fetus and Newborn. Perinatal herpes simplex virus infection. Paediatrics 1980; 66: 147–48.

57 Anonymous. Virological screening for herpes simplex virus during pregnancy. Lancet 1988; ii: 722–23.

58 Prober CG, Hensleigh PA, Boucher FD, Yasukawa LL, Au DS, Arvin AA. Use of routine viral cultures at delivery to identify neonates exposed to herpes simplex virus. N Engl J Med 1988; 318: 887–91.

59 Anonymous. B-virus infection in humans – Pensacola, Florida. MMWR 1987; 36: 289–96.

60 Postlethwaite R. Molluscum contagiosum: a review. Arch Environ Health 1970; 21: 423–52.

61 PHLS Communicable Disease Surveillance Centre and the Communicable Disease (Scotland) Unit. Orf paravaccinia infections, British Isles: 1975–81. Br Med J 1982; 284: 1958.

62 Hunskaar S. A case of ecthyma contagiosum (human orf) treated with idoxuridine. Dermatologica 1984; 168: 207.

63 Pether JVS, Guerrier CJW, Jones SM, Adam AE, Kingsbury WN. Giant orf in a normal individual. Br J Dermatol 1986; 115: 497–99.

64 Savage J, Black MM. 'Giant' orf of a finger in a patient with lymphoma. Proc Roy Soc Med 1972; 65: 766–68.

65 Gassman U, Wyler R, Wittek R. Analysis of parapox genomes. Arch Virol 1985; 83: 17–23.

66 Bennett M, Gaskell CJ, Gaskell RM, Baxby D, Gruffyd-Jones TJ. Poxvirus infection in the domestic cat: some clinical and epidemiological observations. Vet Rec 1986; 118: 387–90.

67 Eis-Hubinger AM, Gerritzen A, Schneweis KE, et al. Fatal cowpox-like virus infection transmitted by cat. Lancet 1990; 336: 880.

68 Downie AW, Taylor-Robinson CH, Caunt AE, Nelson GS, Manson-Bahr PEC, Matthews TCH. Tanapox: a new disease caused by a poxvirus. Br Med J 1971; 1: 363–68.

69 Poiesz BJ, Ruscetti FW, Gazdar AF, Bunn PA, Minna JD, Gallo RC. Detection and isolation of type C retrovirus particles from fresh and cultured lymphocytes of a patient with cutaneous T-cell lymphomas. Proc Nat Acad Sciences USA 1980; 77: 7415–19.

70 Hinuma Y, Komoda H, Chosa T, et al. Antibody to adult T-cell leukemia virus associated antigen (ATLA) in sera from patients with ATL and controls in Japan. Int J Cancer 1982; 29: 631–35.

71 Catovsky D, Greaves MF, Rose M, et al. Adult T-cell lymphoma–leukemia in blacks from the West Indies. Lancet 1982; i: 639–43.

72 LaGrenade L, Hanchard B, Fletcher V, Cranston B, Blattner W. Infective dermatitis of Jamaican children: a marker for HTLV-1 infection. Lancet 1990; 336: 1345–47.

73 Ali NJ, Sillis M, Andrewes BE, Jenkins PF, Harrison BDW. The clinical spectrum and diagnosis of *Mycoplasma pneumoniae* infection. Quart J Med 1986; 58: 241–51.

74 Knobler RM. Human immunodeficiency virus infection. Dermatol Clin 1989; 7: 369–85.

75 Penneys NS. Cutaneous signs of AIDS. Dermatol Clin 1989; 7: 571–77.

76 Cockerell CJ. Cutaneous manifestations of HIV infection other than Kaposi's sarcoma: clinical and histologic aspects. J Am Acad Dermatol 1990; 22: 1260–69.

77 Garcia E, Silver L, Gardner PS. Pityriasis rosea – a virological study. Br J Derm 1968; 80: 514–15.

78 Morgan-Capner P, Hodgson J, Pattison J, Hehir M, Du Vivier A. Case clustering in pityriasis rosea: support for role of an infective agent. Br Med J 1982; 284: 977.

79 Beral V, Peterman TA, Berkelman RL, Jaffe HW. Kaposi's sarcoma among persons with AIDS: a sexually transmitted infection? Lancet 1990; 335: 123–28.

13

Viral skin disease in animals

D. H. LLOYD

Introduction

The range of viral skin disease in animals is very wide and involves many agents which also have significant systemic effects. Comprehensive consideration of all of these infections is beyond the scope of this review and attention will therefore be concentrated on infections of terrestrial mammals and on diseases of the general body surface. Diseases in which the skin signs form a minor part will only be mentioned briefly. Zoonotic infection is not considered here but readers are referred to the CRC handbook on viral zoonoses.[1]

Virus infections of the skin may be divided into those in which the skin disease is the principal feature (Tables 13.1–13.3 below) and those where skin lesions form a subsidiary part of the generalized disease[2] (Tables 13.4 and 13.5 below). Although this division is arbitrary and does not allow for diseases in which severe skin and systemic infections coexist, it provides a framework for consideration of the large and diverse range of viral skin diseases.

The great majority of virus infections in which skin signs predominate are caused by DNA viruses and, in particular, the poxviruses (Table 13.1). RNA viruses are represented only by the retroviruses (feline sarcoma and feline leukaemia viruses), which are responsible for neoplastic disease (see Table 13.3).

Poxvirus infections

The poxviruses are composed of two subfamilies, of which only one, the *Chordopoxvirinae*, affects vertebrates. Five genera and a number of unclassified agents affect domestic animals (Table 13.1), causing diseases that vary from mild, localized papular lesions to severe, life-threatening systemic disease. Host specificity is also quite variable. The majority of pox diseases occur in

Table 13.1. *Dermatoses of domestic animals caused by DNA viruses: the poxviruses*

Pox genus	Skin disease (virus)	Species	Dermatological signs
Orthopox	Cowpox	Cattle	Pocks on teats and udder develop thick crusts and typically heal in about 3 weeks. More severe infections involve perineum, vulva, scrotum and medial thighs. May affect mouths of sucking calves
	(Feline poxvirus infection)	Cats	Crusted papules, plaques, nodules and crateriform lesions usually on face, limbs, paws and dorsal lumbar region
	Vaccinia	Cattle, pigs, horses	Signs are identical to the respective species' pox diseases (cowpox, pig pox, horse pox)
	Buffalopox	Buffaloes	Localized to generalized pox lesions affecting particularly the udder, teats, medial thighs, muzzle and lips
	Camelpox	Camels	Typical pock-like vesicular eruptions with loss of condition and fall in milk production
	Horsepox	Horses	Vesicles, pustules and crusts form in the mouth, on the pastern and fetlocks or on the vulva (coital exanthema)
		Cattle	Signs in cattle are identical to cowpox
Parapox	Pseudocowpox	Cattle	Focal, painful erythematous lesions of the teats and udder develop into small papules which extend and form crusts that fall away leaving characteristic crusty circular or arciform margins. Perineum, medial thighs and scrotum are sometimes affected
	Bovine papular stomatitis	Cattle	Maculopapular, erythematous lesions of the lips, muzzle and nostrils become centrally necrotic and crusted or papillomatous. Teats, prepuce, scrotum, ventral and lateral trunk may also be affected

	Disease	Host	Clinical features
Capripox	Contagious pustular dermatitis (orf)	Sheep, goats, cattle	Typical pock lesions arise on lips, nostrils, muzzle and eyelids and may form thick scabs. Secondary infection may cause necrotic ulcers. Severe infections may involve interdigital spaces, distal limbs, perineum, genitals and udder. Wounds, e.g. docking and ear marking sites, may be infected
	Lumpy skin disease (LSI)	Cattle	Sudden appearance of papules and nodules (< 5 cm diameter) at various sites, and oedema of limbs and ventral trunk. The nodules may become necrotic and resolve in 1–3 months or persist for years. Necrotic lesions ('sitfasts') are sloughed leaving ulcers that heal by scarring
	Sheep-pox	Sheep	Pocks develop at sites including head, neck, ears, axillae, groin, udder, genitals, perineum and under the tail
	Goatpox	Goats	Lesions at the same sites as in sheep-pox but some outbreaks only involve lips and muzzle. Can affect sheep
Suipox	Swinepox	Pigs	Pocks usually develop on ventrolateral trunk and medial surfaces of limbs but may affect head, udder, teats and back
Leporipox	Myomatosis	Rabbits	Oedema of the eyelids, lips, nose, ears and vent, then fibrotic nodules develop on nose, ears and forefeet and genitals
	Shope fibroma	Rabbits	One or more mobile, firm, subcutaneous masses are formed
Unclassified	Ovine viral ulcerative dermatosis	Sheep	Granulating, oedematous, circumscribed ulcers containing pus and with adherent crusts form on the lips, face, feet and distal parts of the limbs and genitalia. Healing is associated with scarring and alopecia
	Equine viral papular dermatitis	Horses	Papules appear over much of the body, sparing the head, followed by crusting, hair loss and scaling. There are no other signs
	Equine molluscum contagiosum	Horses	Circumscribed, greyish, waxy papules, up to 2 mm in diameter, appear on udder, groin, scrotum, prepuce, penis, axilla and muzzle. A central pore develops in each papule and a caseous plug is extruded

farm animals and particularly ruminants;[3] pox diseases of the dog have not been described, although feline poxvirus infection is now well recognized.[4,5]

Normal skin is resistant to topical infection and acquisition of infection generally occurs via skin abrasions, as in orf, or by the respiratory route, as in human smallpox, although mechanical transmission by arthropods is known to be important in swinepox and myxomatosis of rabbits.[2,6] Systemic spread may occur via the lymphatics or, following local multiplication in the skin, as a viraemia. Both degenerative and proliferative lesions are produced. Epithelial breakdown after virus replication results in the formation of typical vesicles in the skin, whilst vascular damage and ischaemia may cause dermal lesions. The characteristic sequence of development of poxvirus lesions in animal skin resembles that in man.

Orthopoxvirus infections
Cowpox

This is an uncommon orthopoxvirus infection of cattle that occurs only in Europe. The epidemiological aspects of the condition are not understood but it has been suggested that there may be a rodent host reservoir.[7] Once infection is introduced into a susceptible herd, it spreads rapidly and there is a high morbidity, particularly amongst milking cattle in which transmission on dairy equipment and by the dairy workers probably occurs. Typical pock lesions develop (Table 13.1) and the disease lasts 3–4 weeks in the absence of complicating factors. Affected animals develop lifelong immunity. An identical clinical syndrome develops after infection of cattle with vaccinia (bovine vaccinia mamillitis) and horsepox virus. However, with discontinuation of human vaccination against smallpox, vaccinia infection in animals has ceased to occur.

Buffalopox

Buffalopox virus is closely related antigenically to cowpox and vaccinia viruses and affects water buffaloes in the Indian subcontinent; it has also been reported in the Soviet Union, Egypt and Italy.[8] It causes localized to generalized pox lesions (Table 13.1) and may also cause teat stenosis and mastitis. Infections in other domestic ruminants have not been reported.

Camelpox

Camelpox virus (Table 13.1), which is closely related to the variola (smallpox) and vaccinia viruses, causes a highly infectious generalized disease in camels in the Middle East and in northern and eastern Africa. Death usually only occurs in young animals.[9]

Catpox

Feline poxvirus infection (catpox) is a sporadic problem in both domestic and wild felidae in Europe, caused by a virus that is believed to be identical to that of cowpox.[10] In domestic cats it occurs in animals of 2–12 months of age, which normally recover within 2 months. There may be mild systemic signs including malaise, pyrexia, dyspnoea, vomiting, diarrhoea and jaundice.

Horsepox

Horsepox virus is also closely related to cowpox and vaccinia. It causes three disease syndromes affecting the distal parts of the limbs, the vulva and the buccal cavity, respectively (Table 13.1). In cattle this agent causes a syndrome identical to cowpox, and the bovine and equine diseases confer reciprocal immunity against each other. The disease is seen in Europe but is rare and seems to be less common than it was in the early part of the century.[3, 5, 11]

Parapoxvirus infections

Pseudocowpox

This parapoxvirus disease is a common, cosmopolitan infection that affects the bovine udder, causing a generally mild and very variable clinical picture (Table 13.1). Vesicle formation is uncommon but the characteristic arciform 'horseshoe' scab of mature lesions is pathognomonic for the disease.[12] In fully susceptible cattle, introduction of the virus results in an acute and more severe syndrome that rapidly spreads to most animals. The disease is endemic in many herds and immunity following infection is short lived (4–6 months). There are cycles of infection and these may coincide with stress factors such as calving or bad weather. Mature mammary lesions of pseudocowpox and bovine herpes mamillitis (see below) may be indistinguishable from those of cowpox.[12]

Bovine papular stomatitis and contagious pustular dermatitis

Two other parapoxvirus infections cause skin problems in domestic animals. Bovine papular stomatitis is a common disease of young cattle in Europe, Africa and North America (Table 13.1). The disease is usually subclinical or mild and is of little economic significance. Contagious pustular dermatitis, 'orf', occurs worldwide and commonly causes skin disease in young sheep and goats of 3–6 months of age[13] (Table 13.1). The virus is highly epitheliotropic and causes lesions, usually restricted to the nostrils and lips, characterized by the formation of thick, dense scabs that heal after about 4 weeks. Recovered animals are typically immune to reinfection for about 2–3 years. The virus survives well in dried scabs falling from affected skin and the disease tends to become endemic on premises. In endemically infected farms, vaccination of lambs and kids with suspensions of live virus prepared from scabs is carried out by scarification into the hairless skin, usually on the medial surface of the thigh, causing localized infection. An attenuated cell-culture vaccine is also made.[14]

Capripoxvirus infections
Sheep and goatpox

The capripoxvirus group includes two viruses causing severe pox diseases in small ruminants. Sheep-pox occurs in North Africa, the Middle East, southern and eastern Europe and in the Indian subcontinent, and is particularly severe in young animals. Infection leads to fever, malaise and abdominal pain followed 24–48 h later by a generalized pox eruption on the skin. Lesions also occur in the trachea, lungs, pharynx and abomasum, and fatalities may reach 50 per cent. Inactivated and attenuated virus vaccines are used to control the disease in enzootic areas.[3, 15]

Goatpox causes a similar syndrome in goats. It occurs in the same regions as sheep-pox but has also been reported in Scandinavia, Australia and the United States.[16] Goatpox immunizes sheep against sheep-pox and cattle against lumpy skin disease.[17, 18]

Lumpy skin disease

Unlike most poxvirus infections, lumpy skin disease is characterized by the formation of papules and nodules (Table 13.1). Systemic signs include pyrexia, oedema and lymphadenopathy. The extent of morbidity and mortality is very variable but may each reach as high as 50 per cent. The disease occurs in much of Africa and appears to be transmitted by biting insects. It also arises in wild ruminants and it is thought that the African buffalo (*Syncerus caffer*) may act as a reservoir of infection in some areas.[16] Vaccination with strains of sheep-pox and an attenuated strain of lumpy skin disease virus have been used to control the disease.[16] A similar clinical syndrome, 'pseudo-lumpy skin disease', can be caused by bovine herpesvirus-2 (see Table 13.2).

Swinepox

Swinepox virus is the only member of the genus *Suipoxvirus*. It causes a mild disease (Table 13.1) with some malaise and a slight pyrexia. The pocks can be quite extensive but healing occurs in about 2 weeks. Recovery may be delayed by concurrent skin infections or systemic diseases, such as bronchopneumonias or gastroenteritis, which reduce the pigs' resistance. The virus can be transmitted by direct contact but the pig sucking louse, *Haematopinus suis*, is believed to act as a mechanical vector and to cause skin damage, which is essential to permit access of the virus to susceptible layers of the epidermis.[6]

Leporipoxvirus infections
Myxomatosis

Myxomatosis is a very contagious disease caused by myxomavirus. It is highly lethal to domestic rabbits but wild breeds in Brazil and the United States are strongly resistant. In Europe, the appearance of resistant strains of wild rabbits has been reported.[19] In susceptible animals, the disease (Table 13.1) has an acute course leading to death in 7–15 days. It is spread by contact and is also transmitted by the rabbit flea, *Spilopsyllus cuniculi*. Animals that survive myxomatosis become solidly immune and vaccination with the Shope fibromavirus (Table 13.1) also gives protection, although large tumours sometimes result from vaccination of young rabbits.[20] In Angora rabbits, Shope vaccine-induced immunity is reduced in plucked areas of skin, which may then develop myxomas locally.[21]

Unclassified poxvirus infections
Ovine viral ulcerative dermatosis

This condition is caused by a virus similar to that of orf but which is antigenically distinct.[22] It occurs in Europe, the United States and South Africa, and causes balanoposthitis, vulvitis and ulcers of the limbs, lips and faces of sheep. It is transmitted at coitus, by contact and on fomites but penetration appears to require damage to skin or mucous membranes.[23] No vaccine is available. A similar condition, ulcerative posthitis and vulvitis ('sheath rot', 'pizzle rot') is associated with *Corynebacterium renale* infection.[5]

Equine papular poxvirus infections

Equine viral papular dermatosis This is caused by a virus resembling cowpox and vaccinia, which has been reported in Africa, Australasia and the United States.[24–26] The disease is mild (Table 13.1), there are no systemic signs and recovery occurs in 4–6 weeks.

Molluscum contagiosum This disease resembles that in man and occurs in horses (Table 13.1) and occasionally in non-domesticated animals. It is self-limiting and mildly contagious.[26]

Herpesvirus infections

Of the three herpesvirus subfamilies, only the *Alphaherpesvirinae* is associated with skin disease in domestic animals.

Bovine mamillitis and pseudo-lumpy skin disease

Bovine herpesvirus-2 (BHV-2), which is also known as bovine mamillitis virus (BMV), causes two dermatological syndromes, bovine herpes mamillitis and pseudo-lumpy skin disease.[5] Bovine herpes mamillitis is a disease principally of the teats (Table 13.2). There is much morbidity in primary herd infections but in previously exposed herds only first-calf heifers tend to be affected. There is a lymphadenitis and mastitis occurs in about 20 per cent of affected animals. Transmission is mechanical during milking or by means of flies. The disease can be controlled by the use of an unmodified virus strain given intramuscularly.[12, 27]

Pseudo-lumpy skin disease is very similar to the condition caused by lumpy skin disease virus (Table 13.1) but is milder and does not cause systemic signs.

Coital exanthema and similar conditions

Coital exanthema, caused by equine herpesvirus-3, is a venereal disease (Table 13.2) which may also be transmitted by contact or via fomites, insects and inhalation.[26] Uncomplicated lesions heal in about 10–14 days but the virus may persist and there may be recurrence, particularly in relation to stress. Similar skin signs are seen in cattle infected with bovine herpesvirus-1 (BHV-1), which causes infectious bovine pustular vulvovaginitis (see Table 13.4) and may cause penile or preputial damage preventing mating. BHV-1 also causes infectious bovine rhinotracheitis, a disease that can be mild or subclinical but in its acute forms causes severe systemic signs and significant economic loss.[5, 28]

Other herpesvirus-related skin signs

Three other herpesvirus infections are associated with skin lesions as minor signs (see Table 13.4). Bovine malignant catarrh is a sporadic disease with very high fatality that principally affects cattle.[29] Aujeszky's disease (pseudorabies, 'mad itch') is a disease principally of pigs but affecting a wide range of other mammalian hosts. Fatality is high in all but adult pigs, which show no skin signs. In other species, intense itching leading to severe self-inflicted wounds, neurological signs simulating rabies or sudden death occur.[5] Feline herpesvirus infection is the cause of feline viral rhinotracheitis, which has also been reported as a cause of skin lesions in cats.[30]

Papovavirus infections

The genus *Papillomavirus* contains a variety of agents, most of which affect the skin but have different sites of predilection and give rise to both true epithelial papillomas and fibropapillomas (Table 13.2).[31-33] In cattle, six serotypes have been described and are divided into subgroups A (fibropapillomas; bovine papillomavirus (BPV)-1, -2, -5) and B (epithelial papillomas; BPV-3, -4, -6).

Papillomas and papillomatoses

Bovine Bovine papillomatosis is a common disease, particularly in animals under 2 years of age and on the head. Warts often appear at sites of trauma and are prevalent especially in the winter when animals are housed in close proximity. Spontaneous remission often occurs in the spring. Inactivated vaccines, including autogenous vaccines, are used with some success in treatment and control.

Sheep, goats, pigs Papillomas are much less common in sheep and goats (Table 13.2). In sheep, they tend to affect the haired rather than woolly skin.[34] In goats, the udder and teat may be affected and transmission during milking may occur.[35] Papillomas are rare in pigs but a transmissible agent, presumed to be a papillomavirus, has been demonstrated in porcine genital papilloma.[26, 36]

Rabbit skin papillomas These are caused by the Shope papillomavirus,[37] the type species of the genus *Papillomavirus*. These papillomas are common in and readily transmitted between wild rabbits in the midwestern United States.[31] However, when transmitted to domestic rabbits (*Oryctolagus cuniculus*) or to hares, the initially benign papillomas tend to develop into carcinomas.[38]

Dogs In dogs, viral papillomatosis particularly occurs in young animals, affecting the lips and mouth, but may also involve the skin (Table 13.2). It is a highly infectious condition but resolves spontaneously after 1–5 months in most cases.[39] A second canine papillomavirus causes cutaneous papillomas that are more common in older animals.[5] In rare cases, cutaneous papillomas develop into carcinomas and therapeutic use of a live-virus vaccine prepared from oral papillomata has been followed by the occurrence of squamous cell carcinomata at the inoculation sites.[40]

Equine sarcoids

These are the most common skin tumours of horses. They have a very variable clinical appearance (Table 13.2) including verrucous, fibroplastic, mixed and

Table 13.2. *Dermatoses of domestic animals caused by DNA viruses: herpesviruses, papillomaviruses and parvoviruses*

Virus family	Genus	Skin disease (virus)	Species	Dermatological signs
Herpes	Alpha	Bovine herpes mamillitis	Cattle	Vesicles appear suddenly on swollen, painful teats and the epithelium sloughs leading to exudation and crust formation. In severe cases, bluish discoloration, necrosis and ulceration may occur. Lesions may extend to the udder and perineal region. Sucking calves may develop lesions of the muzzle
		Pseudo-lumpy skin disease (BHV-2, BMV)		Lesions as in lumpy skin disease but are more superficial
		Equine herpes coital exanthema (EHV-3)	Horses	Papules, vesicles and pustules develop into crusted erosions and ulcers Prepuce and penis or vulva and perineum are affected in stallions and mares. Lesions may also occur on lips and nostrils
Papova	Papilloma	Bovine papillomavirus (BPV-1–6)	Cattle	BPV-1, fibropapillomas of teat and penis; BPV-2, fibropapillomas of head, neck, dewlap, sometimes teats and legs, of cattle under 2 years old; BPV-3, atypical warts; BPV-5, 'rice grain' fibropapillomatous warts on the teats of cattle of any age: BPV-6, mammary gland skin papillomas; BPV-4, principally affects the gut
		Ovine papillomavirus	Sheep	Fibropapillomas on the hairy skin of face and legs
		Caprine papillomavirus	Goats	Fibropapillomas on udder, teats and other areas of skin
		Porcine papillomavirus	Pigs	Affecting genital regions
		Shope rabbit papillomavirus	Rabbits	Single or multiple, grey-black horny tumours particularly affecting the neck, shoulders, abdomen and medial surfaces of the thighs; tend to develop into carcinomas in domestic rabbits
		Canine viral papillomavirus	Dogs	Multiple flat to pedunculated and cauliflower-like lesions (<2 cm diameter) affecting the lips and oral cavity, eyelids, conjunctiva and skin of young dogs
		Equine sarcoid (BPV?)	Horses	Typically, multiple verrucous lesions on muzzles, also genitals and distal parts of limbs, of horses less than 4 years old. Also causes plaques on the ears (aural plaques) and perineum
Parvo		Swine parvovirus vesicular disease	Pigs	Vesicles and erosions of coronets, interdigital spaces, snout and mouth

Table 13.3. *Dermatoses of domestic animals caused by RNA viruses*

Virus family	Genus	Skin disease (virus)	Species	Dermatological signs
Retro	Onco	Feline leukaemia virus (FeLV)	Cats	Cutaneous lymphosarcoma. Generalized or multifocal, rarely solitary, often pruritic lesions presenting as nodules, plaques, ulcers, erythroderma and exfoliative dermatitis
		Feline sarcoma virus (FeSV)	Cats	Multicentric fibrosarcomas in cats < 4 months old; benign, spontaneously regressing in older cats

Table 13.4. *Viral diseases with skin signs as a minor feature : DNA viruses*

Virus family	Genus	Disease (virus)	Species	Dermatological signs
Herpes	Alpha	Infectious bovine rhinotracheitis and infectious bovine pustular vulvovaginitis (BHV-1)	Cattle	Pustules, ulceration and necrosis of the muzzle and/or vulva, penis and prepuce. Perineum, scrotum and udder may be affected
		Bovine malignant catarrh (BHV-3, possibly others)	Cattle, other ruminants	Crusting, ulceration, necrosis of muzzle, periocular skin and sometimes vulva, scrotum, udder, teats. Coronitis may occur
		Aujeszky's disease	Pigs, ruminants, carnivores	Intense, localized pruritus ('mad itch'), self-inflicted lesions
		Feline herpesvirus infection (FHV-1)	Cats	Multiple, superficial ulcers over all parts of the body
Irido		African swine fever	Pigs	Hyperaemia, cyanosis, subcutaneous haemorrhage, haematomas of ears, haunches; localized areas of skin necrosis.

occult forms.[26] Transmission can be by contact and they often arise in areas subjected to injury. Epizootic spread has been described.[41] Although papova-virus and in particular, BPV, is believed to be the causative agent, this is unconfirmed and genetic predilection associated with the major histocompati-bility complex may be involved.[26]

Parvovirus infections

The only parvovirus infection affecting the skin of domestic animals is a vesicular disease of pigs (Table 13.2), reported in the United States in 1985.[42] Morbidity and mortality were up to 100 per cent and 58 per cent, respectively. The disease could be reproduced in normal pigs.

Retrovirus infections

This group of RNA viruses contains two members causing tumours in cats. Feline leukaemia virus (FeLV) is a typical C-type oncovirus and is the cause of most forms of lymphosarcoma in the cat (Table 13.3). It is also an underlying factor in feline cutaneous horns; liposarcoma can be induced by injection of this agent.[40, 43] Feline sarcoma virus is believed to be a recombinant form of FeLV, incorporating chromosomal DNA, which arises in individual cats and induces the formation of fibrosarcomas (Table 13.3). It does not appear to be contagious.[44]

Viral diseases with minor skin signs

A variety of other DNA and RNA viruses induce the formation of skin lesions as a minor part of the disease syndromes that they cause (Tables 13.4 and 13.5). Detailed consideration of these conditions is beyond the scope of this review.

Scrapie agent

Scrapie is an insidious, chronic, afebrile disease of sheep and goats caused by a 'slow virus', the nature of which is as yet unknown.[45] Initial signs of unease and unsteadiness are followed by pruritus, with rubbing and nibbling leading to progressive loss of the coat. At this stage a papular rash and serous exudation of areas of hairy skin may occur. Subsequently, progressive wasting and incoordination occur. Mortality approaches 100 per cent.

Table 13.5. *Viral diseases with skin signs as a minor feature: RNA viruses*

Virus family	Genus	Disease (virus)	Species	Dermatological signs
Toga	Pesti	Bovine virus diarrhoea (BVD, MD)	Cattle	Focal erosions may coalesce causing necrosis of lips, muzzle, nostrils, prepuce, vulva, interdigital region and coronet
		Border disease	Sheep	Lambs are born with a hairy coat and nervous abnormalities ('hairy shakers')
		Swine fever (hog cholera)	Pigs	Patchy erythema then purple discoloration of medial thighs, abdomen, snout, ears. Necrosis of vulva, tail and pinnae of ears
		Equine viral arteritis	Horses	Oedema of ventrum, sheath, scrotum and distal parts of limbs
Calici	Calici	Feline calicivirus (FCV)	Cats	Swollen painful feet, blisters of interdigital skin and ulcers of footpads with oral ulceration ('Paw and mouth disease') (?FCV)
Picorna	Aptho	Foot and mouth disease	Ruminants, pigs	Vesicular bullous and painful erosive lesions of nostrils, muzzle, interdigital spaces, coronets, teats and udder. Exungulation may occur, particularly in pigs
	Calici	Vesicular exanthema	Pigs	As for foot and mouth disease
	Entero	Swine vesicular disease	Pigs	As for foot and mouth disease
Rhabdo	Vesiculo	Vesicular stomatitis	Cattle, pigs, horses	As for foot and mouth disease
Paramyxo	Morbilli	Rinderpest	Ruminants	Erythema, papules and exudation of skin; erosions of muzzle, lips and teats; later crusting and hair loss
		Peste des petits ruminants (PPR)	Sheep	As for rinderpest; buccal lesions like orf
		Canine distemper	Dogs	Hyperkeratosis of the footpads and planum nasale ('hardpad')
Reo	Orbi	Blue tongue	Sheep, goats	Oedema of buccal mucosa, face, ears and throat; erosions of muzzle lips and teats; coronitis and lameness; ocular discharge
		Blue tongue, epizootic haemorrhagic disease (EHDV), Ibaraki disease	Cattle	Erosions and crusting of teats; coronitis; skin thickening, cracking and peeling particularly of neck and perineum
	Unclassified	Caprine viral dermatitis	Goats	Papules, nodules and ulcers giving rise to crusts
Retro	Lenti	Feline T-lymphotropic lentivirus	Cats	Causes immunodeficiency and secondary pustular dermatitis, gingivitis and stomatitis

References

1 Beran GW. Section B: Viral zoonoses. In: Steele JH, Beran GW, eds. CRC handbook series in zoonoses. Boca Raton, FA: CRC Press; 1981.

2 Gibbs EPJ. Differential diagnosis of virus infections of the skin. In: Howard JL, ed. Current veterinary therapy: food animal practice. Philadelphia: WB Saunders; 1981: 1161–66.

3 Tripathy DN, Hanson LE, Crandell RA. Poxviruses of veterinary importance: diagnosis of infections. In: Kurstak E, Kurstack C, eds. Comparative diagnosis of viral diseases, vol 3. New York: Academic Press; 1981: 267–346.

4 Thomsett LR. Feline poxvirus infection. In: Kirk RW, ed. Current veterinary therapy IX. Philadelphia: WB Saunders; 1986: 605.

5 Timoney JF, Gillespie JH, Scott FW, Barlough JE. Hagan and Bruner's microbiology and infectious diseases of domestic animals. 8th ed. Ithaca: Comstock Publishing; 1988.

6 Kasza L. Swine pox. In: Leman AD, Straw B, Glock RD, Mengeling WL, Penny RHC, Scholl E, eds. Diseases of swine. 6th ed. Ames: Iowa State University Press; 1986: 315–20.

7 Baxby D. Poxvirus hosts and reservoirs. Arch Virol 1977; 55: 169–79.

8 Lal SM, Singh IP. Buffalopox – a review. Trop Anim Hlth Prod 1977; 9: 107.

9 Lane JM, Steele JH, Beran GW. Pox and parapoxvirus infections. Volume 2: viral zoonoses. In: Steele JH, Beran GW, eds. Handbook series in zoonoses. Boca Raton, FA: CRC Press; 1981: 365–85.

10 Bennett AM, Gaskell CJ, Baxby D, Gaskell RM, Kelley DF, Naidoo J. Feline cowpox virus infection. J Small Anim Pract 1990; 31: 167–73.

11 De Jong DA. The relationship between contagious pustular stomatitis of the horse, equine variola (horse-pox of Jenner), and vaccinia (cow-pox of Jenner). J Comp Pathol Ther 1917; 30: 242–62.

12 Gibbs EPJ. Viral diseases of the bovine teat and udder. Vet Clin North Am [Large Anim Pract] 1984; 6: 187–202.

13 Robinson AJ, Balassu TC. Contagious pustular dermatitis (orf). Vet Bull 1981; 51: 771–82.

14 Mayr A, Herlyn M, Mahnel H, Danco A, Zach A, Bosted H. Control of ecthyma contagiosum (pustular dermatitis) of sheep with a new parenteral cell culture vaccine. Zentralbl Veterinarme B 1981; 28: 535–52.

15 Solyom F, Perenlei L, Roith J. Sheep-pox vaccine prepared from formaldehyde inactivated virus adsorbed to aluminium hydroxide gel. Acta Microbiol Acad Sci Hung 1982; 29: 69–75.

16 Davies FG. Sheep and goat pox. In: Gibbs EPJ, ed. Virus diseases of food animals, vol 2. London: Academic Press; 1981: 733–49.

17 Sharma NS, Dhands MR. Studies on the interrelationship between sheep and goat pox viruses. Indian J Anim Sci 1971; 41: 267–72.

18 Capstick PB, Brydie J, Coakley W, Burdin ML. Protection of cattle against the virus of lumpy skin disease. Vet Rec 1959; 71: 422–23.

19 Ross J, Sanders MF. The development of genetic resistance to myxomatosis in wild rabbits in Britain. J Hyg Camb 1984; 92: 255–61.

20 Ritchie JN, Hudson JR, Thompson HV. Myxomatosis. Vet Rec 1954; 66: 796–804.

21 Ganiere J-P, Gourreau J-M, Montabord D, Rive M, Chantal J. Myxomatosis of the depilated Angora rabbit. A preliminary study. Vet Dermatol 1991; 2: 1–16.

22 Trueblood MS, Chow TL. Characterization of the agents of ulcerative dermatosis and contagious ecthyma. Am J Vet Res 1963; 24: 42.

23 Morin ML, Baas EJ. Ulcerative dermatosis of sheep. In: Howard JL, ed. Current veterinary therapy: food animal practice. Philadelphia: WB Saunders; 1981: 630–1.

24 Kaminjolo JS, Nyaga PN, Gicho JN. Isolation, cultivation and characterisation of a poxvirus from some horses in Kenya. Zentralbl Veterinarmed B 1974; 21: 592–601.

25 Pascoe RR. A colour atlas of equine dermatology. London: Wolf Publishing; 1990.

26 Scott DW. Large animal dermatology. Philadelphia: WB Saunders, 1988.

27 Gibbs EPJ, Rweyemamu MM. Bovine herpesvirus: I. bovine herpesvirus 1. II. bovine herpesvirus 2 and 3. Vet Bull 1977; 47: 411–25.

28 Crandell RA. Infectious bovine rhinotracheitis. In: Howard JL, ed. Current veterinary therapy: food animal practice. Philadelphia: WB Saunders, 1981: 543–46.

29 Plowright W. Malignant catarrhal fever virus: a lymphotropic herpesvirus of ruminants. In: Wittman G, Gaskell R, Rhiza H, eds. Latent herpes virus infections in veterinary medicine. Boston: Martinus Nijhoff; 1984: 270–305.

30 Flecknell PA, Wright AI, Gaskell RM, Kelly DF. Skin ulceration associated with herpes virus infection in cats. Vet Rec 1979; 104: 313–15.

31 Lancaster WD, Olsen C. Animal papillomaviruses. Microbiol Rev 1982; 46: 191–207.

32 Hunt E. Infectious skin diseases of cattle. Vet Clin North Am [Large Anim Pract] 1984; 6: 155–74.

33 Jarrett WF, Campo MS, O'Neil BW, Laird HM, Coggins LW. A novel bovine papillomavirus (BPV-6) causing true epithelial papillomas of the mammary gland skin: a member of a proposed new BPV subgroup. Virol 1984; 30: 255–64.

34 Mullowney PC. Skin diseases of sheep. Vet Clin North Am [Large Anim Pract] 1984; 6: 131–42.

35 Mullowney PC, Baldwin EW. Skin diseases of goats. Vet Clin North Am [Large Anim Pract] 1984; 6: 142–54.

36 Parish WE. An immunological study of the transmissible genital papilloma of pigs. J Pathol 1962; 83: 429–42.

37 Shope RE. Infectious papillomatosis of rabbits: a virus disease. J Exp Med 1933; 58: 607–24.

38 Kidd JG, Rouse P. A transplantable rabbit carcinoma originating in a virus-induced papilloma and containing the virus in masked or altered form. J Exp Med 1940; 71: 813–38.

39 Calvert CA. Canine viral and transmissible neoplasms. In: Green CE, ed. Clinical microbiology and infectious diseases of the dog and cat. Philadelphia: WB Saunders; 1984: 461–78.

40 Muller GH, Kirk RW, Scott DW. Small animal dermatology. 4th ed. Philadelphia: WB Saunders; 1989.

41 Ragland WL, et al. An epizootic of equine sarcoid. Nature 1966; 210: 1399.

42 Kresse JL, et al. Parvovirus infection in pigs with necrotic and vesicle-like lesions. Vet Microbiol 1985; 10: 525–31.

43 Barton CL. The feline leukemia virus: pathogenesis of disease. In: Scott FW, ed. Contemporary issues in small animal practice, vol 3: infectious diseases. New York: Churchill Livingstone; 1986: 109–28.

44 Hardy WD. The feline sarcoma viruses. J Am Anim Hosp Assoc 1981; 17: 981–87.

45 Carp RI, Merz PA, Kascsak RJ, Merz GS, Wisniewski HM. Nature of the scrapie agent: current status of facts and hypotheses. J Gen Virol 1985; 66: 1357–68.

14

Microbial interactions on skin

R. P. ALLAKER & W. C. NOBLE

Metabolic interactions

The physical and chemical interactions between bacteria and fungi on the skin of man and animals remain inadequately understood. Many such interactions have been demonstrated under experimental conditions; however, their contribution to maintaining the stability of the ecosystem on the skin under natural circumstances remains unclear. Such inherent stability is thought to be a major factor in preventing the establishment of pathogens.[1]

In 1928 Papacostas and Gate[2] first described the main forms of interaction between microorganisms on the skin as: unilateral and reciprocal antagonism ('interference'), unilateral enhancement ('satellitism'), reciprocal enhancement (symbiosis or synergism), and neutral or indifferent association. This has provided a useful classification; however, most reports have focused only on the first of these interactions. Here, attention will be concentrated on the aspects of antagonism and growth enhancement.

Antagonism

One of the earliest reports of this was by Pasteur and Joubert in 1877, who described the in vitro inhibition of *Bacillus anthracis* by an unidentified airborne bacterium.[3] This observation led them to suggest the application of bacterial antagonism to the treatment of infection. However, the precise mechanisms by which an antagonist creates unfavourable growth conditions for another organism remain poorly understood. Antagonism may result from the production of certain inhibitors, exhaustion of nutrient, creation of unfavourable pH or redox potential, or the modification or masking of tissue receptors.

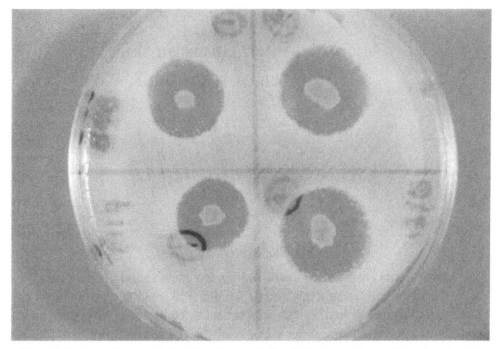

Fig. 14.1. Agar plate seeded with a lawn of *Staph. hyicus* and spot inoculated with
Staph. epidermidis.

Inhibitory compounds

A wide range of inhibitors produced by members of the skin microflora, from
the low molecular-weight end-products of metabolism to the large, complex
protein molecules such as bacteriocins, are known to exist. The production of
certain of these inhibitors is readily demonstrated in the laboratory (Fig. 14.1).
The major types of inhibitor are considered here.

Small metabolic end-products Microorganisms may produce gaseous inhibitors. King and coworkers[4] described the inhibition of dermatophytes by
carbon dioxide evolved by *Candida albicans* and suggested that this might
account for the apparent absence of dermatophytes in lesions infected with
C. albicans. However Moore-Landecker and Stotsky[5] reported that many
bacterial species, including *Micrococcus luteus* from the skin, would inhibit
several fungal species, but considered that carbon dioxide was not wholly
responsible for this.

Other simple compounds may act as inhibitors, for example hydrogen
peroxide formed by streptococci, aerococci and lactobacilli. Indeed it was
reported that hydrogen peroxide formed by lactobacilli will inhibit the growth
of *Staphylococcus aureus* despite the production of catalase by staphylococci.[6]

It is also suggested that the accumulation of short-chain carboxylic acids to toxic levels on the skin – for example, propionic acid produced by members of the genus *Propionibacterium* – will lead to the growth inhibition of neighbouring bacteria.[7]

Bacteriolytic enzymes Strains of *Propionibacterium acnes* have been found to lyse pregrown cells of both staphylococci and other propionibacteria, presumably through the action of bacteriolytic enzymes.[8] Other such enzymes include the proteases of *Bacillus* spp.[9] and lysozyme secreted by staphylococci,[10] both of which are thought to protect the skin against invasion by certain pathogens.

Lipolysis products Sebaceous lipids and their breakdown products have attracted interest as potential inhibitory agents. The production of fatty acids by bacterial lipolysis is probably of significance against streptococci and Gram-negative bacteria, but not against staphylococci on the skin surface.[11] It is also thought that the inhibition of dermatophytes by the yeast *Malassezia furfur*[12] is possibly due to the action of lipolysis products.

Antibiotics Antibiotics are a major class of inhibitory compounds produced by many members of the skin microflora. These are defined as products of secondary metabolism, which are active at low concentrations to cause bacteriostatic or bactericidal effects.

The dermatophytes produce a wide range of antibiotics, including penicillin and compounds closely related to streptomycin, fusidic acid, actinomycin and azalomycin.[13–16] Antibiotic production has readily been detected in artificial media; in skin cultures, evidence of antibiotic activity has been obtained in morphological studies using scanning electron microscopy.[17] The production of antibiotics by dermatophytes in vivo has been demonstrated indirectly; for example, an increased frequency of antibiotic-resistant bacteria is found in the vicinity of tinea lesions.[18,19] Experimentally explanted pieces of skin from human or animal dermatophyte infection have also been used to demonstrate penicillin production.[20,21]

It is also well recognized that bacteria produce antibiotics; however, the proportion that actually produce these on the skin remains unknown. Two main classes of substances are produced. One is the group of peptides with molecular weights of 800–1200, these probably being cyclic in configuration and similar to the commercially available gramicidin. The other group comprises high molecular-weight substances. Many workers have reported the in vitro production of 'antibiotics' but have failed properly to identify the compounds involved. A number of non-antibiotic compounds such as peroxides or simple organic acids may account for some of the activity observed.

The staphylococci are known to produce antibiotics[22-24] which are chiefly effective against other Gram-positive bacteria. Antibiotics are produced by the coryneforms; however, these are more restricted in their range of activity than those from staphylococci. In a detailed study by Holland and coworkers[25] it was shown that although 40 per cent of *P. acnes* strains would inhibit others of the same species, inhibition was restricted when compared to the extent of species inhibited by the micrococcaceae. The *Brevibacterium* spp. appear to be exceptional among coryneforms in producing relatively broad-spectrum polypeptide antibiotics and this activity may be responsible for the suppression of other bacteria in tinea pedis.[26]

Bacteriocins Many bacteriocins act like antibiotics but tend to have a narrower spectrum of action and generally prevent the growth only of members of the same or closely related species as the producer. Bacteriocins are a diverse group of substances, usually proteins and frequently of high molecular weight.

Bacteriocins are known to be produced by the Gram-positive bacteria.[27] The bacteriocin produced by some strains of *S. aureus* is of particular interest because of its wide spectrum of activity and the demonstration of in vivo activity.[28] The production of bacteriocins by coryneforms isolated from the skin has not been studied in detail, although Somerville[29] did report production by some of the aerobic coryneforms, and activity of the bacteriocin produced by *Corynebacterium jeikeium* has been demonstrated in mouse models of skin colonization.[30]

In vitro studies of microbial antagonism

A number of model systems have been used to study microbial interactions in vitro. Selwyn and his colleagues[31,32] completed an extensive study of the production of a peptide antibiotic by a strain of *S. epidermidis* (S6+) under a range of experimental conditions. The antagonistic activity of S6+ was studied in a semiquantitative method on solid media and quantitatively in liquid batch culture.[31] On solid media, S6+ unilaterally inhibited members of all the Gram-positive species tested, but had limited activity against Gram-negative species. In liquid cultures, S6+ was usually able to inhibit other competing strains; however, more complex interactions were sometimes observed. Milyani and Selwyn[32] clearly demonstrated that the inhibitory effect of S6+ was more pronounced on solid than in liquid media, and that this could be attributed to dilution of the antibiotic in the liquid. However, the inhibition of certain indicator strains on solid media was shown to depend on the absolute and relative size of the S6+ inoculum; if this was too low, the indicator grew normally. Such studies emphasize the inadequacies of certain in vitro model systems to study the possible interactions on the skin. Therefore, conditions in which organisms grow on the skin must be adequately reproduced in vitro before the importance of antagonistic strains in the skin microenvironment can be properly assessed. A number of attempts have been made to develop a medium that would closely resemble the chemical composition of the epidermis.[33, 34] For example, Ryall and colleagues[35] used a medium containing skin keratin as the major nutrient to study antibiotic production by dermatophytes. The physical distribution of test strains used in vitro models should also be considered. Malcolm and Hughes,[36] using scanning electron microscopy, were able to demonstrate the location of bacteria on and within the stratum corneum of the human foot. The bacteria of the skin surface were widely scattered in small colonies, a spatial relationship that may affect antibiotic sensitivity on the skin. Indeed, Milyani and Selwyn[32] showed that antibiotic production would be insufficient to suppress the growth of sensitive strains if the producer strain was too widely dispersed.

There remains the problem of whether bacterial inhibitors are produced on the skin of the natural host as distinct from experimental studies. If production occurred in vivo it would seem to imply that producer organisms should be the dominant form, because producer strains should outgrow non-producers. The work of Wright and Terry[37] showed that inhibitory strains do not necessarily dominate numerically on healthy skin but they may control the population densities of sensitive resident organisms. In contrast, Selwyn[38] demonstrated that inhibitory strains did predominate in the lesions of dermatological patients and he associated their presence with protection against secondary infection. However, Noble and Willie[39] were unable to confirm these results and observed that carriage of inhibitory strains was not associated with protection against colonization by *S. aureus* (Table 14.1).

In vivo studies: the use of antagonism to control microbial skin disease

The role of microbial interactions as a major mechanism in controlling colonization of the skin is of particular therapeutic interest. Antagonistic interaction that may enhance the host's capacity to resist infection by bacteria is often referred to as 'bacterial interference'. Interest in bacterial interference has been accelerated because of the limited usefulness of antibiotics as prophylactic agents and the increased prevalence of antibiotic resistance exhibited by some strains. Two main types of interference are thought to

Table 14.1. *Relapse in chronic staphylococcal skin infection in patients treated with antibiotics with or without nasal implantation of* S. aureus *502A*

	Number of families	Number of individuals	Number (%) relapse
Controls	27	85	31 (36)
502A treated	33	118	11 (9)

Based on Steele[47] and Boris and coworkers.[48]

operate. The first is 'colonization resistance', in which the antagonist occupies available niches and utilizes the nutrient supply, thereby excluding the pathogen. The second type would use organisms that produce inhibitors active against the pathogen.

In vivo models for examining interactions on the skin have used the hairless obese mouse[40] and the rabbit.[41] Such studies suggested that inhibition was caused by bacteria that produce inhibitors acting against the pathogen *S. aureus* on the skin surface. These two systems required cultures applied to the skin to be occluded with plastic film, which emphasizes the difficulty of establishing a new flora on skin with an established microbial flora. In studies of subcutaneous infection,[40] inhibitor-producing bacteria were unable to suppress the growth of *S. aureus*. This failure might have been due to the poor ability of certain inhibitor-producing strains to survive subcutaneously.

A mouse model developed by Noble and coworkers[28] was used to study the interactions of antibiotic-producing staphylococci and the cattle pathogen *Dermatophilus congolensis*. It was observed that lesion formation by *D. congolensis* could be suppressed by inhibitor-producing cocci, including the *S. epidermidis* strain S6+, applied to the skin in cetomacrogol cream.

Other in vivo models have included those of Wickman,[42] who reported that *S. epidermidis* applied to burns would prevent subsequent infection with *S. aureus*, and Dajani and Wannamaker,[43] who described the suppression of streptococci by *S. aureus* in a hamster model of impetigo.

Bacterial interference and the control of staphylococcal skin disease
S. aureus 502 A and human infections During outbreaks of staphylococcal sepsis among newborn infants in the 1960s it was observed that early colonization with non-pathogenic staphylococci could protect against virulent strains. Subsequently Shinefield and colleagues[44] used the *S. aureus* strain 502A as a prophylactic agent; 502A had been isolated from the nose of a nurse and could readily colonize babies both by natural transmission and after

Table 14.2. *Carriage of inhibitor-producing organisms in relation to lesion colonization with* S. aureus: *data from two studies*

	Number (%) of lesions colonized with *S. aureus*			
	Colonized	Not colonized[a]	Colonized	Not colonized[b]
Patients with inhibitors	8 (16)	43 (84)	9 (38)	15 (63)
Without inhibitors	84 (40)	128 (60)	118 (42)	166 (58)

[a] Based on Selwyn[38] and [b] on Noble.[39]

artificial inoculation. During epidemics of neonatal infections with *S. aureus* strains of phage type 80/81, babies colonized with 502A had considerably fewer infections than those not colonized by the antagonist.[45] Unfortunately, 502A was found to be capable of producing occasional severe infections in infants[46] and its use in non-epidemic situations is contraindicated except in the control of chronic furunculosis, where it provides an effective measure[47-49] (Table 14.2).

Nasal colonization with 502A in adults was more difficult to achieve than in neonates and required a much larger bacterial inoculum. Also, in contrast to infants, who needed no antibacterial preparation, the pre-existing microflora of the anterior nares had to be suppressed by both topical and systemic agents; successful colonization then gave a more limited protection against staphylococcal cross-infection than in neonates.[50]

No antibacterial substance seems to be produced by 502A[51] and therefore its mode of interference does not appear to be by the production of a bacteriocin or other inhibitor. It is thought that the interference observed with strain 502A is due to colonization resistance; perhaps tissue receptors are masked or modified by 502A.

Exudative epidermitis of pigs Studies have been undertaken to evaluate the prospects of using bacterial interference in the control of exudative epidermitis of piglets caused by *Staphylococcus hyicus*. A reproducible model of *S. hyicus* infection in the germ-free piglet has been developed[52] to enable the interaction of individual organisms to be studied in isolation. Precolonization with certain inhibitor-producing bacteria can delay the onset of exudative epidermitis[53,54] and antagonism by an avirulent variant of *S. hyicus* can completely prevent the disease (Fig. 14.2).[55]

Competition for available niches in the ecosystem is thought to be an important interference factor in the experimental prevention of exudative

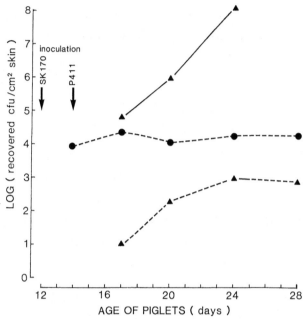

Fig. 14.2. Mean counts (cfu, colony-farming units) of avirulent *Staph. hyicus* (SK170)
and virulent *Staph. hyicus* (P411) on the skin of gnotobiotic piglets. Colonization with
P411 (▲--------▲) two days after colonisation with SK170 (●-------●); P411
(▲———▲) alone.

epidermitis. However, the relative contribution of inhibitory substances has
yet to be established. It has not been possible to detect inhibitor in concentrated
skin washings obtained from gnotobiotic piglets colonized with inhibitor-
producing staphylococci.[53]

Investigations to determine the use of antagonistic bacteria in the control of
S. hyicus infection of pigs under farming conditions have been undertaken.[56]
Studies have shown that the normal skin flora of the pig is created almost
immediately at birth and a rise in the number of staphylococci and coryneforms
within the sow's vulva and vagina immediately before parturition appears to
promote this. Once the flora is established it is difficult to introduce other
bacteria. Thus it may be necessary to insert potentially antagonistic organisms
into the vulval flora of the sow before parturition to ensure that they are
inoculated on to and become established in the piglet skin flora at the earliest
opportunity. In a similar situation in man it has been shown that at birth the
organisms arriving first will generally prevail.[57]

Bovine mastitis Although current preventative measures, including sanitation
and dry-cow therapy, in the control of bovine mastitis have been partially
successful, the disease remains a costly problem to the dairy industry. A factor

contributing to differences in the susceptibility of individual animals to mastitis may be differences in the ecology of the normal flora on the teat ends.[58] Woodward and coworkers[59] attempted to colonize teat ends with organisms previously shown to inhibit *S. aureus* and other mastitis pathogens in vitro. However, the inhibitor-producing bacteria used were only able to persist for a limited time on the teats and the ability of such organisms to increase resistance to infection remains to be properly evaluated.

Other staphylococcal diseases Bacterial interference appears to be particularly useful in the control of certain staphylococcal skin diseases in both man and animals. Its use may therefore be of value in the treatment of other skin conditions involving staphylococci. Interference mechanisms may well be able to prevent and control canine pyoderma, one of the most common diseases of the skin encountered in veterinary practice. The principal causative organism of canine pyoderma is *Staphylococcus intermedius* and it is possible that an avirulent variant[60] may interfere with colonization by virulent strains.

Growth enhancement

The converse of antagonistic interactions, growth synergy or enhancement, has attracted little attention by comparison. In contrast to the many antimicrobial factors produced by the skin microflora directly or indirectly from epidermal substrates, only a relatively small number of products are able to enhance microbial growth. These include certain lipids, some amino acids and other nutrients, and a specific growth factor related to coenzyme A.[33]

The laboratory stimulation of certain skin bacteria by others can easily be demonstrated and indeed is frequently seen in routine skin cultures. Examples of enhancement relevant to skin ecology include the growth stimulation of dermatophytes by micrococci,[17] perhaps as a result of fungal attraction to a gradient of bacteria-processed skin nutrients, and the aerobic growth of *P. acnes*,[61] possibly as a result of other bacteria lowering the oxygen tension.

The possible importance of growth enhancement in vivo is indicated by several reports of the potentiation of clinical infection, especially for a number of anaerobic skin infections.[62] Staphylococci are known to promote anaerobic infections, as in progressive synergistic gangrene. It is thought that the hyaluronidase from *S. aureus*, together with an unidentified growth factor, enables anaerobic cocci to invade the tissues.

In a mouse model of *D. congolensis* infection, Lloyd and Noble[63] demonstrated that some strains of staphylococci were associated with enhanced formation of lesions. This increased pathogenicity may involve chemotropic attraction of the zoospores of *D. congolensis* towards carbon dioxide[64] produced by the staphylococci or perhaps the production of a probiotic factor.

The role of growth enhancement in the microbial ecology of skin has yet to be studied systematically and could well prove to be a significant factor both in the promotion and prevention of disease.

Comment

Many fascinating problems of the cutaneous ecosystem remain to be elucidated, apart from the obvious antibiotic and probiotic mechanisms of interaction. The importance of more complex interactions, including the competition for essential growth substrates, the production of accessory growth factors and the production of enzymes that destroy inhibitors, remains to be determined.

The use of natural antibiosis as a therapeutic tool is an obvious application developed from our understanding of both the antagonism and growth enhancement aspects of interactions between microorganisms on the skin. It does appear that the use of avirulent variants to reduce the colonization of virulent organisms may be the most effective method of interference. However, the possibility that avirulent strains may acquire a capacity for virulence must be thoroughly examined before more extensive use. The alternative and perhaps safer method is offered by the use of non-pathogenic inhibitor producing organisms, but this too requires further evaluation. It is possible that microorganisms could be designed, using genetic manipulation, to meet given stipulations if a naturally occurring one is not available.

Genetic interactions

There is a well-established relationship between antibiotic usage in hospital and the appearance of resistant strains in patients treated in that hospital. This has been well documented for staphylococci and neomycin,[65] gentamicin[66-68] and erythromycin.[69] Among outpatients, treatment with erythromycin for acne has been shown to result in the appearance of resistant strains, which may result in therapeutic failure[70,71] and a similar phenomenon may have occurred in patients treated with erythromycin for cutaneous diphtheria.[72] In such cases the overwhelming probability is for selection of pre-existing resistant strains and elimination of sensitive organisms.

However, the prevalence of plasmids in microorganisms argues for transfer mechanisms that operate in vivo. Conjugative mechanisms of gene transfer seem inherently more likely to operate on the relatively dry surface of the skin than do transformation or transduction (but see below) and it has generally been assumed, as a result of parallel experiments in vitro, that it is conjugative transfer that operates on the skin.

Acquisition of antibiotic resistance plasmids by *Staphylococcus aureus* under natural conditions has been recorded.[73] Two patients in a hospital for skin disease carried different, single strains of *S. aureus* on admission to hospital. During therapy with topical gentamicin both strains, together with a third strain acquired by one of these patients during her hospital stay, became resistant to gentamicin by acquisition of a plasmid. In one case, a *S. hominis* strain also resistant to gentamicin and recovered from the patient's skin was shown to be capable of transferring a conjugative gentamicin-resistance plasmid to the two strains of *S. aureus* carried by the patient (Fig. 14.3) and is assumed to have been the original source of the resistance plasmid. Conversely, loss of antibiotic resistance in a single strain of *S. aureus* has also been reported.[74] It is thought that therapy with cloxacillin was responsible for the loss of penicillin plus fusidic acid resistance or loss of streptomycin plus neomycin sometimes linked to loss of erythromycin resistance. The location of the genes on plasmid or chromosome was not determined.

Staphylococci

The similarity of specific resistance plasmids in coagulase-positive and -negative staphylococci in hospital outbreaks and in the staphylococci generally has been described by several groups. Thus tetracycline-resistance plasmids in staphylococci of human origin have been described as belonging to a closely related group when studied by restriction endonuclease analysis[75, 76] and some, though not all, tetracycline-resistance plasmids from animal staphylococci also belong to this group.[77-80] Similarly, plasmids mediating resistance to streptomycin in strains of human and animal origin share the same structural group.[81] Apparently identical trimethoprim-resistance determinants have been shown to occur in coagulase-positive and -negative cocci[82] and the same is true for chloramphenicol-resistance plasmids.[83] No particular transfer mechanism has been suggested for these plasmids but the conjugative mode of transfer has been invoked by several groups to account for the similarity of gentamicin plasmids.[84-88]

Conjugative transfer in staphylococci in vitro requires the cells of donor and recipient to be in intimate contact. Experimental systems that would permit the transfer of phage but not cell-to-cell contact do not result in conjugative transfer. The presence of DNAase does not prevent transfer, apparently eliminating transformation, and removal of calcium ions, which are usually

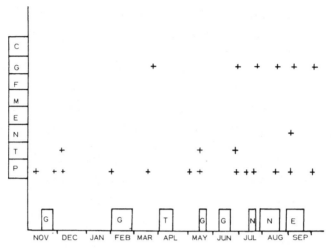

Fig. 14.3. Acquisition of antibiotic resistance during therapy. Therapy (see key below) is shown as blocks on the base line; crosses represent resistance to the antibiotic. This patient carried a single strain of *Staph. aureus*, which acquired resistance to neomycin and gentamicin. P = penicillin, T = tetracycline, N = neomycin, E = erythromycin, M = methicillin, F = fusidic acid, G = gentamicin, C = clindamycin. (Based on Naidoo and Noble.[73])

needed for phage activity, also has no effect on conjugation.[89, 90] Nevertheless, two types of transfer may occur in vitro; one without phage but one that is best described as phage-mediated conjugation in which cell-bound phages are proposed to account for the results observed.[91]

In vitro conjugative transfer is achieved by placing donor and recipient on a filter and incubating this on agar without antibiotic. Transconjugants are then recovered by diluting and inoculating the consequent growth on media containing two or more antibiotics. In vivo, donor and recipient strains are inoculated on intact human, mouse or dog skin under occlusion for 6 h, after which transconjugants are recovered as described above.[92, 93] Table 14.3 shows that transfer is frequently more efficient on skin than on filters or in broth. Transfer is rarely very efficient in vivo but some strains may give excellent transfer rates.[94-99] Conjugative gentamicin-resistance plasmids have been shown to transfer between strains of *S. aureus*, bidirectionally between *S. aureus* and coagulase-negative staphylococci, and extensively within the coagulase-negative cocci.[100] Gentamicin and also mupirocin-resistance plasmids transfer between *S. aureus* and *S. intermedius* on filters and on canine and murine skin.[100, 101] The ability to demonstrate in vivo transfers that exactly parallel those achieved on filters leads to an assumption that data from these experiments are essentially interchangeable.

It is interesting that transfer is best between taxonomically closely related

Table 14.3. *Transfer of plasmids from* S. epidermidis *J724 to* S. aureus *80CR5 in vitro and in vivo (results from a single experiment are shown); transconjugants were selected on agar containing rifampicin and gentamicin only*

	Resistance transfers per 10^{10} recipients			
	Gm^a	Tc	Em	Cm
Broth	20	2	0	300
Filter	7 000	200	1 000	10 000
Mouse skin	1 200 000	3500	46 500	860 000

^{a} Gm, gentamicin (plasmid is conjugative); Tc, tetracycline; Em, erythromycin; Cm, chloramphenicol.
Based on Naidoo.[100]

Table 14.4. *Cotransfer of resistance during filter mating experiments*

Resistance transfer selected	Percentage of recipients resistant to:			
	Gm^a	Tc	Em	Cm
Gm	(100)	4	41	50
Tc	2	(100)	2	59
Em	38	3	(100)	29

^{a} Cm, chloramphenicol; Em, erythromycin; Gm, gentamicin; Tc, tetracycline.
Based on Naidoo and Lloyd.[93]

Table 14.5. *Effect of the presence of a conjugative gentamicin plasmid on the transfer rates of other resistance plasmids in a single donor*

Skin surface	Resistance plasmids possessed by donor				Plasmid transfers per 10^{10} recipients		
					Tc^a	Em	Cm
Mouse	Tc	Em	Cm		0	0	0
	Tc	Em	Cm	Gm^a	900	20 000	40 000
Human 1	Tc	Em	Cm		0	0	0
	Tc	Em	Cm	Gm	40 000	50 000	50 000
Human 2	Tc	Em	Cm		0	0	0
	Tc	Em	Cm	Gm	400	30 000	50 000

^{a} Gm, gentamicin (plasmid is conjugative); Tc, tetracycline; Em, erythromycin; Cm, chloramphenicol.
Based on Naidoo.[100]

strains, so that *S. hominis*, *S. epidermidis* or *S. haemolyticus* exchange gentamicin-resistance plasmids more efficiently amongst themselves than to the more distant *S. saprophyticus* group.[100]

The conjugative method of transfer in some, but not all, plasmids has an additional property. Some conjugative plasmids are able to mobilize other plasmids within the donor cell and effect their transfer to a recipient. Thus a donor strain possessing separate plasmids for tetracycline, erythromycin or chloramphenicol resistance, together with a conjugative gentamicin-resistance plasmid may transfer any combination of these plasmids to a recipient, in which they will also exist as separate plasmids. On occasion the conjugative plasmid itself may not appear in the recipient.[102] Table 14.4 shows typical cotransfer data and Table 14.5 shows the effect of the presence or absence of the conjugative plasmid in the donor strain. Similar cotransfer results have been obtained in vitro.

Conjugative plasmids mediating gentamicin resistance were the first conjugative plasmids to be described in staphylococci but have been followed by others. These are: (a) the group of plasmids mediating production of a diffusible pigment and carrying a hitch-hiking erythromycin-resistance transposon – some also mediate resistance to kanamycin, neomycin and streptomycin;[103] (b) some of the diversity of mupirocin-resistance plasmids are conjugatively transferable.[104] Plasmids from these two groups do not apparently mobilize other plasmids, however. The most recently described class of conjugative plasmid is able to mobilize other plasmids but does not itself carry a resistance determinant.[105] These four classes of conjugative plasmid are all distinct. The scope for movement of plasmids within the genus *Staphylococcus* under natural conditions is clearly large and validates the idea of a gene pool available, in principle, to all members.

Streptococci

Conjugative mechanisms are well described, especially in the enterococci;[106] these include conjugative plasmids and conjugative transposons, replicons that may excise to form a plasmid-like structure before reintegration in a chromosome or plasmid (see below).

Conjugative plasmids in *Enterococcus faecalis* that mediate resistance to erythromycin have been shown to be transferable bidirectionally to *S. aureus* in vitro. *Enterococcus faecalis* plasmid pAM β1 mobilizes other plasmids into *S. aureus*, which then expresses resistance to chloramphenicol, clindamycin, erythromycin and tetracycline.[107] Conjugative plasmids will also transfer from *E. faecalis* to *S. aureus* and *S. intermedius* in vivo.[101] It is not clear whether these plasmids are able to mobilize vancomycin resistance in *E. faecalis* or whether some other mechanism operates, but resistance to vancomycin is transferred to about one-tenth of *E. faecalis* recipients to which erythromycin resistance is transferred in vitro.[108] The conjugative transposon that resembles Tn916 and mediates tetracycline resistance will transfer between strains of *E. faecalis* on filters and on human and murine skin.[101]

The genes for aminoglycoside resistance in enterococci and staphylococci have been shown to be remarkably homogeneous, despite differing expression as measured by minimal inhibitory concentrations of antibiotic in the two species.[109]

Conjugative transposons

Conjugative transposons appear not to have yet been described in staphylococci but there is some evidence that natural transfer may occur by this route. Erythromycin transposons are well established in *S. aureus* and may appear in plasmids as well as in the chromosome where transposon mutagenesis has shown that insertion of a transposon may alter host characteristics.[110] The presence of erythromycin transposons at several sites in wild-type strains presupposes their ability to achieve transfer. However, examples of apparent transfer of resistance markers during filter mating without plasmids being demonstrable by conventional gel electrophoresis[111] may be examples of the hidden plasmids of the type reported to mediate mupirocin resistance,[112] in which apparently relaxed plasmids are not seen in conventional gels or in caesium-chloride gradients but may be demonstrated by pulsed gel electrophoresis. There are similar reports in *Streptococcus pyogenes* of erythromycin resistance transfer in the apparent absence of plasmid DNA;[113] such reports require a thorough evaluation of the transfer mechanism.

Coryneforms

Although many resistance plasmids have been described in coryneforms of human origin,[114-118] it has not yet proved possible to find a transfer mechanism that operates in vivo. Conjugative-type mechanisms have been described for *Rhodococcus fascians*, a plant pathogenic coryneform,[119] and it seems improbable that a mechanism does not exist for strains of human or animal origin. Erythromycin resistance mediated by plasmids appeared in *Corynebacterium diphtheriae* strains after therapy with this antibiotic but were not the same as those found in skin coryneforms in the same group of patients,[114] although all may have had a distant common origin.

Although the role of phage in transfer on skin has usually been discounted or ignored, there is evidence that pharyngeal diphtheria may result from in vivo lysogenization of pre-existing strain at a carrier site.[120] The more fluid environment of the throat makes phage transfer seem more inherently likely than on skin but there is tantalizing evidence that phage transfer may have occurred between *C. diphtheriae* strains on skin.[121] On rare occasions, plasmid transfer mediated by phage may occur during filter mating; a plasmid mediating production of the epidermolytic toxin B has been transferred in this way but at very low frequency.[122] As propionibacterium phage can readily be demonstrated in sebaceous glands, this may occur in vivo more readily than we can at present demonstrate.

Other organisms

We do not yet have any real appreciation of the extent of gene transfer that can occur on the skin or other epithelial surfaces but it probably ranges, to varying degrees, throughout the taxonomically related Gram-positive group comprising staphylococci, streptococci including enterococci, lactococcus[123] and clostridia.[124] *Bacillus* spp. are well-explored tools in laboratory genetic studies and gene exchange probably also takes place, though more rarely, with this genus in vivo. Experimentally the conjugative enterococcal transposon Tn916 has also been shown to transfer to Gram-negative bacilli including *Escherichia coli* during filter mating, indicating the probability that this could occur in vivo.[125]

Selective agents on skin

No antibiotics are added to the skin or filter in the experiments described above and the impression is gained that gene transfer between at least the staphylococci on skin is a natural event but one generally occurring at a low level. The action of prescribing antibiotic selects a minority population of pre-existing transconjugants. There are, however, conditions on the skin surface where a natural selective agent may act. The most obvious of these is the complex ecosystem of the human toe web, where dermatophytes may produce antibiotics including penicillins and fusidanes and in consequence select an antibiotic-resistant bacterial flora[14, 15, 18] (Table 14.6). Staphylococci and coryneforms also produce antibiotics, often of a cyclic peptide nature such as gramicidin,[23, 24, 126] and most recently, ulcers contaminated or infected with *Pseudomonas* spp. have been suggested as the origin of mupirocin resistance in staphylococci, as the antibiotic is a natural product of some pseudomonads. Less evident is the selection of staphylococci bearing certain penicillinase plasmids by the presence of lipids similar to those of skin, as the plasmid appears to protect the strain against the inhibitory action of lipid.[127] This mechanism is more evident at skin pH (5.5) than at nasal pH (7), suggesting a

Table 14.6. *Selection of antibiotic-resistant bacteria in lesions caused by penicillin-producing or non-producing dermatophytes in humans*

	Percentage resistant to:			
	Pc[a]	Tc	Fc	Sm
Penicillin producer	84	68	56	36
Non-producer	47	26	26	16

[a] Fc, fusicid acid; Pc, penicillin; Sm, streptomycin; Tc, tetracycline.
Based on Youssef and coworkers.[18]

Table 14.7. *Ratio of penicillin-resistant* S. aureus *in the skin versus nose of dermatological patients*

Proportion of resistant strains (skin:nose)			
< 1:1	1:1–2:1	2:1–5:1	> 5:1
4	12	7	5

Based on Noble.[128]

rationale for the observation that patients with skin disease may have resistant staphylococci on their skins but sensitive variants of the same strain in the anterior nares.[128] In Table 14.7 are shown the ratios of resistant to sensitive staphylococci of the same phage type. It can be seen that an excess of sensitive isolates on the skin was not encountered. Isolates from the perineum of dermatological patients were also more likely to be resistant than those of the same phage type in the anterior nares of these patients. A similar phenomenon has been observed in a population of normal women outside hospital[129] where 11.5 per cent of nasal *S. aureus* were resistant to two or more antibiotics compared with 22 per cent of perineal strains.

Continued research on the ecological genetics of the skin reveals that there is yet more to be learned.

References

1 Mims CA, ed. The pathogenesis of infectious disease. 3rd ed. London: Academic Press; 1988: 30–3.
2 Papacostas G, Gate J, eds. Les associations microbiennes, leurs applications therapeutiques. Paris: Doin; 1928.
3 Pasteur L, Joubert JF. Charbon et septicemie. Compt Rend Acad Sci 1877; 85: 101–28.
4 King RD, Dillavou CL, Greenberg JH, Jeppsen JC, Jaegar JS. Identification

of carbon dioxide as a dermatophyte inhibitory factor produced by *Candida albicans*. Can J Microbiol 1976; 22: 1720–27.

5 Moore-Landecker E, Stotsky G. Inhibition of fungal growth and sporulation by volatile metabolites from bacteria. Can J Microbiol 1972; 18: 957–62.

6 Dahiya RS, Speck ML. Hydrogen peroxide formation by lactobacilli and its effect on *Staphylococcus aureus*. J Dairy Sci 1968; 51: 1568–72.

7 Eady EA, Holland KT. Inhibitors produced by propionibacteria and their possible roles in the ecology of skin bacteria. Proc Roy Soc Edinb 1980; 79B: 193–99.

8 Eady EA. Antimicrobiosis by members of the resident bacterial flora of normal and acne skin [PhD thesis]. University of Leeds; 1979.

9 Kingali JM, Heron ID, Morrow AN. Inhibition of *Dermatophilus congolensis* by substances produced by bacteria found on the skin. Vet Microbiol 1990; 22: 237–40.

10 Woodroffe RCS, Shaw DA. Natural control and ecology of microbial populations on skin and hair. In: Skinner FA, Carr JA, eds. The normal microbial flora of man. London: Academic Press; 1974: 13–34.

11 Heczko PB, Kasprowicz A. Epidemiological and ecological studies on mechanisms of staphylococcal carriage. In: Jeljaszewicz J, ed. Staphylococci and staphylococcal diseases. Stuttgart: Fischer-Verlag; 1976: 935–40.

12 Weary PE. *Pityrosporum ovale*: observation on some aspects of host–parasite interrelationship. Arch Dermatol 1968; 98: 408–22.

13 Youssef N, Wyborn CHE, Holt G, Noble WC, Clayton YM. Antibiotic production by dermatophyte fungi. J Gen Microbiol 1978; 105: 105–11.

14 Noble WC. Antibiotics as mediators of interaction between cutaneous microorganisms. In: Aly R, Shinefield HR, eds. Bacterial interference. Boca Raton, FA: CRC Press; 1982: 91–98.

15 Perry MJ, Hendricks-Gittins A, Stacey LM, Adlard MW, Noble WC. Fusidane antibiotics produced by dermatophytes. J Antibiot 1983; 36: 1659–63.

16 Lappin-Scott HM, Rogers ME, Adlard MW, Holt G, Noble WC. High-performance liquid chromatographic identification of beta-lactam antibiotics produced by dermatophytes. J Appl Bacteriol 1985; 59: 437–41.

17 Bibel DJ, Smiljanic RJ. Interactions of *Trichophyton mentagrophytes* and micrococci on skin culture. J Invest Dermatol 1979; 72: 133–37.

18 Youssef N, Wyborn CHE, Holt G, Noble WC, Clayton YM. Ecological effects of antibiotic production by dermatophyte fungi. J Hyg Camb 1979; 82: 301–07.

19 Bibel DJ, Leburn JR. Effect of experimental dermatophyte infections on cutaneous flora. J Invest Dermatol 1975; 64: 119–23.

20 Uri J, Szathmary S, Herpay Z. Production of an antibiotic by dermatophytes living in horn products. Nature 1957; 179: 1029–30.

21 Smith JMB, Marples MJ. A natural reservoir of penicillin resistant strains of *Staphylococcus aureus*. Nature 1964; 201: 844.

22 Allaker RP, Lloyd DH, Noble WC. Studies on antagonism between porcine skin bacteria. J Appl Bacteriol 1989; 66: 507–14.

23 Hsu C-Y, Wiseman GM. The nature of epidermidins, new antibiotics from staphylococci. Can J Microbiol 1972; 18: 121–25.

24 Marsh PD. In vitro studies of antagonism among human skin bacteria [PhD thesis]. University of London; 1975.

25 Holland KT, Cunliffe WJ, Eady EA. Intergeneric and intrageneric inhibition between strains of *Propionibacterium acnes* and micrococcaceae, particularly *Staphylococcus epidermidis*, isolated from normal and acne lesions. J Med Microbiol 1979; 12: 71–82.

26 Al-Admawy AM, Noble WC. Antibiotic production by cutaneous *Brevibacterium* sp. J Appl Bacteriol 1981; 51: 535–40.

27 Tagg JR, Dajani AS, Wannamaker LW. Bacteriocins of gram positive bacteria. Bacteriol Rev 1976; 40: 722–56.

28 Noble WC, Lloyd DH, Appiah SN. Inhibition of *Dermatophilus congolensis* in a mouse model by antibiotic-producing staphylococci. Br J Exp Pathol 1980; 61: 644–47.

29 Somerville DA. The microbiology of the cutaneous diphtheroids. Br J Dermatol 1972; 86 (Supp 8): 16–20.

30 Noble WC. Activity of *Corynebacterium jeikeium* bacteriocin *in vivo*. Micro Ecol Hlth Dis 1988; 1: 201–03.

31 Marsh PD, Selwyn S. Studies on antagonism between human skin bacteria. J Med Microbiol 1977; 10: 161–69.

32 Milyani RM, Selwyn S. Quantitative studies on competitive activities of skin bacteria growing on solid medium. J Med Microbiol 1978; 11: 379–86.

33 Murphy CT. Nutrient materials and the growth of bacteria on human skin. Trans St Johns Hosp Dermatol Soc 1975; 61: 51–57.

34 Milyani RM. Studies on interactions of human skin microorganisms on solid surfaces [PhD thesis]. University of London; 1976.

35 Ryall C, Holt G, Noble WC. Production of a penicillin like antibiotic by *Trichophyton mentagrophytes* on an agar based medium containing skin keratin as the major nutrient. J Appl Bacteriol 1980; 48: 359–65.

36 Malcolm SA, Hughes TC. The demonstration of bacteria on and within the stratum corneum using scanning electron microscopy. Br J Dermatol 1980; 102: 267–75.

37 Wright P, Terry CS. Antagonism within populations of microorganisms from normal human skin. J Med Microbiol 1981; 14: 271–78.

38 Selwyn S. Natural antibiosis among skin bacteria as a primary defence against infection. Br J Dermatol 1975; 93: 345–49.

39 Noble WC, Willie JA. Carriage of inhibitor producing organisms on human skin. J Med Microbiol 1980; 13: 329–32.

40 Noble WC, Willie JA. Interactions between antibiotic producing and non-producing staphylococci in skin surface and sub-surface models. Br J Exp Pathol 1980; 61: 339–43.

41 Selwyn S, Marsh PD, Sethna TN. *In vitro* and *in vivo* studies on antibiotics from skin *Micrococcaceae*. In: Williams JD, Geddes AM, eds. Chemotherapy: proceedings of the 9th international congress. 1976; 5: 391–96.

42 Wickman K. Studies of bacterial interference in experimentally produced burns in guinea pigs. Acta Pathol Microbiol Scand 1970; 78B: 15–28.

43 Dajani AS, Wannamaker LW. Experimental infection of the skin in the hamster simulating human impetigo. 3. Interaction between staphylococci and group A streptococci. J Exp Med 1971; 134: 588–99.

44 Shinefield HR, Ribble JC, Boris M, Eichenwald HF. Bacterial Interference: its effect on nursery acquired infections with *Staphylococcus aureus*; 1, 2, 3, 4. Am J Dis Child 1963; 105: 646–82.

45 Light IJ, Walton RL, Sutherland JM, Shinefield HR, Brackvogel V. Use of

bacterial interference to control a staphylococcal nursery outbreak: deliberate colonisation of all infants with the 502A strain of *Staphylococcus aureus*. Am J Dis Child 1967; 113: 291–300.

46 Houck PW, Nelson JD, Kay JL. Fatal septicemia due to *Staphylococcus aureus* 502A: report of a case and review of the infectious complications of bacterial interference programs. Am J Dis Child 1972; 123: 45–48.

47 Steele RW. Recurrent staphylococcal infection in families. Arch Dermatol 1980; 116: 189–90.

48 Boris M, Shinefield HR, Romano P, et al. Bacterial interference: protection against recurrent intrafamilial staphylococcal disease. Am J Dis Child 1968; 115: 521–29.

49 Maibach HI, Strauss WG, Shinefield HR. Bacterial interference: relating to chronic furunculosis in man. Br J Dermatol 1969; 81 (Suppl 1): 69–72.

50 Boris M, Sellers TF, Eichenwald HF, Ribble JC, Shinefield HR. Bacterial interference: protection of adults against nasal *Staphylococcus aureus*: infection after colonisation with a heterologous *S. aureus* strain. Am J Dis Child 1964; 108: 252–61.

51 Anthony BF, Wannamaker LW. Bacterial interference in experimental burns. J Exp Med 1967; 125: 319–36.

52 Lloyd DH, Allaker RP, Smith IM, Mackie A. Colonisation of gnotobiotic piglets by *Staphylococcus hyicus* and the development of exudative epidermitis. Microb Ecol Hlth Dis 1990; 3: 15–18.

53 Allaker RP, Lloyd DH, Lamport AI. Interaction of *Staphylococcus hyicus* and an inhibitor producing strain of *Staphylococcus chromogenes* on the skin of gnotobiotic piglets. Vet Derm 1990; 1: 93–95.

54 Allaker RP, Lloyd DH, Smith IM, Noble WC. Interactions of *Staphylococcus hyicus* with inhibitor producing bacteria on the skin of gnotobiotic piglets. Microb Ecol Hlth Dis 1990; 3: 19–24.

55 Allaker RP, Lloyd DH, Smith IM. Prevention of exudative epidermitis in gnotobiotic piglets by bacterial interference. Vet Rec 1988; 123: 597–98.

56 Allaker RP, Lloyd DH, Lamport AI. Bacterial interference in the control of exudative epidermitis of pigs. In: Von Tscharner C, Halliwell REW, eds. Advances in veterinary dermatology, vol 1. London: Bailliere Tindall; 1990: 327–34.

57 Mackowiak MD. The normal microbial flora. New Engl J Med 1982; 307: 83–93.

58 Neave FK, Oliver J. The relationship between the number of mastitis pathogens placed on the teats of dry cows, their survival and the amount of intramammary infection caused. J Dairy Res 1962; 29: 79–83.

59 Woodward WD, Ward ACS, Fox LK, Corbeil LB. Teat skin normal flora and colonisation with mastitis pathogen inhibitors. Vet Microbiol 1988; 17: 357–65.

60 Allaker RP, Lamport AI, Lloyd DH, Noble WC. Production of 'virulence factors' by *Staphylococcus intermedius* isolates from cases of canine pyoderma and healthy carriers. Microb Ecol Hlth Dis 1991; 4: 169–73.

61 Evans CA, Mattern KL. The aerobic growth of *Propionibacterium acnes* in primary cultures from skin. J Invest Dermatol 1979; 72: 103–06.

62 Willis AT, ed. Anaerobic bacteriology: clinical and laboratory practice. 3rd ed. London: Butterworths; 1977: 223–24.

63 Lloyd DH, Noble WC. Interaction between antibiotic producing bacteria and

Dermatophilus congolensis: a potential therapeutic tool? In: Woodbine M, ed. Antimicrobials and agriculture. London: Butterworths; 1984: 277–83.

64 Roberts DS. Dermatophilus infection. Vet Bull 1967; 37: 513–21.

65 Alder VG, Gillespie WA. Influence of neomycin sprays on the spread of resistant staphylococci. Lancet 1967; 2: 1062–63.

66 Wyatt TD, Ferguson WP, Wilson TS, McCormick E. Gentamicin resistant *Staphylococcus aureus* associated with the use of topical gentamicin. J Antimicrob Chemother 1977; 3: 213–17.

67 Schaberg DR, Power G, Betzold J, Forbes BA. Conjugative R plasmids in antimicrobial resistance of *Staphylococcus aureus* among nosocomial infections. J Infect Dis 1985; 152: 43–49.

68 Naidoo J, Noble WC, Weissmann A, Dyke KGH. Gentamicin-resistant staphylococci: genetics of an outbreak in a dermatology department. J Hyg Camb 1983; 91: 7–16.

69 Westh H, Jensen BL, Rosdahl VT, Prag J. Development of erythromycin resistance in *Staphylococcus aureus* as a consequence of high erythromycin consumption. J Hosp Infect 1989; 14: 107–15.

70 Eady EA, Cove JH, Holland KT, Cunliffe WJ. Erythromycin resistant propionibacteria in antibiotic treated acne patients: association with therapeutic failure. Br J Dermatol 1989; 121: 51–57.

71 Leyden JJ, McGinley KJ, Cavalieri S, Webster GF, Mills OH, Kligman AM. *Propionibacterium acnes* resistant to antibiotics in patients. J Am Acad Dermatol 1983; 8: 41–45.

72 Coyle MB, Minshew BH, Bland JA, Hsu PC. Erythromycin and clindamycin resistance in *Corynebacterium diphtheriae* from skin lesions. Antimicrob Ag Chemother 1979; 16: 525–27.

73 Naidoo J, Noble WC. Acquisition of antibiotic resistance by *Staphylococcus aureus* in skin patients. J Clin Pathol 1978; 31: 1187–92.

74 Lacey RW, Lewis E, Grinsted J. Loss of antibiotic resistance in *Staphylococcus aureus* probably resulting from cloxacillin therapy. J Med Microbiol 1973; 6: 191–99.

75 Groves DJ. Interspecific relationships of antibiotic resistance in *Staphylococcus* species: isolation and comparison of plasmids determining tetracycline resistance in *S. aureus* and *S. epidermidis*. Can J Microbiol 1979; 25: 1468–75.

76 Cooksey RC, Baldwin JN. Relatedness of tetracycline resistance plasmids among species of coagulase negative staphylococci. Antimicrob Ag Chemother 1985; 27: 234–38.

77 Schwarz S, Blobel H. Isolation and restriction endonuclease analysis of a tetracycline resistance plasmid from *Staphylococcus hyicus*. Vet Microbiol 1990; 24: 113–22.

78 Schwarz S, Cardosa M, Grolz-Krug S, Blobel H. Common antibiotic resistance plasmids in *Staphylococcus aureus* and *Staphylococcus epidermidis* from human and canine infections. Zbl Bakt 1990; 273: 369–77.

79 Noble WC, Rahman M, Lloyd DH. Plasmids in *Staphylococcus hyicus*. J Appl Bacteriol 1988; 64: 145–49.

80 Schwarz S, Cardoso M, Blobel H. Plasmid mediated chloramphenicol resistance in *Staphylococcus hyicus*. J Gen Microbiol 1989; 135: 3329–36.

81 Rahman M, Kent L, Noble WC. Streptomycin and tetracycline resistance plasmids in *Staphylococcus hyicus* and other staphylococci. J Appl Bacteriol 1991; 70: 211–15.

82 Tennent JM, Young H-K, Lyon Br, Amyes SGB, Skurray RA. Trimethoprim resistance determinants encoding a dihydrofolate reductase in clinical isolates of *Staphylococcus aureus* and coagulase negative staphylococci. J Med Microbiol 1988; 26: 67–73.

83 Tennent JM, May JM, Skurray RA. Characterization of chloramphenicol-resistance plasmids of *Staphylococcus aureus* and *S. epidermidis* by restriction enzyme mapping techniques. J Med Microbiol 1986; 22: 79–84.

84 Goering RV, Ruff EA. Comparative analysis of conjugative plasmids mediating gentamicin resistance in *Staphylococcus aureus*. Antimicrob Ag Chemother 1983; 24: 450–52.

85 McDonnell RW, Sweeney HM, Cohen S. Conjugal transfer of gentamicin resistance plasmids intra- and inter-specifically in *Staphylococcus aureus* and *Staphylococcus epidermidis*. Antimicrob Ag Chemother 1983; 23: 151–60.

86 Archer GL, Johnson JL. Self-transmissible plasmids in staphylococci that encode resistance to aminoglycosides. Antimicrob Ag Chemother 1983; 24: 70–77.

87 Forbes BA, Schaberg DR. Transfer of resistance plasmids from *Staphylococcus epidermidis* to *Staphylococcus aureus*: evidence for conjugative exchange of plasmids. J Bacteriol 1983; 153: 627–34.

88 Schaberg DR, Zervos MJ. Intergeneric and interspecies gene exchange in Gram positive cocci. Antimicrob Ag Chemother 1986; 30: 817–22.

89 Townsend DE, Bolton S, Ashdown N, Grubb WB. Transfer of plasmid borne aminoglycoside resistance determinants in staphylococci. J Med Microbiol 1985; 20: 169–85.

90 Al-Masaudi SB, Russell AD, Day MJ. Factors affecting conjugative transfer of plasmid pWG613 determining gentamicin resistance in *Staphylococcus aureus*. J Med Microbiol 1991; 34: 103–07.

91 Lacey RW. Evidence for two mechanisms of plasmid transfer in mixed cultures of *Staphylococcus aureus*. J Gen Microbiol 1980; 119: 423–35.

92 Naidoo J, Noble WC. Transfer of gentamicin resistance between strains of *Staphylococcus aureus* on skin. J Gen Microbiol 1978; 107: 391–93.

93 Naidoo J, Lloyd DH. Transmission of genes between staphylococci on skin. In: Woodbine M, ed. Antibiotics in agriculture. London: Butterworth; 1984: 285–92.

94 Meijers JA, Winkler KC, Stobberingh EE. Resistance transfer in mixed cultures of *Staphylococcus aureus*. J Med Micribiol 1981; 14: 21–39.

95 Witte W. Transfer of drug resistance plasmids in mixed cultures of staphylococci. Zent Bakt I Abt A 1977; 237: 147–59.

96 Evans J, Dyke KGH. Characterization of the conjugation system associated with the *Staphylococcus aureus* plasmid pJE1. J Gen Microbiol 1988; 134: 1–8.

97 Lacey RW, Lord VL. Transfer of gentamicin resistance between cultures of *Staphylococcus aureus* in nutrient broth, serum and urine. J Med Microbiol 1980; 13: 411–21.

98 Cohen ML, Wong ES, Falkow S. Common R plasmids in *Staphylococcus aureus* and *Staphylococcus epidermidis* during nosocomial *Staphylococcus aureus* outbreak. Antimicrob Ag Chemother 1982; 21: 210–15.

99 Townsend DE, Bolton S, Ashdown N, Annear DI, Grubb WB. Conjugative staphylococcal plasmids carrying hitch-hiking transposon similar to Tn554: intra and inter-species dissemination of erythromycin resistance. Aust J Exp Biol Med Sci 1986; 64: 367–79.

100 Naidoo J. Interspecific co-transfer of antibiotic resistance plasmids *in vivo*. J Hyg Camb 1984; 93: 59–66.

101 Kent L, Petts DN, Noble WC. [Unpublished observations].

102 Naidoo J, Noble WC. Skin as a source of transferable antibiotic resistance in coagulase negative staphylococci. Zent Bakt (Suppl 16). Stuttgart: Fischer; 1987: 225–34.

103 Townsend DE, Ashdown N, Annear DI, Grubb WB. A conjugative plasmid encoding production of a diffusible pigment and resistance to aminoglycosides and macrolides in *Staphylococcus aureus*. Aust J Exp Biol Med Sci 1985; 63: 573–86.

104 Rahman M, Connolly S, Noble WC, Cookson B, Phillips I. Diversity of staphylococci exhibiting high-level resistance to mupirocin. J Med Microbiol 1990; 33: 97–100.

105 Udo EE, Grubb WB. A new class of conjugative plasmid in *Staphylococcus aureus*. J Med Microbiol 1990; 31: 207–12.

106 Clewell DB, Fitzgerald GF, Dempsey L, et al. Streptococcal conjugation, plasmids, sex pheromones, and conjugative transposons. In: Molecular basis of oral adhesion. Bethesda, MD: Am Soc Microbiol; 1985: 194–203.

107 Schaberg DR, Clewell DB, Glatzer L. Conjugative transfer of R plasmids from *Streptococcus faecalis* to *Staphylococcus aureus*. Antimicrob Ag Chemother 1982; 22: 204–07.

108 Uttley AHC, George RC, Naidoo J, et al. High level vancomycin-resistant enterococci causing hospital infection. Epidem Infect 1989; 103: 173–81.

109 Ounissi H, Derlot E, Carlier C, Courvalin P. Gene homogeneity for aminoglycoside-modifying enzymes in Gram-positive cocci. Antimicrob Ag Chemother 1990; 34: 2164–68.

110 Luchansky JB, Pattee PA. Isolation of transposon Tn551 insertions near chromosomal markers of interest in *Staphylococcus aureus*. J Bacteriol 1984; 159: 894–99.

111 ElSolh N, Alligret J, Bismuth R, Buret B, Fouace J-M. Conjugative transfer of staphylococcal antibiotic resistance markers in the absence of detectable plasmid DNA. Antimicrob Ag Chemother 1986; 30: 161–69.

112 Rahman M, Noble WC, Cookson B. Transmissible mupirocin resistance in *Staphylococcus aureus*. Epidem Infect 1989; 102: 261–70.

113 Scott RJD, Naidoo J, Lightfoot NF, George RC. A community outbreak of group A beta haemolytic streptococci with transferable resistance to erythromycin. Epidem Infect 1989; 102: 85–91.

114 Schiller J, Groman N, Coyle MB. Plasmids in *Corynebacterium diphtheriae* and diphtheroids mediating erthromycin resistance. Antimicrob Ag Chemother 1980; 18: 814–21.

115 Serwold-Davies TM, Groman NB. Mapping and cloning of *Corynebacterium diphtheriae* plasmid pNG2 and characterization of its relatedness to plasmids from skin coryneforms. Antimicrob Ag Chemother 1986; 30: 69–72.

116 Kerry Williams SM, Noble WC. Plasmids in group JK coryneform bacteria from a single hospital. J Hyg Camb 1986; 97: 255–63.

117 Kerry Williams SM, Noble WC. Plasmids in coryneform bacteria of human origin. J Appl Bacteriol 1988; 64: 475–82.

118 Kono M, Sasatsu M, Aoki T. R plasmids in *Corynebacterium xerosis* strains. Antimicrob Ag Chemother 1983; 23: 506–08.

119 Desomer J, Dhaese P, van Montague M. Conjugative transfer of cadmium

resistance plasmids in *Rhodococcus fascians* strains. J Bacteriol 1988; 170: 2401–05.

120 Pappenheimer AM Jr, Murphy JR. Studies on the molecular epidemiology of diphtheria. Lancet 1983; ii: 923–26.

121 Coyle MB, Groman NB, Russell JQ, Harnisch JP, Rabin M, Holmes KK. The molecular epidemiology of three biotypes of *Corynebacterium diphtheriae* in the Seattle outbreak 1972–1982. J Infect Dis 1989; 159: 670–79.

122 Rogolsky M, Beall BW, Wiley BB. Transfer of the plasmid for exfoliative toxin B synthesis in mixed culture on nitrocellulose membrane. Infect Immun 1986; 54: 265–68.

123 van der Lelie D, Wosten HAB, Bron S, Oskam L, Venema G. Conjugative mobilization of streptococcal plasmid pMV158 between strains of *Lactococcus lactis* subsp. *lactis*. J Bacteriol 1990; 172: 47–52.

124 Hachler H, Berger-Bachi B, Kayser FH. Genetic characterization of a *Clostridium difficile* erythromycin–clindamycin resistance determinant that is transferable to *Staphylococcus aureus*. Antimicrob Ag Chemother 1987; 31: 1039–45.

125 Bertram J, Stratz M, Durre P. Natural transfer of conjugative transposon Tn916 between Gram-positive and Gram-negative bacteria. J Bacteriol 1991; 173: 443–48.

126 Selwyn S, Marsh PD, Sethna TN. *In vitro* and *in vivo* studies on antibiotics from skin micrococcaceae. Chemotherapy 1976; 5: 391–96.

127 Naidoo J. Effect of pH on inhibition of plasmid carrying cultures of *Staphylococcus aureus* by lipids. J Gen Microbiol 1981; 124: 173–79.

128 Noble WC. Variation in the prevalence of antibiotic resistance of *Staphylococcus aureus* from human skin and nares. J Gen Microbiol 1977; 98: 125–32.

129 Dancer SJ, Noble WC. Nasal, axillary and perineal carriage of *Staphylococcus aureus* among antenatal women: identification of strains producing epidermolytic toxin. J Clin Pathol 1991; 44: 681–84.

15

Adherence of skin microorganisms and the development of skin flora from birth

R. ALY & D. J. BIBEL

Among the various known ecological factors that determine host–parasite relationships is the specific binding of microorganisms to cells and tissues. This important process is called adherence; the microbe-borne molecule that connects with a host receptor is an 'adhesin'. Like those tenacious microorganisms inhabiting streams and other marine environments, the flora indigenous to skin and mucosa has the selective advantage of being able to stick to substrates, resisting the abrasive forces of air and fluid currents that would otherwise wash it away.[1,2] Furthermore, like the attachment of viruses to their target cells, microbial adherence is a significant, if not crucial, step in infectivity and in subsequent infectious disease.[3] Indeed, the molecular principles previously established for specific viral attachment have been found appropriate for bacteria and fungi as well.

The macroscopic perspective

Although recognized as early as 1908 when G. Guyot observed attachment of bacteria to erythrocytes, medical interest in adherence stems from the research of Gibbons and colleagues on the microbial ecology of the oral cavity.[4] Their analyses of the general phenomenon of adherence were soon verified with intestinal, vaginal, and nasal mucosal cells.[5] Reflecting the relative proportions of flora observed in the mouth, *Streptococcus salivarius* adhered poorly to teeth, moderately to buccal cells, but in high numbers to epithelial cells of the tongue, while *Strep. mitis* attached well to teeth and cheek but only moderately so to tongue.[4,6] In contrast, *Enterococcus faecalis* and *Escherichia coli*, named for their normal intestinal habitat, were infrequently detected on oral surfaces and had a correspondingly low adherence. Host species specificity was also demonstrated by experiments in which *Strep. salivarius* from human tongue

355

was unable to adhere to rat tongue, while rat *E. faecalis*, which attached well to rat tongue, failed to adhere to human tongue.[7]

Aly and coworkers[8] observed similar specificity in microbial adherence on nasal mucosal cells. *Staphylococcus aureus* and *Staph. epidermidis*, *Strep. pyogenes* and *Pseudomonas aeruginosa*, but not *Klebsiella pneumoniae* or alpha-haemolytic streptococci, attached to collected nasal cells. Adherence selectivity on labium majus cells was nearly the same; however, an alpha-haemolytic streptococcus attached as well as did *Strep. pyogenes*, and *Ps. aeruginosa*, which equalled the adherence of *Staph. aureus* on nasal cells, was substantially inferior in adherence on labial cells.[9] Adherence of *Staph. aureus* to the outermost labium majus cells was superior to adherence to cells taken from the labium minus and the vagina, and matched the findings for fully keratinized nasal cells.

Utilizing members of the axillary flora and cultured, differentiated and undifferentiated epidermal cells, Romero-Steiner and colleagues[10] tested various coryneforms. Good adherence was found with *Corynebacterium minutissimum*, *C. xerosis* and groups F-1, G-2, C, and JK. *Corynebacterium diphtheriae* was the least able to attach. In their assay, *E. coli* attached to about the same degree as most coryneforms. However, the adherence counts of *Propionibacterium acnes* were meagre. Differentiated cells generally allowed greater adherence, which was also observed by Bibel and colleagues[11] with nasal cells undergoing keratinization.

Alkan and coworkers[12] reported differences in adherence on oral and cutaneous cells between *Strep. pyogenes* isolated from the pharynx and from the skin. This site affinity may be related to the proclivity of certain serotypes of pathogenic isolates. Strain distinctions associated with site were also observed in the adherence of *C. diphtheriae*.[13] While all throat isolates adhered well to buccal cells, with a mean of 50 adherent bacteria per cell, only some 30 per cent of isolates from skin lesions showed moderate levels of adherence, the mean being less than 8 bacteria per cell. There was no correlation with toxin production, that is, the presence of lysogenic bacteriophage.

Adherence of fungi indigenous to the skin has also been investigated. Kimura and Pearsall[14] showed the importance of candidal germ-tube formation, which occurs in saliva but not in saline. Adherence was two- to five-fold greater in saliva. They eliminated the possibility of a coating adhesin in saliva by finding reduced adherence (and no germination) in saliva incubated at 25 °C rather than at 37 °C and also by assaying heat- or formalin-killed yeast. However, once germ tubes were formed, formalin killing did not reduce the number of adherent cells.

Bibel and coworkers[9] reported that *Candida albicans* adhered better to labium majus cells than to cells from the labium minus, vagina, cheek, forearm, and nose. Adherence counts on labium majus cells were similar to those of streptococci.

That there is a strong relationship between pathogenicity and adherence was the conclusion of Ray and colleagues[15] when they mixed various candidal species with corneocytes or buccal cells. While *C. albicans* and *C. stellatoidea* were the only two species that adhered to buccal cells, a gradation in affinity was seen on corneocytes, whose order was *C. albicans, C. stellatoidea, C. parapsilosis, C. tropicalis, C. krusei,* and *C. guilliermondii.* Adherence of dermatophytes can also be ranked. Zurita and Hay[16] found that on keratinocytes from palm, dorsum of hand, or knee *Trichophyton quinckeanum* was superior in adherence to *T. interdigitale,* which in turn produced a higher degree of attachment than did *T. rubrum.* Keratinocytes from the sole favoured the adherence of *T. interdigitale.* Quantitatively, they found that the greatest adherence tallied with keratinocytes from the sole, followed in order by palm, dorsum of hand, forearm, and knee.

Malassezia furfur (*Pityrosporum orbiculare*) is the agent of tinea versicolor, which typically affects the neck and trunk. Tests of adherence showed increases with incubation time and elevated temperature; however, no statistically significant differences were found among keratinocytes taken from forearm, back, and chest.[17] Adherence to nasal cells was substantially lower.

The microscopic perspective

Clues to the structures of adherence have been sought by scanning and transmission electron microscopy. Clinical isolates, but usually not laboratory strains that have undergone a long series of subcultures, have a surrounding fibrillar network called a glycocalyx.[18] This network was once largely ignored or even, when at first regarded as debris or artefact, assailed by vigorous washes for obscuring the microorganisms; however, it is now clear that this covering naturally enmeshes microbe and host cell alike. Indeed, a glycocalyx is also synthesized by many epithelial cells exposed to environmental surfaces. However, the glycocalyx may not be the specific adhesive substance, but, rather, the non-specific physical means by which microorganisms can cling to, say, a rock, the hull of ships, or an inert surgical device in a hospitalized patient. Microbial 'adhesion', as distinct from 'adherence', is the term commonly applied to the formation of such biofilms.

By electron microscopy, streptococci have a distinct, 'fuzzy' fibrillar coat that can be removed by trypsin.[19] Similar fibrillar elements have been seen on the wall of most other bacteria that have been recently isolated from their natural environment.

By scanning electron microscopy of the early stages of epidermal colonization and infection of mice by several candidal species, Ray and Payne[20] described the formation of amorphous strands from blastoconidia of only *C. albicans* and *C. stellatoidea*. The material, which linked blastoconidia as well as blastoconidia and corneocytes, was not synthesized on nylon filter surfaces and was not found with heat-killed blastoconidia or latex particles; the bridging strands, hence, are a result of interactive induction. As reported by Bibel and colleagues,[21] agar-cultured mycelia of *T. mentagrophytes* can develop a thick fibrillar coating under 8 per cent CO_2 incubation (which leads to arthrospore formation) but not under normal aerobic conditions. Zurita and Hay[16] noticed a webbing of fibrils on microconidia of *T. interdigitale* attached to keratinocytes.

Some bacterial species produce flagella and fimbriae (pili). These appendages have been associated with adherence because of their obvious potential to enmesh, to enter crevices, and to overcome electrostatic barriers (both bacteria and host cells are charged negatively). They are not constituents of *Staphylococcus* and *Micrococcus* spp., but fimbriae have been reported in *Corynebacterium* spp.[22] Found chiefly on Gram-negative enteric bacilli, pseudomonads, and *Neisseria* spp., their importance may be evident on the nasal or other mucosal surface.[23, 24] Sato and Okinaga,[25] using four mutants with or without each appendage, established that fimbriae, not flagella, are responsible for the adherence of *Pseudomonas aeruginosa* to mouse epidermal cells.

The molecular perspective

The most common tactic used to ascertain the composition of adhesins and receptors is the introduction of a known microbial or epithelial molecule into the adherence assay; inhibition of adherence indicates that the molecule at least shares stereochemical features with one of the binding sites. Other evidence can be attained with mutants of microorganisms known to lack a given surface component. Enzymatic treatments, antibody interference, and antibiotics have also yielded information.

Because a glycocalyx, by definition, consists in part of polymeric sugar, the interfering capacity of mannose, galactose, fucose, and other disaccharides has been examined, sometimes with equivocal results. The adherence of coryneforms to undifferentiated cultured epithelial cells was retarded by mannose, galactose, fucose, and *N*-acetylglucosamine, as well as the protein, fibronectin.[10] Mannose clearly interfered the best at some 90 per cent reduction compared to approximately 25–65 per cent. However, in assays with differentiated epidermal keratinocytes, results were nearly equivalent, with all giving about 80 per cent reduction in adherent bacteria.

Bibel and colleagues,[11] working with *Staphylococcus aureus*, also obtained suggestive evidence that multiple adhesins and receptors are involved in microbe–keratinocyte interactions. Teichoic acid is apparently one adhesin of *S. aureus* for nasal, labial, and vaginal cells.[9, 26] On investigating its inhibition of staphylococcal adherence on spinous, granular, and fully keratinized cells, they observed that teichoic acid is effective only on the keratinocytes; the number of attached bacteria on cells from the lower, less differentiated layers remained the same.

Cole and Silverberg[27] found that the protein A-deficient Wood strain of *Staph. aureus* adhered less well to cutaneous cells than the protein A-rich Cowan 1 strain; when the assay tube included added protein A, adherence was diminished by the competition. The difference in type of host cell may be the key. This conclusion is also apparent in the work of Bibel and coworkers.[28] Protein A did not inhibit adherence of the staphylococcus to nasal cells.

Furthermore, fibronectin, which is absent on keratinocytes but present in plasma, basement membranes, and on connective tissue, binds *Staph. aureus*.[29] Ribitol teichoic acid, which can compete with *Staph. aureus* in adherence assays, was itself neutralized by preincubation with fibronectin. The wall components protein A, N-acetyl muramic acid, N-acetyl-glucosamine, adonitol (ribitol) and ribose, or ribose-1-phosphate, could not block the coupling of fibronectin and *Staph. aureus*. However, others reported that a protein A-deficient strain could not bind fibronectin[30] but that a teichoic acid-deficient strain could.[31] It is possible that the teichoic acid preparation of Bibel and colleagues was insufficiently purified, as a fibronectin-binding protein has been isolated from *Staph. aureus*.[32, 33] (To confuse matters still further, *Strep. pyogenes* lipoteichoic acid is the microorganism's primary adhesin, and it apparently binds fibronectin; see below.) Nevertheless, in all cases no tested staphylococcal cell-wall component or host fibronectin prevented adherence completely. Clearly, *Staph. aureus* has several adhesins for keratinized epithelial cells.

Lipoteichoic acid was among the first adhesins identified on Gram-positive bacteria. It is the adhesin by which *Strep. pyogenes* attaches to oral mucosal cells.[34] Neither M protein nor C carbohydrate had appreciable blocking ability. Furthermore, antilipoteichoic-acid antiserum interfered with adherence, and purified lipoteichoic acid could attach to the outer membranes of erthryocytes and oral epithelial cells. Alkan and coworkers[12] later found through inhibition studies that this wall substance is also involved in streptococcal adherence to human stratum corneum cells. The oral epithelial cells of newborn infants carry less than half the receptors for *Strep. pyogenes* of adults; however, within 3 days, adherence counts reach adult levels.[35] Adult buccal cells constituted some 5×10^9 binding sites for lipoteichoic acid.[36]

As with *Staph. aureus*, the adhesin of *Strep. pyogenes* has also been regarded as a protein. Ellen and Gibbons,[37] using strains with and without M protein, found that *Strep. pyogenes* lacking the protein (a recognized virulence factor) adhered relatively poorly to buccal cells. Trypsin treatment of the M protein-containing strain reduced its ability to attach to epithelial cells. However, as noted earlier, Ofek's group introduced M protein to their assay without significant effect on adherence.[34] They did notice that lipoteichoic acid and M protein can form soluble complexes and that these molecules possibly anchor each other to the bacterium. The exposed lipid portion was shown to be the active moiety that interacts with host cell receptors. One such receptor is fibronectin, which has two separate binding sites for both streptococci and staphylococci.[38, 39]

Adherence of *Candida albicans* to buccal and cutaneous cells is probably related to a glycoprotein receptor. Pretreatment of the yeast with various polysaccharides inhibited adherence. In increasing order of interference, these components or analogues were galactose, maltose, galactosamine, glucosamine and mannosamine.[40] While all these carbohydrates were effective in buccal cell assays, only galactosamine, glucosamine, and mannosamine gave statistically significant reductions with corneocytes. Testing adherence of *C. albicans* on corneocytes, Kahana and coworkers[41] found that chitin-soluble extract was inhibitory when introduced into the test solution. Chitin is a polymer of *N*-acetyl glucosamine. Again, adherence was not completely eliminated, indicating the existence of multiple adhesins and receptors in this microbe–epithelial cell interaction. Furthermore, the aminosugars did not inhibit candida from binding fibronectin.[42]

One other molecular aspect needs to be mentioned: the correlation of adherence with plasmids. A specific protein adhesin in an enteropathogenic strain of *E. coli* was linked with R factors and with genes for producing a colicin, but could be separated by interrupted conjugation with *E. coli* strain K-12.[43] Moreover, the ability to adhere to mucosal cells of human small intestine was significantly reduced by treatment with ethidium bromide. Another plasmid linkage of antibiotic resistance and apparent adhesin production was found in a strain of *Staph. aureus*.[44] The adhesin was not established; however, increased adherence to HeLa cells in different strains could be achieved by transferring the plasmid to protoplasts by transformation.

Correlation with pathology

Altered adherence has been associated with certain pathological conditions and infectious diseases. Apparently, epithelial cells of some individuals are predisposed to greater numbers of receptors or undergo unmasking or development of receptors with the rise of the local or systemic disorder.

Skin and nasal cells of patients with atopic dermatitis allow substantially greater adherence of *Staph. aureus* than those of normal subjects.[11, 27, 45] Granular cells, rather than fully keratinized nasal cells, were responsible for the increase in bacterial counts. When nasal and cutaneous epithelial cells from psoriatic patients were tested against normal cells, no difference was found. Nasal keratinocytes from healthy nasal carriers of *Staph. aureus* also bound more staphylococci than cells from normal noncarriers.[8]

Kurono and colleagues[46] reported that *Strep. pyogenes* attached more plentifully to nasal cells of patients with chronic sinusitis than to cells of normal subjects. These patients also had lower levels of anti-M protein secretory IgA.

The oral use of synthetic retinoids in the treatment of certain keratinization disorders has been correlated with an increase in staphylococcal infections. To explore whether the drug could influence adherence and thereby contribute to the opportunistic infections, Lianou and colleagues[47] incubated nasal cells with acitretin before introducing an inoculum of *Staph. aureus*. They observed a statistically significant enhancement of adherence over controls. The retinoid apparently directly affected the nasal epithelial cells, as they found no alteration of adherence with an inoculum of *Staph. aureus* grown in presence of acitretin.

Little is known about the effects of immunodeficiency on microbial ecology and particularly on adherence. In a pilot study of AIDS patients and subjects infected with the human immunodeficiency virus (HIV), Bibel and coworkers[48] determined that nasal cells of HIV-infected subjects bound more *Staph. aureus* than did cells from HIV-negative subjects. This enhancement included those patients and control subjects who were carriers of *Staph. aureus*. Moreover, adherence was greater on stratum corneum cells of HIV-positive subjects; the degree of adherence was related to the progression of AIDS, as indicated by decreases in CD4 (T4 helper) lymphocytes.

Prospects for novel therapy

The modern approach to therapy has become the stereochemical molecular understanding of ligand–receptor interactions and the application of competitors. These interlopers may be the purified soluble units themselves, the reactive binding portion of the molecules, or synthesized analogues. One example of current therapeutic use of a competitive inhibitor is the CD4 cell-membrane receptor to the gp120 glycoprotein of the HIV in AIDS.[49] Produced by recombinant DNA techniques, soluble CD4 is injected to bind HIV before the virus reaches the cell-bound receptor.

Antibody is the first recognized inhibitor of ligand–receptor binding, and at present it remains the only means clinically involved in preventing specific adherence, although it does not have that specific purpose. However, in an animal model, vaccination has been attempted to hinder the formation of dental caries through the reduction of adherent *Strep. mutans*.[50,51]

Raja and coworkers[52] have suggested that various peptide analogues to a fibronectin receptor might be used to block the attachment of *Staph. aureus* to plasma clots and fibronectin-coated prosthetic implants. Methyl α-D-mannose-pyranoside, which inhibits adherence of *E. coli* to epithelial cells in vitro, was tested in the prevention of experimental urinary tract infections in mice.[53] The inoculum included the mannose analogue. Both cellular adherence counts and bacteriuria rates were less than in control animals.

Competition and interference

No adherence inhibitors to prevent colonization of indigenous nasal and cutaneous flora have yet been examined in vivo. However, the phenomena of competition and bacterial interference do have attributes related to adherence. If one microorganism can block the adherence of another, a benign member of the normal flora could prevent an important early step in colonization with a virulent pathogen.

Competitive adherence or colonization has been investigated by sequential or simultaneous exposure of a host, or its isolated cells, to two microorganisms of the same or different species. The first such study was by Bibel and colleagues,[54] who tested in vitro the adherence of *Staph. aureus* and a nasal coryneform; *Staph. aureus* and *Ps. aeruginosa*; and two strains of *Staph. aureus* on nasal cells. After standardizing the inoculum to equivalent colony-forming units, these researchers determined the adherence of each bacterium alone, in mixed culture, and in alternating sequences of presentation. They observed that in all instances the bacterium first to adhere to the epithelial cells was able to interfere with the colonization of the subsequently added bacterium. This secondary adherence was reduced, not eliminated. The sum of independent adherence was always greater than the adherence of mixed inocula, indicating competition for the same binding sites or, more probably, stereometric blockage. In simultaneous inocula, the coryneform had higher adherence counts than those of *Staph. aureus*, but the staphylococcus adhered better than *Ps. aeruginosa*; the virulent strain of *Staph. aureus* was superior in adherence to the weakly pathogenic strain.

In their study of plasmid-linked adherence, Dunkle and coworkers[44] compared the ability of isolated and mixed strains of *Staph. aureus* with and without the plasmid to adhere to HeLa cells. The adherence index of the plasmid-containing strain was not reduced by competition from the strain lacking the plasmid, and the plasmidless strain did not affect adherence of the plasmid strain. These results indicated that the plasmid coded for a unique adhesin for a different epithelial-cell receptor. Upon transfer of the plasmid, the former plasmidless strain showed increased adherence, and the strains now containing two plasmids could interfere with each other.

Abraham and colleagues[55] interacted *Strep. pyogenes* and *E. coli* or *Ps. aeruginosa* with buccal cells. They sought to examine the role of fibronectin, which does not bind Gram-negative bacteria. While they were more interested in their discovery of three populations of buccal cells, which could bind one, the other, or both bacteria depending on the presence of fibronectin, their data keenly demonstrated the importance of specificity and the variety of membrane-binding sites in competitive adherence. It is worthwhile to add that Mertz and colleagues,[56] in their model for studying adherence to skin wounds, observed a reduction in adherence of *Ps. aeruginosa* in the presence of fibronectin wash or of fibronectin-containing serum and wound fluids; they found no change in the adherence of *Staph. aureus*.

In conclusion, the recent recognition and investigation of microbial adherence have been a major advance in our understanding of the ecological principles leading to the establishment of a normal flora and the onset of infectious disease. Of course, this field is still fresh, particularly in dermatobiology, with much more research needed in the determination of the molecular composition and arrangement of adhesins and cell receptors, their respective production and distribution, and the physicochemical aspects of the interaction. Forthcoming discoveries will almost certainly ensure the development of new ecologically based forms of therapy or prophylaxis.

Neonatal skin

The normal fetus is microbiologically sterile until shortly before birth, as long as the amniotic membrane remains intact. Microorganisms do not cross the placenta unless it has been damaged by some pathological process.[57] At birth, relatively few organisms are found on human skin and mucous membranes. The host defence mechanisms are not well developed at this age, and some of the resident flora, as opportunistic pathogens, can initiate disease, particularly in compromised infants admitted to hospital for the treatment of certain conditions. Skin infections, mainly of the umbilical cord stump and the circumcision site, were at one time a major medical problem and still occur sporadically. *Staphylococcus aureus* is often the predominant organism, but *Staph. epidermidis*, haemolytic streptococci other than *Strep. pyogenes*, coliforms, *Proteus* spp, *Pseudomonas* spp., and yeasts also are likely transients.[58, 59] As such colonization seldom results in umbilical infections, recent concern has focused on the cord as a reservoir of nursery-acquired staphylococcal infection.

The skin of the newborn at birth is physiologically different from that of the adult because, in part, it is coated with the vernix caseosa. The coating is from fatty degeneration of epidermal cells and has a pH of 7.4. Whether it has any nutritional properties for bacteria is not known; however, its neutral pH may be more conducive to microbial multiplication than the skin of older children and adults, which is acidic. With the disappearance of vernix, the skin pH reaches the acid level of 3.0–5.9 found in adults.[60] Besides the vernix coating, the infant skin is thinner, less hairy, has weaker intercellular attachments, and produces fewer sweat and sebaceous gland secretions than adult skin.[61] In addition, the biochemical and physical properties of skin and respiratory mucosa may inhibit bacterial growth. Skin surface lipids of adult skin are antimicrobial.[62]

As mentioned earlier, adherence of microorganisms to the skin surface is another important factor that determines their colonization. Ofek and colleagues[35] reported that the adherence capacity of group A and B streptococci to buccal mucosal cells at birth (day 1) was minimal and rapidly increased toward the adult level on day 3. Aly and coworkers[63] investigated the adherence of *Staph. aureus* to nasal mucosal cells in newborns, and compared the level to the binding capacity of the adult epithelial cells. A comparison of attachment of *Staph. aureus* is shown in Table 15.1. The binding of *Staph. aureus* to nasal epithelial cells is markedly low during the first 4 days of life, reaching adult level by the fifth day. The decreased adherence of bacteria to mucosal membranes may be due to immature receptor sites or other host factor. Some investigators have suggested that the reduced binding of group A and B streptococci to buccal mucosal cells is specifically a result of the diminished capacity of neonatal epithelial cells to bind lipoteichoic acid found on the surface of streptococci.[64] We believe that teichoic acid, which is the

Table 15.1. *Percentage adherence of* Staph. aureus *to nasal epithelial cells*

	Age of infants (h)	% adherence[a]
1	24 ($\pm$3)	22
2	48 ($\pm$4)	25
3	72 ($\pm$4)	38
4	96 ($\pm$3)	35
5	120 ($\pm$4)	98

[a] Level of adherence of *Staph aureus* to adult mucosal cells was considered to be 100 %

major cell-wall component of staphylococci, may play the same role for staphylococcal binding to neonatal and adult epithelial cells. A better understanding of the mechanisms involved in the attachment of bacteria to infant epithelial cells should provide useful information about the colonization of mucous membranes of newborns and help clarify how this differs from that of the older infant and adult.

The development of bacterial flora after birth

Umbilical cord

After 72 h, the most significant bacteria isolated were *E. coli*, *Klebsiella aerogenes*, and *Enterococcus faecalis*.[65] *Staphylococcus aureus* was detected in only 2 per cent of neonates, a result attributed to the use of hexachlorophane. Dugdale and coworkers[66] reported that staphylococcal colonization does not interfere with Gram-negative colonization and that the two types of organisms colonize the skin independently. They observed *Staph. aureus* colonization as early as within 24 h, even when antistaphylococcal agents were used. Bhatia and colleagues[67] noticed that *E. coli* and *Klebsiella* were more commonly found than *Staph. aureus* and *Staph. epidermidis*.

Nose

The nose was sterile at birth in 90–100 per cent of the preterm and full-term babies of both sexes.[67, 68] However, after 72 h, 40 per cent of the examined infants became colonized with *Staph. aureus* and 22 per cent with Gram-negative bacteria.[67] Evans and colleagues[68] also described higher nasal colonization with *Staph. aureus*, and this finding was attributed to routine use of hexachlorophane and other antimicrobial agents. Hurst[69] reported a colonization rate as high as 99 per cent with *Staph. aureus* at discharge; half of these babies continued to be carriers of this organism at the end of their first year of life. The prevalence of overall colonization was greater at the umbilicus than the nares during the first 3 days of life,[68] but by day 5 these differences were not obvious.

Oral cavity

The throat is sterile in 91 per cent of the infants at birth and in 14 per cent after 72 h.[67] The major isolate was *Strep. viridans*.[65,70] Rotimi and Duerdan[70] reported that about 65 per cent of neonates were colonized by viridans streptococci on the first day and that nearly all were colonized by these organisms by the sixth day. *Streptococcus salivarius* was also common, and was isolated from most neonates by the sixth day (Table 15.2). *Staphylococcus epidermidis* and anaerobic cocci comprised 14 and 12 per cent of the total flora, respectively. Perhaps oxygen utilization by the aerobic flora is sufficient to permit growth of anaerobes, as found in this study.

On examining bacterial adherence to cheek and tongue cells of 1-day-old newborns, Long and Swenson observed the same selectivity as found in adults.[71] *Streptococcus mitis* and *Strep. salivarius* but not *Strep. mutans* showed strong attraction to these cells. The ability of buccal cells to support adherence of *Candida albicans* seemed to increase in newborns between 3 h and 10 days after birth.[72] Although differences in average adherence counts were not statistically significant in age-related groups of children, the proportion of cells with 10 or more yeasts significantly increased over time. The authors of this study speculated on the incidence rate of thrush with the maturation of binding sites.

Rectum

The rectal area is devoid of bacteria at birth. Ninety-six per cent of rectal swabs were sterile at 0 h, compared to 10 per cent at 72 h[67]. McAllister and colleagues[65] reported a higher colonization rate by day 3, almost reaching 87 per cent. The predominant organisms were *E. coli*, *Enterobacter cloacae*, *K. aerogenes*, and *Enterococcus faecalis*. Dugdale and colleagues[66] isolated *Proteus* spp. (38 per cent) from the rectum on day 3, while Ericksson and coworkers[73] reported *Staph. aureus* in 32 per cent of faecal specimens in 7-day-old neonates.

Skin

The development of a resident skin flora from birth to adulthood has not been systematically studied, but the child's flora probably begins to resemble that of the adult fairly early. Most studies on the bacterial flora of skin have been concerned with the organisms that are the primary cause of neonatal infections, such as *Staph. aureus* and *C. albicans*. Leyden's[74] investigations

Table 15.2. *Development of the oral flora in 23 neonates*

Species/group	Number of neonates colonized				Cumulative % of total isolates
	Day 1	Day 2	Day 3	Day 6	
Viridians streptococci	15	17	20	22	30.9
Strep. salivarius	8	14	18	19	25.3
Staph. epidermidis	6	7	12	8	14.2
Anaerobic cocci	0	7	10	12	12.4
Haemophilus influenzae	0	3	3	3	4.3
Bifidobacteria	0	2	3	5	4.3
Neisseria spp.	1	2	3	3	3.8
Enterobacteriaceae	0	1	2	2	2.6
Enterococci	0	1	2	2	2.2

involved quantitative cultures using the detergent scrub technique on the axilla, groin, forehead, and antecubital fossa. Twenty-five newborns were sampled within 2 h of birth, on days 1, 2, and 5, and then 6 weeks later. At birth, an aerobic flora was commonly found (76–80 per cent of sites), but the total number of organisms was very low (36–51 colony-forming units (cfu)/cm^2). Within 24 h, bacteria were recovered from all sites. The axilla and groin had 10^3 cfu/cm^2 compared to 540 cfu for the scalp. At 48 h, the scalp had 525 cfu/cm^2; the axilla and groin had 10^4 cfu/cm^2. The same number of organisms was found in the groin and axilla at day 5, while the bacteria on the scalp increased to an average of 2.7×10^3 cfu/cm^2. By 6 weeks, the total number of organisms for each site was comparable to that found in adults, with 1.8×10^5 cfu/cm^2 on the scalp, 9.8×10^4 cfu/cm^2 in the axilla, and 3.2×10^5 cfu/cm^2 on the groin. *Staphylococcus epidermidis* was the most commonly isolated organism. The paucity of bacteria found in the first few hours of life on the skin indicates that skin is essentially sterile at birth. The few organisms taken from the skin could come from either contact with nursery personnel, contact with the mother, or contamination during the passage through the vagina. The dense population in the axilla and groin at 48 h possibly reflects the onset of eccrine sweating and the effect of semiocclusion in the intertriginous area.[74]

At 6 weeks, the flora was qualitatively that of adults. However, Gram-negative bacilli are rarely found on the skin of adults, but are frequently isolated from the skin of children.[75] The relative dryness of most of the skin surface is thought to be a major factor in limiting colonization of these organisms. Gram-negative bacilli require more moisture for their growth than does the Gram-positive flora.[76] Similarly, colonization of *Staph. aureus* is higher on infant skin than on adult. It is not known why the newborn skin has greater affinity for *Staph. aureus*. Skin surface lipids are said to prevent survival of this organism in adult skin;[62] the skin of the neonate may be deficient in these secretions. How long infant skin remains colonized with *Staph. aureus* is not certain, but there is some evidence that the condition persists for a long time. Hurst[69] obtained *Staph. aureus* from the groin of 46 per cent and from the axilla of 12 per cent of 18-month-old children.

In general, the age of individuals influences the bacterial flora of the skin. Coagulase-negative staphylococci and micrococci occur frequently in all sites and at all ages. Streptococci were reported to be more prevalent in infants; diphtheroids were dominant in adults.[75]

References

1 Beachey EH. Bacterial adherence: adhesion–receptor interactions mediating the attachment of bacteria to mucosal surfaces. J Infect Dis 1981; 143: 325–45.

2 Rusch VC. The concept of symbiosis: a survey of terminology used in description of associations of dissimilarly named organisms. Microecol Ther 1989; 19: 33–59.

3 Ofek I, Beachey EH. General concepts and principles of bacterial adherence in animals and man. In: Beachey EH, ed. Bacterial adherence. London: Chapman and Hall; 1980: 1–29.

4 Gibbons RJ, van Houte J. Bacterial adherence in oral microbial ecology. Ann Rev Microbiol 1975; 29: 19–44.

5 Beachey EH, ed. Bacterial adherence. London: Chapman and Hall; 1980: 466.

6 Gibbons RJ, van Houte J. Selective bacterial adherence to oral epithelial surfaces and its role as an ecological determinant. Infect Immun 1971; 3: 567–73.

7 Gibbons RJ, Spinell DM, Skobe Z. Selective adherence as a determinant of the host tropisms of certain indigenous and pathogenic bacteria. Infect Immun 1976; 13: 238–46.

8 Aly R, Shinefield HR, Strauss WG, Maibach HI. Bacterial adherence to nasal mucosal cells. Infect Immun 1977; 17: 546–49.

9 Bibel DJ, Aly R, Lahti L, Shinefield HR, Maibach HI. Microbial adherence to vulvar epithelial cells. J Med Microbiol 1987; 23: 75–82.

10 Romero-Steiner S, Witek T, Balish E. Adherence of skin bacteria to human epithelial cells. J Clin Microbiol 1990; 28: 27–31.

11 Bibel DJ, Aly R, Shinefield HR, Maibach HI, Strauss WG. Importance of the keratinized epithelial cell in bacterial adherence. J Invest Dermatol 1982; 79: 250–53.

12 Alkan M, Ofek I, Beachey EH. Adherence of pharyngeal and skin strains of group A streptococci to human skin and oral epithelial cells. Infect Immun 1977; 18: 555–57.

13 Deacock SJ, Steward KA, Carne HR. The role of adherence in determining the site of infection by *Corynebacterium diphtheriae*. J Hyg Camb 1983; 90: 415–24.

14 Kimura LH, Pearsall NN. Adherence of *Candida albicans* to human buccal epithelial cells. Infect Immun 1978; 21: 64–68.

15 Ray TL, Digre KB, Payne CD. Adherence of *Candida* species to human epidermal corneocytes and buccal mucosal cells: correlation with cutaneous pathogenicity. J Invest Dermatol 1984; 83: 37–41.

16 Zurita J, Hay RJ. Adherence of dermatophyte microconidia and arthroconidia to human keratinocytes in vitro. J Invest Dermatol 1987; 89: 529–34.

17 Faergemann J, Aly R, Maibach HI. Adherence of *Pityrosporum orbiculare* to human stratum corneum cells. Arch Dermatol Res 1983; 275: 246–50.

18 Costerton JW, Geesey GG, Cheng K-J. How bacteria stick. Sci Am 1978; 238: 86–95.

19 Liljemark WF, Gibbons RJ. Proportional distribution and relative adherence of *Streptococcus miteor* (*mitis*) on various surfaces in the human oral cavity. Infect Immun 1972; 6: 852–59.

20 Ray TL, Payne CD. Scanning electron microscopy of epidermal adherence and cavitation in murine candidiasis: a role for *Candida* acid proteinase. Infect Immun 1988; 56: 1942–49.

21 Bibel DJ, Crumrine DA, Yee K, King RD. Development of arthrospores of *Trichophyton mentagrophytes*. Infect Immun 1977; 15: 958–71.

22 Pearce WA, Buchanan TM. Structure and cell membrane-binding properties of bacterial fimbriae. In: Beachey EH, ed. Bacterial adherence. London: Chapman and Hall; 1980: 289–344.

23 Eden CS, Hansson HA. *Escherichia coli* pili as possible mediators of attachment to human urinary tract epithelial cells. Infect Immun 1978; 21: 229–37.

24 Duguid JP, Cold DC. Adhesive properties of Enterobacteriaceae. In: Beachey EH, ed. Bacterial adherence. London: Chapman and Hall; 1980: 187–217.

25 Sato H, Okinaga K. Role of pili in the adherence of *Pseudomonas aeruginosa* to mouse epidermal cells. Infect Immun 1987; 55: 1774–78.

26 Aly R, Shinefield HR, Litz C, Maibach HI. Role of teichoic acid in the binding of *Staphylococcus aureus* to nasal epithelial cells. J Infect Dis 1980; 141: 463–65.

27 Cole GW, Silverberg NL. The adherence of *Staphylococcus aureus* to human corneocytes. Arch Dermatol 1986; 122: 166–69.

28 Bibel DJ, Aly R, Shinefield HR, Maibach HI. The *Staphylococcus aureus* receptor for fibronectin. J Invest Dermatol 1983; 80: 494–96.

29 Kuusela P. Fibronectin binds to *Staphylococcus aureus*, Nature 1978; 276: 718–20.

30 Doran JE, Raynor RH. Fibronectin binding to protein A-containing staphylococci. Infect Immun 1981; 33: 683–89.

31 Verbrug HA, Petgerson PK, Smith DE, et al. Human fibronectin binding to staphylococcal surface protein and its relative inefficiency in promoting phagocytosis by human polymorphonuclear leukocytes, monocytes, and alveolar macrophages. Infect Immun 1981; 33: 811–19.

32 Espersen F, Clemmensen I. Isolation of a fibronectin-binding protein from *Staphylococcus aureus*. Infect Immun 1981; 37: 526–31.

33 Froman G, Switalski LM, Speziale P, Hook M. Isolation and characterization of a fibronectin receptor from *Staphylococcus aureus*. J Biol Chem 1987; 262: 6564–71.

34 Ofek I, Beachey EH, Jefferson W, Campbell GL. Cell membrane binding

properties of group A streptococcal lipoteichoic acid. J Exp Med 1985; 141: 990–1003.

35 Ofek I, Beachey EH, Eyal F, Morrison JC. Postnatal development of binding of streptococci and lipoteichoic acid by oral mucosal cells of humans. J Infect Dis 1977; 135: 267–74.

36 Simpson WA, Ofek I, Sarasohn C, Morrison JC, Beachey EH. Characteristics of the binding of streptococcal lipoteichoic acid to human oral epithelial cells. J Infect Dis 1980; 141: 457–64.

37 Ellen RP, Gibbons RJ. M protein-associated adherence of *Streptococcus pyogenes* to epithelial surfaces: prerequisite for virulence. Infect Immun 1972; 5: 826–30.

38 Simpson WA, Beachey EH. Adherence of group A streptococci to fibronectin on oral epithelial cells. Infect Immun 1983; 39: 275–79.

39 Kuusela P, Vartio T, Vuento M, Myhre EB. Binding sites for streptococci and staphylococci in fibronectin. Infect Immun 1984; 45: 433–36.

40 Collins-Lech C, Kalbfleisch JH, Franson TR, Sohnle PG. Inhibition by sugars of *Candida albicans* adherence to human buccal mucosal cells and corneocytes in vitro. Infect Immun 1984; 46: 831–34.

41 Kahana M, Segal E, Millet MS, Gov Y. In vitro adherence of *Candida albicans* to human corneocytes. Acta Dermatol Venerol Stockh 1988; 68: 98–101.

42 Skerl KG, Calderone RA, Sega E, Sreevalsan T, Scheld WM. In vitro binding of *Candida albicans* yeast cells to human fibronectin. Can J Microbiol 1984; 30: 221–27.

43 Williams PH, Sedgwick MI. Evans N, Turner PJ, George RH, McNeish AS. Adherence of an enteropathogenic strain of *Escherichia coli* to human intestinal mucosa is mediated by a colicinogenic conjugative plasmid. Infect Immun 1978; 22: 393–402.

44 Dunkle LM, Blair LL, Fortune KP. Transformation of a plasmid encoding an adhesin of *Staphylococcus aureus* into a nonadherent staphylococcal strain. J Infect Dis 1986; 153: 670–75.

45 Aly R, Shinefield HR, Maibach HI. Staphylococcus adherence to nasal epithelial cells: studies of some parameters. In: Maibach HI, Aly R, eds. Skin microbiology: relevance to clinical infection. New York: Springer-Verlag; 1981: 171–79.

46 Kurono Y, Fujiyoshi T, Mogi G. Secretory IgA and bacterial adherence to nasal mucosal cells. Ann Otol Rhinol Laryngol 1989; 98: 272–77.

47 Lianou P, Bassaris H, Vlachodimitropoulos D, Tsambaos D. Acitretin induces an increased adherence of *S. aureus* to epithelial cells. Acta Dermato-Venereol 1989; 69: 330–32.

48 Bibel DJ, Aly R, Conant MA, Shinefield HR. From HIV infection to AIDS: changes in the microbial ecology of skin and nose. Microb Ecol Health Dis 1990; 4: 9–17.

49 Smith DH, Byrn RA, Marsters SA, Gregory T, Groopman JE, Capon DJ. Blocking of HIV-1 infectivity by a soluble, secreted form of the CD4 antigen. Science 1987; 238: 1704–07.

50 Olson GA, Bleiweis AS, Small PA Jr. Adherence inhibition of *Streptococcus mutans*: an assay reflecting a possible role of antibody in dental caries prophylaxis. Infect Immun 1972; 5: 419–27.

51 Evans RT, Emmings FG, Genco RJ. Prevention of *Streptococcus mutans*

infection of tooth surfaces by salivary antibody in Irus monkeys (*Macaca fascicularis*). Infect Immun 1975; 12: 293–302.

52 Raja RH, Raucci G, Hook M. Peptide analogous to a fibronectin receptor inhibits attachment of *Straphylococcus aureus* to fibronectin-containing substances. Infect Immun 1990; 58: 2593–98.

53 Aronson M, Medalia O, Schori L, Mirelman D, Sharon N, Ofek I. Prevention of colonization of the urinary tract of mice with *Escherichia coli* by blocking of bacterial adherence with methyl α-D-mannosepyranoside. J Infect Dis 1979; 139: 329–32.

54 Bibel DJ, Aly R, Bayles C, Strauss WG, Shinefield HR, Maibach HI. Competitive adherence as a mechanism of bacterial interference. Can J Microbiol 1983; 29: 700–03.

55 Abraham SN, Beachey EH, Simpson WA. Adherence of *Streptococcus pyogenes*, *Escherichia coli*, and *Pseudomonas aeruginosa* to fibronectin-coated and uncoated epithelial cells. Infect Immun 1983; 41: 1261–68.

56 Mertz PM, Patti JM, Marcin JJ, Marshall DA. Model for studying bacterial adherence to skin wounds. J Clin Microbiol 1987; 25: 1601–04.

57 Bass MH. Viral and parasitic diseases of the pregnant woman affecting the fetus. Clin Obstet Gynecol 1959; 2: 627–38.

58 Fairchild JP, Graber CD, Vogel EH, Ingersoll RL. Flora of the umbilical stump. J Pediatr 1958; 53: 538–42.

59 Laursen H. Bacteriological colonisation of infants and mothers in a maternity unit. Acta Obstet Gynecol Scand 1963; 42: 43–64.

60 Aly R, Shirley C, Cunico B, Maibach HI. Effect of prolonged occlusion on the microbial flora, pH, CO_2 and transepidermal water loss. J Invest Dermatol 1978; 71: 378–81.

61 Hurtwitz S. Clinical pediatric dermatology: a textbook of skin disorders of childhood and adolescence. Philadelphia: WB Saunders; 1981.

62 Aly R, Maibach HI, Shinefield HR, Strauss WG. Survival of pathogenic microorganisms on human skin. J Invest Dermatol 1972; 58: 205–10.

63 Aly R, Shinefield HR, Maibach HI. Adherence of *Staphylococcus aureus* to infant nasal epithelial cells. Am J Dis Child 1980; 134: 522–23.

64 Beachey EH. Binding of group A streptococci to human oral mucosal cells by lipoteichoic acid. Trans Assoc Am Physicians 1978; 88: 285–92.

65 McAllister TA, Given J, Black A, Turner MJ, Kerr MM, Hutchison JH. The natural history of bacterial colonization of the newborn in a maternity hospital [1]. Scot Med J 1974; 19: 119–23.

66 Dugdale AE, Harper J, Tiernan JR. Colonization of the neonates with staphylococci and gram negative bacilli. Acta Paediatr Scand 1967; 56: 455–60.

67 Bhatia BD, Chung S, Narang P, Singh MN. Bacterial flora of newborns at birth and 72 hours of age. Indian Pediatr 1989; 25: 1058–65.

68 Evans HE, Akpata SO, Baki A, Glass L. Bacterial flora of newborn infants in the external auditory canal and other sites. NY State J Med 1973; 73: 1071–72.

69 Hurst V. Transmission of hospital staphylococci among newborn infants: colonization of the skin and mucous membranes of the infants. Pediatr 1960; 25: 204–08.

70 Rotimi VO, Duerdan BI. The development of the bacterial flora in normal neonates. J Med Microbiol 1981; 14: 51–62.

71 Long SS, Swenson RM. Determinants of the developing oral flora in normal newborns. Appl Environ Microbiol 1976; 32: 494–97.

72 Davidson S, Brish M, Rubinstein E. Adherence of *Candida albicans* to buccal epithelial cells of neonates. Mycopathologia 1984; 85: 171–73.

73 Eriksson M, Melen B, Myrback KE, Winbladh B. Bacterial colonization of newborn infants in a neonatal intensive care unit. Acta Paediatr Scand 1982; 71: 779–83.

74 Leyden JJ. Bacteriology of newborn skin. In: Maibach HI, Boisits TV, eds. Neonatal skin: structure and function. New York: Marcel Dekker; 1982: 167–81.

75 Somerville DA. The normal flora of the skin in different age groups. Br J Dermatol 1969; 81: 248–58.

76 Aly R, Maibach HI. Aerobic microbial flora of intertriginous skin. Appl Environ Microbiol 1977; 33: 97–100.

16

Skin disinfection

H. KOBAYASHI

The purpose of skin disinfection is the removal of both transient and resident skin bacteria. The transient skin flora, which just happens to be deposited on the skin but does not multiply there, is removed rather easily, even with soap and water. The resident skin bacteria, which colonize and multiply on the skin, mostly persist after washing. Residents form microcolonies which are difficult to eradicate; these may contain between 100 and 1000 viable cells but can be reduced to smaller numbers with disinfectant (antiseptic). Resident skin bacteria are normally harmless to a surgical patient unless a prosthesis or catheter is inserted but may, on rare occasions, include pathogens such as methicillin-resistant *Staphylococcus aureus* (MRSA). Some transient bacteria on the skin, such as *Clostridium perfringens*, present as a result of faecal contamination from the buttocks, may resemble the resident flora in their persistence after washing with soap and water.[1] During washing, but not disinfection, bacteria rubbed on to the skin are more persistent than those applied without rubbing.[2]

The removal or killing of transient bacteria on the hands is often described as hygienic hand disinfection and the killing of resident bacteria as surgical hand disinfection.[3] The disinfection of operating sites is also intended to kill the resident flora. The characteristics of six antimicrobial ingredients designed for topical application to the skin have been reported by Larson[4] (Table 16.1).

Surgical hand disinfection

For surgical hand disinfection, the removal and killing of resident bacteria is necessary. Washing with an antiseptic detergent preparation such as 4 per cent chlorhexidine detergent solution (Hibiscrub®) or 7.5 per cent povidone–iodine detergent solution (Betadine®, Isodine®) is effective for this purpose.

Lowbury and coworkers,[5] in their study on alternative methods for the

Table 16.1. Characteristics of six topical antimicrobial ingredients[a]

Agent	Mode of action	Gram-positive bacteria	Gram-negative bacteria	M.tb[b]	Fungi	Viruses	Rapidity of action	Substantivity	Recommended concentrations	Affected by organic matter?	Comments
Alcohols	Denaturation of protein	+++	+++	++	++	++	Most rapid	0	70–92%	Yes	Drying, volatile
Chlorhexidine	Cell wall disruption	+++	++	+	++	±	Intermediate	+++	4%; 2% in detergent base; 0.5% in alcohol	Minimal	Formula-dependent efficacy
Hexachlorophane	Cell wall disruption	+++	±	±	±	±	Slow–intermediate	+++	3% by prescription only	Minimal	Neurotoxicity
Iodine/iodophors	Oxidation substitution by free iodine	+++	+	++	++	++	Intermediate	+	10%, 7.5%, 2%, 0.5%	Yes	Absorption from skin with possible toxicity; skin irritation more common
PCMX (chloroxylenol)	Cell wall disruption	++	+	+	+	+	Slow–intermediate	±	0.5–3.75%	Minimal	Formula dependent
Triclosan (Irigasan, DP-300)	Cell wall disruption	++	++[c]	+	±	±	Intermediate	+++	0.3–2.0%	Minimal	More efficacy data needed

[a] Based on Larson.[4]
[b] M.tb = Mycobacterium tuberculosis.
[c] Except for Pseudomonas spp.

removal of the transient flora, reported that povidone–iodine surgical scrub caused a reduction of 99.97 per cent in mean counts of samples from sites experimentally contaminated with *S. aureus*. Connel and Rousselot[6] demonstrated a 98 per cent reduction in mean counts of cultures from fingernail beds and the palmar surfaces of 50 hands after twice scrubbing for 2 min with povidone–iodine surgical scrub. Lowbury and Lilly[7] reported that 2 min of washing with 4 per cent chlorhexidine caused a significantly greater mean immediate reduction (86.7 per cent) in the bacterial count than was found with povidone–iodine surgical scrub (68 per cent). Kobayashi[8] also demonstrated a greater reduction in the number of positive cultures from the fingertips with 4 per cent chlorhexidine detergent solution than with povidone–iodine surgical scrub after 6 min of washing.

The effect of blood on the disinfection of surgeons' hands was also studied by Lowbury and Lilly.[9] Immediately after hand washing with disinfectant, 2 ml of blood or 2 ml of water were spread over the hands and sterile rubber gloves were put on. Viable counts were obtained from the hands before washing and after wearing the gloves for 1 h. Both the mean percentage reduction in viable counts after 1 h of wearing gloves and the mean viable counts of bacteria per ml of glove fluid were evaluated statistically. With povidone–iodine there was a significantly smaller reduction in the skin flora, when blood was present than there was with water, although chlorhexidine did not give a significant reduction. Povidone–iodine also gave a significantly higher viable count with blood than with water in the gloves after 1 h. These results showed that blood significantly interfered with the effectiveness of povidone–iodine detergent solution. Regrowth of resident bacteria on gloved hands after using povidone–iodine was noted by Peterson and colleagues.[10] After a 6-min scrub with 10 ml of the assigned preparation, the left hands were occluded by surgical gloves for 1, 2, 3, 4, 5 or 6 h and their bacterial flora was then tested by the glove fluid technique. They found a significant regrowth on gloved hands that had been washed with 7.5 per cent povidone–iodine but not on gloved hands after scrubbing with 4 per cent chlorhexidine detergent solution.

Single-use sponge/brushes impregnated with surgical scrubbing agents have been compared; the immediate effect in reducing the resident bacterial flora of the hands after two 3-min scrubs, the residual effect in maintaining the bacterial reduction, the influence on residual antimicrobial efficacy and the irritation potential after repeated use were evaluated.[11] In the context of immediate and delayed mean reductions in bacterial counts after washing, the chlorhexidine gluconate (Hibiclens®) sponge/brush was significantly more effective than was povidone–iodine (E-Z Scrub®), both in the absence and presence of blood. There were no significant increases in irritation or other adverse reactions with the use of either product. Kobayashi[8] demonstrated by image analysis of skin replicas before and after three 6-min hand scrubs with single-use brushes that 4 per cent chlorhexidine detergent solution generally caused less damage to the skin.

Mitchell and Rawluk[12] found that the prevalence of skin reactions associated with surgical scrubbing among a representative sample of theatre personnel in Scotland was 37.2 per cent. There were more excessive reactors in the group using soap (31/40, 77.5 per cent) than using chlorhexidine (126/409, 30.8 per cent) or povidone–iodine (47/112, 42.0 per cent), but no statistical difference between the latter two. A statistical difference in the distribution of reactors between different gloves worn during surgery was apparent. Certain surgical gloves were more likely to cause skin reactions than others, but this skin reaction is most likely due to a drying effect from frequent scrubs, so that moisturizing creams are effective in controlling the symptoms. Individuals who have other allergic symptoms appear more likely to develop skin reactions than those with no allergic symptoms. Regular use of moistening hand cream may benefit those individuals.

Ethanol is today the classic[13] but still effective and important surgical disinfectant. Price[14] found that 60–90 per cent of all ethanol solutions proved strongly and rapidly bactericidal, and that much of the killing effect apparently takes place during the first few seconds of contact. Lowbury and coworkers[15] also emphasized the effect of a 2-min application of 0.5 per cent chlorhexidine in 70 per cent ethanol after hand washing in a standard manner. This group later reported[16, 17] that much larger reductions in the microbial skin flora were obtained by vigorous rubbing with 10 ml of 0.5 per cent chlorhexidine in 95 per cent ethanol into the hands, wrists and forearms, allowing the solution to evaporate to dryness whilst rubbing, than by a single, standard, 2-min hand wash with a 4 per cent chlorhexidine detergent solution.

In a survey by King and Zimmerman[18] in 1965, 119 of 195 hospitals (61 per cent) utilized scrub procedures lasting 10 min or more. However, Dineen[19] showed that there was no significant difference in reduction of skin flora between a 5-min and a 10-min scrub assessed in 50 individuals in each group. Ayliffe and coworkers[3] proposed that a wash of only 2 min without scrubbing should be adequate for surgical hand preparation. They also mentioned that repeated scrubbing tends to damage the skin and may be associated with an increase in the numbers of the resident flora, possibly allowing *S. aureus* to colonize the hand (Figs. 16.1 and 16.2).

The residual bactericidal activity of 4 per cent chlorhexidine detergent solution in 50 orthopaedic and vascular surgical operations was demonstrated

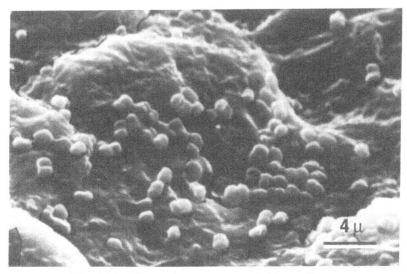

Fig. 16.1. Microcolony on normal skin surface.

by Dahl and colleagues.[20] After a standard 5-min scrub, one hand was randomly rinsed before gloving and the other lightly patted dry with a sterile towel, leaving some foam on the hand. There were statistically fewer bacterial colonies isolated from the hand coated with chlorhexidine than from the other. In vitro, Lilly and coworkers[21] studied the delayed antimicrobial effects of ethanol for aqueous suspensions of *S. aureus* deposited on a Millipore filter. They showed that the mean immediate reduction of 97.6 per cent in viable counts after treatment with 70 per cent ethanol was followed by a further mean reduction of 67.1 per cent during a 3-h holding time; the same bacterial suspensions dried on the filters without exposure to ethanol showed a significantly smaller reduction of 34.3 per cent during the holding time. The further fall in the number of bacteria on hands whilst wearing rubber gloves for 3 h after ethanol disinfection can also be explained by sublethal damage to some of the bacteria, from which they recover only if promptly inoculated on to culture medium. Lilly and coworkers[22] also reported that antiseptic preparations used repeatedly to disinfect the skin caused a reduction in the yield of resident flora to a low equilibrium level beyond which there was no further reduction. This equilibrium level varied with the antiseptic used and, in their findings from 12 experimental hand disinfections over a period of 4 days, 95 per cent ethanol achieved a lower equilibrium level than did 4 per cent chlorhexidine detergent solution.

Disinfection of operating sites

The skin at the operating site may be the source of self-contamination during surgery. The clinical effects of such contamination depend on the virulence of the microorganism, the resistance of the host and the contaminating dose. To prevent infection from the skin at the operating site, microorganisms have to be removed by washing with detergent and water and then, to some extent, destroyed by applying the bactericidal agents. It is possible to decontaminate but not to sterilize skin, as is customary for surgical instruments; it is our inability to sterilize that necessitates aseptic practice in modern surgery. Povidone–iodine was introduced in the 1950s as the iodine antiseptic for skin and mucous membranes[23] and chlorhexidine followed it.[24] Chlorhexidine gluconate (0.5 per cent) in 70 per cent ethanol, 10 per cent povidone–iodine in 70 per cent ethanol, 0.5 per cent aqueous chlorhexidine gluconate and 10 per cent aqueous povidone–iodine are the agents usually used at the operating site. Iodine (1 per cent) in ethanol was also frequently used but has an irritant effect on the skin. Ethanol solutions should be allowed to dry thoroughly before the incision, particularly where electrosurgery is used.

It was shown by Lowbury and Lilly[25] that 0.5 per cent chlorhexidine gluconate in 95 or 70 per cent ethanol, or 0.5 per cent aqueous chlorhexidine solution, caused a significantly greater mean reduction in skin bacteria when rubbed by a gloved hand on to the skin of the hand for 2 min than when applied to the same area with the traditional gauze used at operating sites.

Davies and coworkers[26] reported the effect of several preparations on the disinfection of abdominal skin of 106 staff and 358 patients using contact plates 5 min and 2 h after disinfection. Povidone–iodine (10 per cent) in 30 per cent ethanol, 0.5 per cent chlorhexidine in either 85 or 70 per cent ethanol, 70 per cent ethanol alone, aqueous 10 per cent povidone–iodine or 0.5 per cent chlorhexidine showed more than 90 per cent reduction 5 min after disinfection. They found a 1.19–1.40 $\log_{10}$ reduction even 2 h after disinfection. Goldblum and colleagues[27] compared the effects of repeated applications of 4 per cent chlorhexidine detergent solutions and povidone–iodine for skin preparation of haemodialysis patients and personnel. The chlorhexidine reduced total bacterial counts and eradicated *S. aureus* at both 2 and 4 h after disinfection to a significantly greater extent than did the povidone–iodine.

In a randomized study of preoperative skin preparation techniques in 178 thoracic and general surgical patients analysed by Geelhoed and colleagues,[28] no statistically significant differences at skin closure were found between three different groups – a 5-min iodophor scrub followed by cloth drape, a 5-min scrub followed by an alcohol cleansing of the skin and application of an antimicrobial film (Ioban 2 antimicrobial film®) and a 1-min alcohol cleansing of the skin without iodophor followed immediately by application of the antimicrobial film. Ulrich and Beck[29] reported that using a 1-min cleansing with 70 per cent isopropanol followed by application of antimicrobial film provided a significant time advantage and was as effective as a traditional preparative regimen.

Whole-body disinfection

Recently the effectiveness of preoperative whole-body disinfection has been investigated.[30-33] Using contact samples, Davis and coworkers[30] studied the effect on the skin of staff and patients of bathing with different detergent antiseptic preparations. They showed that a reduction in viable counts occurred most frequently with chlorhexidine, particularly 4 h after bathing. Ayliffe and colleagues[34] reported that, in a 60-week cross-over study on 5536 patients in 20 wards of two general and one orthopaedic city hospitals, preoperative bathing with chlorhexidine detergent failed to influence the incidence of postoperative infection in spite of the relatively high incidence of infection with skin organisms. Ayliffe[35] emphasized that alcoholic solutions are always to be preferred, as the maximum effect is required from a single application of the disinfectant at the site of operation.

The efficacy of showering and of scrubbing the incision site with disinfectant was evaluated by Garibaldi and colleagues[36] in a randomized, prospective study of 575 patients undergoing elective surgery. Patients who showered twice with 4 per cent chlorhexidine detergent solution had lower colony counts of skin bacteria at the incision site when sampled in the operating room before the final scrub than did patients who showered with 7.5 per cent povidone–iodine solution or a medicated bar soap. Patients in the chlorhexidine group had no growth on 43 per cent of cultures from the incision site compared with 16 per cent in the povidone–iodine group and 6 per cent in the soap group. Patients who showered and scrubbed with chlorhexidine also had less intraoperative wound contamination. However, the investigators failed to demonstrate a statistically significant difference in the surgery-specific infection rate between the three groups.

In a prospective, randomized, double-blind, placebo-controlled study involving 27 surgical units in six European countries carried out by the European Working Party on Control of Hospital Infection,[37] the effect of preoperative whole-body bathing with a detergent containing chlorhexidine on the incidence of wound infection in elective and clean surgery was compared with that of bathing with the same detergent without chlorhexidine. In the chlorhexidine group, 2.62 per cent of 1413 patients subsequently became

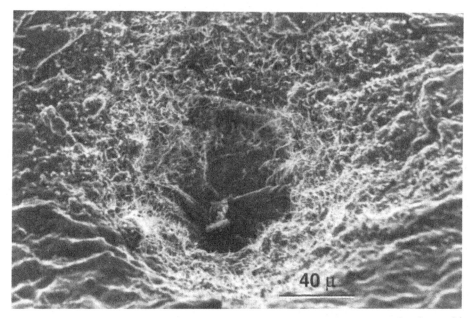

Fig. 16.2. Growth of filamentous bacteria around an eccrine sweat gland on skin occluded for 4 h.

infected compared with 2.36 per cent of 1400 patients in the control group; this difference was not statistically different. The investigator concluded that preoperative whole-body bathing of the patient twice with chlorhexidine detergent solution does not reduce the incidence of clean-wound infection. Earnshaw and coworkers[38] also reported that the beneficial effect of preoperative bathing in vascular surgery remains unproven.

However, in a recent report by Byrne and coworkers,[39] it was stressed that showering three times with chlorhexidine detergent solution was necessary to obtain the maximum level of skin disinfection.

Hygienic hand disinfection

Transient bacteria on the hands of hospital personnel are hazardous to susceptible patients in hospital. As noted by Ayliffe and colleagues,[3] washing with soap or detergent, with or without a disinfectant, is generally effective in removing transient bacteria if done diligently and regularly. An alternative method of hygienic hand disinfection is the application of small amounts of 70 per cent ethanol with an emollient, with or without additional disinfectant, which are then rubbed to dryness. Emollient is important for the prevention of skin damage by ethanol; 70 per cent ethanol with 1 per cent glycerol is useful for this purpose. These methods are a convenient and effective alternative to hand washing where there is no gross soiling of the hands, where a sink is not readily available, or when rapid disinfection is required.[3]

Bannan and Ludge[40] examined several bacteriological tests designed to evaluate the role of bar soap without antibacterial additives in the spread of bacteria. They demonstrated the following: (a) bacteria are not transferred from person to person through the use of bar soaps; (b) bar soaps do not support the growth of bacteria under normal usage; (c) bar soaps are inherently antibacterial as a result of their physicochemical properties; (d) the level of bacterial contamination that may occur on bar soap under extreme conditions (heavy usage, poorly designed non-drainable soap dishes, etc.) does not constitute a health hazard.

Ojajarvi[41] pointed out the considerable differences found in the acceptability of soaps, implying that the choice of a soap acceptable to the nursing staff is important in promoting proper hand hygiene. During the use of five different soaps, only slight differences were found in the numbers of total bacteria or in the occurrence of *S. aureus* and Gram-negative bacilli on the hands.

In the study by Meers and Yeo,[42] particles released into the air by wringing the hands together were collected in a slit sampler before and after washing with bar soap, with three surgical scrubs, and after rubbing the hands with a spirit-based lotion. There was a significant increase, averaging 14-fold, in the number of particles carrying viable bacteria released after washing with bar soap, but washing with surgical scrubs or rubbing with alcoholic lotion suppressed the increase in dissemination. This finding suggests that a surgical scrub should be used more widely in clinical practice, and that a spirit-based hand lotion might, with advantage, become a partial substitute for hand washing, particularly in areas where hand washing is frequent and iatrogenic infection common.

The effectiveness of various hand-washing and disinfection methods in removing transient skin bacteria after dry or moist contamination of the hands when nursing burns' patients in a hospital was examined by Ojajarvi.[43] None of the methods consistently removed all patient-borne bacteria from the hands. *Staphylococcus aureus* was more often completely removed by 4 per cent chlorhexidine detergent solution, or by 70 or 90 per cent ethanol with 3 per cent glycerol, than by liquid soap or iodophor scrub. Gram-negative bacilli were removed more easily by all methods than was *S. aureus*. Ojajarvi emphasized the importance of using gloves when nursing a profuse spreader of bacteria or one who must be protected from infection.

Rotter and coworkers[44] evaluated the efficacy, for hygienic hand disinfection after artifical contamination with *Escherichia coli*, of washing with 4 per cent chlorhexidine detergent scrub or 7.5 per cent povidone–iodine and rubbing 65 per cent isopropanol on the hands for 1 min. The mean $\log_{10}$ reduction obtained with povidone–iodine or chlorhexidine detergent solution was considerably less than with isopropanol. Thus alcohols were shown to be far more effective for the removal of transient bacteria from the hands in hygienic hand disinfection. The effectiveness and harshness of 4 per cent chlorhexidine gluconate, glycol-poly-siloxane gel with methylcellulose (Spectro-Jel®) and a natural liquid soap (Dermapro®) was studied in a special-care baby unit by Webster and Faoagali.[45] Chlorhexidine was the most effective product in reducing the skin microflora but the weekly colonization rate for methicillin-resistant *S. aureus* in neonates on the unit remained unaffected by any of the products tested. Product acceptability was tested with a self-reporting questionnaire, which showed that users preferred the gel preparation. A gloved-hand method was used by Aly and Maibach[46] to compare the antimicrobial effect of 0.5 per cent chlorhexidine gluconate/alcohol/emollient hand wash (Hibistat®) with that of 70 per cent isopropanol on the normal hand flora of 81 subjects. The difference in efficacy immediately after washing between the two products was not statistically significant on the first and second days but on the fifth day the chlorhexidine product showed a larger $\log_{10}$ reduction than did the isopropanol. There was no significant growth of bacteria after the chlorhexidine treatment over a period of 6 h when compared with the baseline counts.

Rotter[47] compared several methods of hygienic hand disinfection with the efficacy of a standard (rubbing the hands twice with 3 ml of 60 per cent isopropanol for 30 s) tested on hands artificially contaminated with *E. coli*. Rubbing twice with 60, 50 or 40 per cent *n*-propanol, 80 or 70 per cent ethanol or 10 per cent povidone–iodine was not statistically significantly different when compared with the standard method. However, rubbing with 60 per cent ethanol or washing with 7.5 per cent povidone–iodine or 4 per cent chlorhexidine were inferior to the standard method.

In a study by Kobayashi and colleagues,[48] povidone–iodine killed methicillin-resistant *S. aureus* the quickest but it was easily inactivated by organic matter; 70 and 50 per cent ethanol or isopropanol gave a killing time of 30 s against this staphylococcus. Chlorhexidine and povidone–iodine had a very short killing time against Gram-negative bacilli but they were also inactivated by organic matter.[49] 'Washing out' or 'removing' any contaminating matter from the hands is therefore essential for hygienic hand disinfection.

Albert and Condie[50] observed the care of 28 patients, all of whom had vascular catheters, in the intensive-care unit of a university hospital. Hand washing occurred after only 41 per cent of a total of 1212 staff–patient contacts. Forty different physicians and 15 nurses had contact with these patients on 326 and 701 occasions, respectively. Physicians washed their hands after 28 per cent of contacts and nurses did so after 43 per cent ($p < 0.001$). In another private hospital, physicians washed after 14 and nurses after 28 per cent of contacts. Respiratory therapists washed most frequently at both hospitals.

The factors affecting hand washing in 193 health care personnel employed at the University Hospital in Seattle were investigated by Larson and Killen[51] through a questionnaire. The main important reasons for hand washing were given as the prevention of spread of infection among patients and the prevention of acquiring an infection oneself. The most important factors against hand washing were being too busy, minimal contact with infectious patients, detriment of hand washing to skin and priority of patient needs. Physicians reported hand washing significantly less frequently than did nurses. Individuals who washed infrequently placed significantly more value on the detrimental effects of frequent hand washing on their own skin. Clearly emphasis should be placed on minimizing deterrents rather than on stressing the importance of hand washing.

McLane and colleagues[52] surveyed medical-surgical nurses by questionnaire and check-list to assess their perceived ability to perform selected clinical procedures. Among 37 errors of medical asepsis in 75 observations on 34 nurses, hand washing not done before or after a procedure was the most frequent (35 per cent). The duration of 180 hand washes by health care personnel and 52 hand washes by non-health care personnel (teaching and non-teaching) was recorded by Guraishi and coworkers.[53] The mean duration of hand washing for health care personnel was 8.62 ± 0.29 s (SEM), which was twice as long as for non-health care personnel. No statistically significant differences were revealed between personnel at teaching and non-teaching hospitals or among those in different occupations. These data indicate that the duration of hand washing among health care personnel is below the standard recommended by authorities in hospital infection.

References

1 Lowbury EJL, Ayliffe GAJ, Geddes AM, Williams JD, eds. Control of hospital infection. 2nd ed. London: Chapman and Hall; 1981.
2 Lilly HA, Lowbury EJL. Transient skin flora. J Clin Path 1978; 31: 919–22.
3 Ayliffe GAJ, Coates D, Hoffman PN. Chemical disinfection in hospital. London: PHLS; 1984.
4 Larson E. Draft guideline for use of topical antimicrobial agents. Am J Hosp Infect 1987; 15: 25A–36A.

5 Lowbury EJL, Lilly HA, Bull JP. Disinfection of hand: removal of transient organisms. Brit Med J 1964; 2: 230–33.

6 Connell JF Jr, Rousselot LM. Povidone–iodine. Am J Surg 1964; 108: 849–55.

7 Lowbury EJL, Lilly HA. Use of 4% chlorhexidine detergent solution (Hibiscrub®) and other methods of skin disinfection. Brit Med J 1973; 1: 510–15.

8 Kobayashi H. Evaluation of surgical scrubbing. J Hosp Infect 1991; 18(Suppl B): 29–34.

9 Lowbury EJL, Lilly HA. The effect of blood on disinfection of surgeons' hands. Br J Surg 1974; 61: 19–21.

10 Peterson AF, Rosenberg A, Alatary SD. Comparative evaluation of surgical scrub preparations. Surg Gynecol Obstet 1978; 146: 63–65.

11 Aly R, Maibach HI. Comparative evaluation of chlorhexidine gluconate (Hibiclens®) and povidone–iodine (E–Z Scrub®) sponge/brushes for pre-surgical hand scrubbing. Curr Ther Res 1983; 34: 740–45.

12 Mitchell KG, Rawluk DJR. Skin reactions related to surgical scrub-up: results of a Scottish survey. Br J Surg 1984; 71: 223–24.

13 Price PB. New studies in surgical bacteriology and surgical technic. JAMA 1938; 111: 1993–96.

14 Price PB. Reevaluation of ethyl alcohol as a germicide. Arch Surg 1950; 60: 492–502.

15 Lowbury EJL, Lilly HA, Bull JP. Method for disinfection of hand and operating site. Brit Med J 1964; 2: 531–36.

16 Lowbury EJL, Ayliffe GAJ. Alcoholic solution and other agents for disinfection of surgeon's hand. J Clin Pathol 1974; 28: 753–54.

17 Lowbury EJL. Lilly HA, Ayliffe GA. Preoperative disinfection of surgeons' hands: use of alcoholic solutions and effects of gloves on the skin flora. Brit Med J 1974; 4: 369–72.

18 King TC, Zimmerman JM. Skin degerming practices: chaos and confusion. Am J Surg 1965; 109: 695–98.

19 Dineen P. An evaluation of the duration of the surgical scrub. Surg Gynecol Obstet 1969; 129: 1181–84.

20 Dahl J, Wheeler B, Mukherjee D. Effect of chlorhexidine scrub on postoperative bacterial count. Am J Surg 1990; 159: 486–88.

21 Lilly HA, Lowbury EJL, Wilkins MD, Zazzy A. Delayed antimicrobial effects of skin disinfection by alcohol. J Hyg Camb 1979; 82: 497–500.

22 Lilly HA, Lowbury EJL, Wilkins MD. Limits to progressive reduction of resident skin bacteria by disinfection. J Clin Pathol 1979; 32: 382–85.

23 Gershenfeld L. Povidone–iodine as a topical antiseptic. Am J Surg 1957; 94: 938–39.

24 Lowbury EJL, Lilly HA, Bull JP. Disinfection of the skin of operation site. Br Med J 1960; 2: 1039–44.

25 Lowbury EJL, Lilly HA. Gloved hand as applicator of antiseptic to operation sites. Lancet 1975; ii: 153–56.

26 Davis J, Babb JR, Ayliffe GAJ, Wilkins MD. Disinfection of the skin of the abdomen. Br J Surg 1978; 65: 855–58.

27 Goldblum SE, Ulrich JA, Goldman RS, Reed WP, Avasthi PS. Comparison of 4% chlorhexidine gluconate in a detergent base (Hibiclens) and povidone–iodine (Betadine) for the skin preparation of hemodialysis patients and personnel. Am J Kidney Dis 1983; 11: 548–52.

28 Geelhoed GW, Sharpe K, Simon GL. A comparative study of surgical skin preparation methods. Surg Gynecol Obstet 1983; 157: 265–68.

29 Ulrich JA, Beck WC. Surgical skin prep regimens: comparison of antimicrobial efficacy. Infect Surg 1984; 3: 569–72.

30 Davis J, Babb DJ, Ayliffe GAJ, Ellis SH. The effect on the skin flora of bathing with antiseptic solutions. J Antimicrob Chemother 1977; 3: 473–81.

31 Seeberg S, Lindberg A, Bergman BR. Preoperative shower bath with 4% chlorhexidine detergent solution: reduction of *Staphylococcus aureus* in skin carrier and practical application. In: Maibach H, Aly R, eds. Skin microbiology. New York: Springer-Verlag; 1981: 86–91.

32 Brandberg A, Andersson I. Preoperative whole body disinfection by shower bath with chlorhexidine soap: effect on transmission of bacteria from skin flora. In: Maibach NI, Aly R, eds. Skin microbiology. New York: Springer-Verlag; 1981: 92–97.

33 Brandberg A, Holm J, Hammarsten, J, Schersten T. Postoperative wound infections in vascular surgery: effect of preoperative whole body disinfection by shower-bath with chlorhexidine soap. In: Maibach HI, Aly R, eds. Skin microbiology. New York: Springer-Verlag; 1981: 98–102.

34 Ayliffe GAJ, Noy MF, Babb JR, Davis JG, Jackson J. A comparison of pre-operative bathing with chlorhexidine-detergent and non-medicated soap in the prevention of wound infection. J Hosp Infect 1983; 4: 237–44.

35 Ayliffe GAJ. Surgical scrub and skin disinfection. Infect Control 1984; 5: 23–27.

36 Garibaldi RA, Skolnick D, Lerer T, et al. The impact of preoperative skin disinfection on preventing intraoperative wound contamination. Infect Control Hosp Epidemiol 1988; 9: 109–13.

37 Rotter ML, Larsen SO, Cooke EM, et al. A comparison of the effects of preoperative whole-body bathing with detergent alone and with detergent containing chlorhexidine gluconate on the frequency of wound infections after clean surgery. J Hosp Infect 1988; 11: 310–20.

38 Earnshaw JJ, Berridge DC, Slack RCB, Markin GS, Hopkinson BR. Do preoperative chlorhexidine baths reduce the risk of infection after vascular reconstruction? Eur J Vasc Surg 1989; 3: 323–26.

39 Byrne DJ, Napier A, Cuschieri A. Rationalizing whole body disinfection. J Hosp Infect 1990; 15: 183–87.

40 Bannan EA, Ludge LF. Bacteriological studies relating to handwashing. Am J Publ Health 1965; 55: 915–22.

41 Ojajarvi J. The importance of soap selection for routine hand hygiene in hospital. J Hyg Camb 1981; 86: 275–83.

42 Meers PD, Yeo GA. Shedding of bacteria and skin squames after handwashing. J Hyg Camb 1978; 81: 99–105.

43 Ojajarvi J. Effectiveness of hand washing and disinfection methods in removing transient bacteria after patient nursing. J Hyg Camb 1980; 85: 193–203.

44 Rotter M, Koller W, Wewalka G. Povidone–iodine and chlorhexidine gluconate-containing detergents for disinfection of hand. J Hosp Infect 1980; 1: 149–58.

45 Webster J, Faoagali JL. An in-use comparison of chlorhexidine gluconate 4% w/v, glycol-poly-siloxane plus methylcellulose and a liquid soap in a special care baby unit. J Hosp Infect 1989; 14: 141–51.

46 Aly R, Maibach HI. Comparative study on the antimicrobial effect of 0.5% chlorhexidine gluconate and 70% isopropyl alcohol on the normal flora of hand. Appl Environ Microbiol 1979; 37: 610–13.

47 Rotter ML. Hygienic hand disinfection. Infect Control 1984; 5: 18–22.

48 Kobayashi H, Tsuzuki M, Hosobuchi K. Bactericidal effects of antiseptics and disinfectant against methicillin-resistant *Staphylococcus aureus*. Infect Control Hosp Epidemiol 1989; 10: 562–64.

49 Kobayashi H, Tsuzuki M, Hosobuchi K. Bactericidal effects of antiseptics and disinfectants against Gram-negative rods. [In Japanese with English summary]. J Jpn Assoc Operating Room Technol 1987; 8: 481–86.

50 Albert RK, Condie F. Hand-washing patterns in medical intensive-care units. N Engl J Med 1981; 304: 1465–66.

51 Larson E, Killen M. Factors influencing hand washing behavior of patient care personnel. Am J Infect Control 1982; 10: 93–99.

52 McLane C, Chenelly S, Sylwestrak ML, Kirchhoff KT. A nursing practice problem: failure to observe aseptic technique. Am J Hosp Infect 1983; 11: 178–82.

53 Guraishi ZA, McGuckin M, Blais FX. Duration of handwashing in intensive care units: a descriptive study. Am J Hosp Infect 1984; 12: 8387.

Index

[Bold numbers denote major mentions]

Acetate as nutrient 48, 54
Acinetobacter spp.
  carriage on animals 265
  carriage on humans **210–11**
  nutrition 38, 39, 43, 51, 53
Acne **125–8**
Actinobacillus spp. 266, 271, 275
Actinomyces 266, 270–3, 276
Acute glomerulonephritis 190–2, 199
Acute guttate psoriasis 193, 195
Acute rheumatic fever 199
Adherence
  bacteria 196, 355, **360–4**
  fungi 250, 360
  physical environment 73, 89
  see also individual microbial species
Aerobic coryneforms 34–40, 43, 63
  see also Brevibacterium, Corynebacterium and
    Dermabacter
Aeromonas spp. 215
AIDS
  and bacteria 141, 217, 223, 361
  and fungi 236–8, 244, 249, 252, 254, 255
Alcaligenes spp. 215
Amino acids, as nutrients 49, 52, **55–8**, 61, 79,
  80
Anaerobic coryneforms, *see Propionibacterium*
Anterior nares, as carrier site 107, 108, 111, 112,
  141
Arginine, as nutrient 52, 54, 58
Aspergillus spp. 257, 283
Atopic dermatitis, as carrier site 77, 164, 173, 185,
  251, 361
Axilla
  as carrier site 107, 108, 111, 112, 114, 141,
    142
  growth conditions 78, 80, 83

Bacillus spp. 221, 269, 331, 333, 346
Bacterial interference **331–9**, 362
Bacteroides spp. 222

Biofilms 87
Biotin, as nutrient 60, 61, 64
Borrelia spp. 222, 276
Brevibacterium spp.
  carriage 105, 110, 111, 123
  interactions 334
  nutrition 39, 43, 48, 50, 54, 61
  physical factors 87
Brucella spp. 213, 277

Candida albicans
  adherence 357, 358, 366
  carriage in animals 281
  carriage in humans **249–51**
  interactions 332
  physical factors 86, 89, 90, 91
Candida spp.
  carriage in animals 281
  carriage in humans 232, 234, 236, 237, 249, 251,
    281
CAPD infections 166, 167
Capripox 317
Cellulitis 184, 277
Citrobacter spp. 214, 215
Clostridium perfringens 221, 269, 373
Conjugative gene transfer **340–6**
Corynebacterium diphtheriae
  adherence 345, 346
  carriage 104, 124
Corynebacterium jeikeium
  carriage **104–11**, 123
Corynebacterium minutissimum
  carriage 104, 106, 111, **118–23**, 334, 356
  nutrition 50, 61
  physical factors 91
Corynebacterium spp.
  adherence 356, 358
  carriage in animals 270, 271
  carriage in humans **106–9**, 124, 129
  nutrition 39, 43
  physical factors 78, 87

Corynebacterium xerosis
  carriage 105, 106, 111, 118, 123
  nutrition 50, 61
Cowpox 294, 309, 316
Cryptococcus neoformans 283

Dandruff 78
Demodex 21
Dermabacter hominis 110
Dermatophilus congolensis
  carriage in animals 268, 271, 272
  carriage in humans 124, 221
  skin structure 25
Dermatophyte infection
  antibiotic production 333, 346
  in animals **278–80**
  in humans **239–44**
  see also Epidermophyton, Microsporum,
    Trichophyton
Diphtheroids
  see Brevibacterium, Corynebacterium,
    Dermabacter, Propionibacterium
Disinfection of the hands 375, 378
Dispersal of skin flora 149

Eccrine sweat 7, **17–19, 33–4**, 83
Ecthyma 183, 189
Enterobacter spp.
  carriage 214, 215
  nutrition 38, 39, 51, 53
Enterococcus spp.
  carriage 174, 175, 365, 366
  gene transfer 344, 345
Epidermolytic toxin 157
Epidermophyton spp.
  in animals 279
  in humans 239, 241
Erysipelas 184, 199
Erysipelothrix spp. 221, 269
Erythema infectiosum 297
Erythrasma 86, **120–2**
Escherichia coli
  adherence 355, 360, 362
  carriage in animals 277
  carriage in humans 213–15
  disinfection 381
  nutrition 38, 39, 43, 49, 51, 53, 63
  physical factors 89–91
Exudative epidermitis, porcine 268

Fatty acids
  as inhibitors 234–5
  as nutrients 41, 49, 54, 62–5
Folliculitis, in animals 266, 268, 277
Forehead, as carrier site 107, 111
Furunculosis **160–2**
Fusobacterium necrophorum 270, 276

Genital herpes 307
Genital warts 303
Gram-negative bacilli
  carriage 214, 215

nutrition 41, 44, 62, 65, 67
physical factor 87
see also individual genera
Groin
  as carrier site 141, 142
  physical factors 78, 80, 83

Hair structure 2, 4
Hair follicles
  structure 8, 11
  physical factors 75, 77
Hand, foot and mouth disease 294, 302
Heat-shock protein 83
Hendersonula toruloidea 248
Herpes simplex virus
  in animals 322, 324, 325
  in humans **291–5**, 298, 305, 306, 308
HIV 299, 310
HLA-DR antigen 141
Hormones 15, 19
Hot-tub dermatitis 86, **211–12**
Human papillomavirus 304
Hyaluronate lyase 46, 52
Hydrophobicity 88
Hygienic hand disinfection 380

'Id' reactions 247
Immersion foot 86, 211
Impetiginization 183, 185, 189
Impetigo 163, 164, 265
Inhibitors 35, 346, 358

JK coryneforms *see Corynebacterium jeikeium*

Keratin 10, 11
Keratinase 42, 61
Klebsiella spp. 214, 277, 365, 366

Lauric acid 65, 66
Legionella spp. 213
Leporipox 317, 321
Light, effect on flora 89, 91
Linoleic acid 65, 66
Linolenic acid 65, 66
Lipase 41, 46
Lipids
  as inhibitors 65, 234, 368
  as nutrients 41, 63, 65
  in structure 15
  see also fatty acids
Lipophilic coryneforms
  nutrition 39, 43, 48, 50, 52, 61, 62
  see also Corynebacterium and *Rhodococcus*
Listeria monocytogenes 221
Lysozyme 75

Malassezia furfur
  adherence 357
  carriage **232–8, 253–6**
  interactions 333
  nutrition 33, 36–44, 61–7
  physical factors 76–8, 90–2

Malassezia pachydermatis (*Pityrosporum canis*) 281
Meat handlers, infections 177, **187–9**
Meningococci 213
Microcolonies 23
Micronutrients 61, 62
Microsporum canis
  in animals 278, 280
  in humans 239, 242, 243
Microsporum spp.
  in animals 278–80
  in humans 239–47
Moraxella spp. 214, 215
Molluscum contagiosum 294, 308, 321
Monkeypox 299
Mycobacterium avium-intracellulare
  in animals 274
  in humans 218, 220
Mycobacterium leprae 218
Mycobacterium marinum 218–20
Mycobacterium spp.
  in animals 273, 274
  in humans 218, 221
Mycobacterium tuberculosis
  in animals 274, 277
  in humans 217, 218
  physical factors 83, 92
Mycoplasma spp. 278, 310
Myristic acid 65, 66

Neisseria spp. 89
Nocardia spp. 221, 271, 273
Nose, *see* anterior nares

Oleic acid 63–5
Orf 293–4, 309, 318, 319
Orthopox 316
Oxygen requirements 7, 48, 87

Papillomavirus
  in animals 323, 324
  in humans 294, 303
Papovavirus 323, 324
Parapoxvirus 309, 316, 319
Parvovirus
  in animals 324, 326
  in humans 294, 297
Pasteurella spp. 212, 270, 277
Peptococcus spp. 222
Perineum, as carrier site 107, 108, 111, 112, 114
Peritonitis, in CAPD 167
pH
  of skin 17, **78–81**, 364
  nutrition 35, 46, 47, 64, 66
  physical factors **78–81**, 86
Phosphate 44, 46
Pitted keratolysis 124, 217, 221
Pityriasis versicolor 237, 253, 254
Pneumocystis spp. 223
Polyalcohols 45, 50, 51
Poxvirus 308, 315
Propionate 48, 54

Propionibacterium acnes
  adherence 356
  carriage **112–14, 125–7**, 148, 222
  interactions 334, 337, 339
  nutrition 33, 39–43, 46, 47, 50–8, 62–7
  physical factors 76–79, 87, 91, 92
Propionibacterium avidum
  carriage **112–14**
  nutrition 46, 47, 50, 54, 57, 58, 62
Propionibacterium granulosum
  carriage **112–14**
  nutrition 39, 43, 46, 47, 50, 54, 57, 58, 62, 65, 66
Protease 41, 46, 54, 61
Protein A of *Staph. aureus* 155, 156, 166
Proteins 15, 41, 83
Proteus spp.
  carriage in animals 276, 277
  carriage in humans 210, 212–16, 364
  nutrition 38, 39, 43, 51, 53
Prototheca spp. 222
Providencia spp., nutrition 38, 39, 43, 51, 53
Pseudomonas aeruginosa
  carriage in animals 270
  carriage in humans 212, 216, 356, 358, 362, 363
  nutrition 39, 51, 53
  physical factors 77, 86, 91
Pseudomonas spp.
  carriage in animals 275, 276
  carriage in humans 123, 211–16, 245, 364
  interactions 346
  nutrition 38, 43, 52
Pyoderma 177, 178, 180, 182, 197, 198

Resident flora 21, 147, 373
Retrovirus 325, 326
Rhodococcus spp. 270, 271, 345
Rickettsia 279
Rubella 294, 296

Scalded skin syndrome 163
Scalp, as carrier site 107, 111, 114, 243
Scarlet fever and toxin 192–194
Scytalidium hyalinum 248
Sebaceous glands 8, 18, 75, 333
Serratia spp.
  carriage in animals 277
  carriage in humans 214
  nutrition 38, 39, 43, 44, 49–53
Squames 4, 23, 149
Staphylococcus aureus
  adherence 356, 359–62
  carriage in animals 265, 267
  carriage in humans 139, **141–144**, 153, **160–163**
  carriage in infants 364, 365
  disinfection 375, 377, 378, 381, 382
  genetic exchange **341–344**
  interaction 332, 339, 344, 346
  nutrition 36–39, 42–48, 54, 56, 58, 60, 64–66
  physical factors 77, 81, 90, 91
  toxic-shock syndrome 36, 37, 46, 81, 156, 194
  with streptococci 182, 185, 199
  502A 336

Staphylococcus epidermidis
  adherence 356
  carriage in animals 266
  carriage in humans **136–38, 144–7**, 159, 165, 167, 217
  carriage in infants 365, 367
  genetic exchange 343, 344
  interaction 334, 336
  nutrition 39, 41–5, 54, 56, 58, 60
  physical conditions 90, 91
Staphylococcus haemolyticus
  carriage in animals 266
  carriage in humans 136, 137, 146, 148, 159, 165, 167, 217
  genetic exchange 344
  nutrition 39, 43, 45, 56, 60
Staphylococcus hominis
  carriage in humans 136, 137, 145–7, 159, 165, 167
  genetic exchange 341, 344
  nutrition 39, 43, 45, 56, 60
Staphylococcus hyicus
  carriage in animals 138, 139, **265–8**
  carriage in humans 136, 144
  interactions 337–8
Staphylococcus intermedius
  carriage in animals 265–7
  carriage in humans 144, 147
  genetic exchange 339, 342, 344
Staphylococcus saprophyticus
  carriage in animals 266
  carriage in humans 136, 137, 144, 148, 159
  genetic exchange 344
  nutrition 52, 56, 58, 60
Staphylococcus spp.
  adherence 358
  carriage in animals 266
  carriage in humans **135–8, 145–8**, 153, 158, 159, 165, 167
  nutrition 38–41, 43, 45, 48–52, 58, 60, 62, 64, 67
  physical conditions 76, 83, 87
Stratum granulosum 9, 10, 158
Streptococcal pyoderma 181, 189
Streptococci
  group A, *see Streptococcus pyogenes*
  group B **174–80**, 184, 195
  group C, G **174–80**, 184, 195
  animal strains 174, 175, 268
Streptococcus pyogenes
  adherence 356, 359–64

carriage in animals 268
carriage in humans 163, 164, **173–86**
genetic exchange 344, 345
infectious sequelae **190–3**, 195, 199
nutrition 65, 66
physical factors 77, 86, 89
Sugars 45, 49–52
Surgical wound disinfection 373
Sweat glands
  apocrine 24
  eccrine 17, 79
  sebaceous 8, 18, 75, 333

Tanapox 309
Temperature of skin 35, 80–84
Tinea lesions 239, 241, 245
Toes and toe-web flora 78, 80, 83, 107–12, 122, 142
Toxic shock, toxin and syndrome 36, 37, 46, 81, 156, 194
Transepidermal water loss 7, 86
Transient flora 25, 147, 373, 380
Trichomycosis axillaris 86, 118–20
Trichophyton interdigitale, see T. mentagrophytes
Trichophyton mentagrophytes
  adherence 358
  carriage in animals 278
  carriage in humans 235, **239–42**, 244, 246
  physical conditions 86, 92
Trichophyton rubrum
  carriage in animals 278–280
  carriage in humans 235, **238–40**, 246, 248
Trichophyton spp.
  adherence 357
  carriage in animals 278–80
  carriage in humans 239–46
  physical conditions 81
Trichosporon spp. 234, 281
Triglycerides 63–7
Tumour necrosis factor 197

Ultraviolet light 90–2

Varicella–zoster virus 293, 294, 300, 302
Vitamins 40, 61, 62

Warts 303, 304

Yersinia spp. 277

Printed in the United States
By Bookmasters